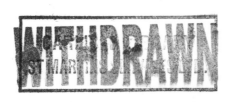

Sociologies of Food and Nutrition

ENVIRONMENT, DEVELOPMENT, AND PUBLIC POLICY

A series of volumes under the general editorship of
Lawrence Susskind, *Massachusetts Institute of Technology,
Cambridge, Massachusetts*

PUBLIC POLICY AND SOCIAL SERVICES

Series Editor: Gary Marx, *University of Colorado, Boulder, Colorado*

Recent Volumes in this Series

**AMERICANS ABROAD: A Comparative Study of Emigrants
from the United States**
Arnold Dashefsky, Jan DeAmicis, Bernard Lazerwitz, and Ephraim Tabory

**THE DIFFUSION OF MEDICAL INNOVATIONS: An Applied
Network Analysis**
Mary L. Fennell and Richard B. Warnecke

DIVIDED OPPORTUNITIES: Minorities, Poverty, and Social Policy
Edited by Gary D. Sandefur and Marta Tienda

HISPANICS IN THE LABOR FORCE: Issues and Policies
Edited by Edwin Melendez, Clara Rodriguez, and Janis Barry Figueroa

INNOVATION UP CLOSE: How School Improvement Works
A. Michael Huberman and Matthew B. Miles

**INTELLIGENCE POLICY: Its Impact on College Admissions
and Other Social Policies**
Angela Browne-Miller

**RACIAL AND CULTURAL MINORITIES: An Analysis of Prejudice
and Discrimination (Fifth Edition)**
George E. Simpson and J. Milton Yinger

SOCIOLOGIES OF FOOD AND NUTRITION
Wm. Alex McIntosh

Other subseries:

ENVIRONMENTAL POLICY AND PLANNING
Series Editor: Lawrence Susskind, *Massachusetts Institute of Technology,
Cambridge, Massachusetts*

CITIES AND DEVELOPMENT
Series Editor: Lloyd Rodwin, *Massachusetts Institute of Technology,
Cambridge, Massachusetts*

Sociologies of Food and Nutrition

Wm. Alex McIntosh

Texas A&M University
College Station, Texas

Plenum Press • New York and London

Library of Congress Cataloging-in-Publication Data

On file

ISBN 0-306-45335-5

© 1996 Plenum Press, New York
A Division of Plenum Publishing Corporation
233 Spring Street, New York, N. Y. 10013

10 9 8 7 6 5 4 3 2 1

Printed in the United States of America

PREFACE

The reasons for writing this book are fairly straightforward. I have long believed that the subjects of food and nutrition offer untapped riches for sociological study. Humans produce, distribute, prepare, and consume foods in collectivities. The groups involved include friendship networks, families, communities, formal organizations, and societies. In addition, the early state depended on food resources for its growth and development, and the modern state maintains an active interest in food production and trade and in the nutritional health of its citizenry. Food and nutrition have also played significant roles in the change and development of society through their effects on resource production and population growth. Finally, food habits and food consumption have not only physiological but social consequences as well. These include microlevel impacts on role performance and more macrolevel effects on societal economic growth.

I am interested in food and nutrition partly for applied reasons: I believe that sociologists can make significant contributions to solving problems associated with access to food and sound nutritional health. However, my chief motivation lies in the further development of sociological theories. As this book attempts to demonstrate, concepts involving food and nutrition have already begun to make contributions to the sociology of the body, the sociology of the family, the sociology of culture, social stratification, the rise and development of the state, societal change, studies of economic development, world systems and dependency theories, and a host of other theoretical perspectives within the various fields of sociology. I also hope to show additional ways that studies of food and nutrition can broaden and deepen these theories.

The intended audience is both graduate students and postgraduates, primarily in sociology and the social sciences. My goal is to persuade others to see the relevance of food and nutrition studies for further development of sociological theory. I also hope that those working in nutrition, dietetics, food science, and related fields will make greater use of sociological theories and models in their work. It is my hope that sociologists will find new issues of both theoretical and empirical importance for sociology and that scientists will discover new frameworks to approach old problems.

All books are social to varying degrees. My book began in graduate school as I interacted with faculty mentors Gerry Klonglan and Les Wilcox and fellow graduate students Kerry Byrnes, John Callaghan, and Dan Tweed about the role sociological theory might play in studies of human nutrition. Susan Evers, a graduate student in nutrition, acted as my mentor in a field in which I had little knowledge or appropriate educational background.

After coming to Texas A&M, I participated in a number of non-food–nutrition research projects, including studies of religious participation, adolescent drug use, and the effects of training on labor force participation. During each of these experiences, I tried to think of how the theories used in these projects might be applied to the study of food and nutrition. I owe many thanks to Jon Alston, Ken Nyberg, and Steve Picou for the opportunities they offered me in this regard.

I also began to search for colleagues in the College of Agriculture that I could enlist as co-investigators in interdisciplinary studies of food and nutrition. I discovered Pat Guseman and her interests in demographic predictions of food consumption trends, and she and I completed several projects together. After many false starts, I also found a dietitian–nutritionist and two biochemists who expressed an interest in sociological approaches to food and nutrition. I owe a great deal to Karen Kubena, Barbara O'Brien, and the late Wendall Landmann for their willingness to take a chance on me.

Many of my colleagues in the Rural Sociological Society and particularly in the Association for the Study of Food and Society and the Agriculture, Food, and Human Values group have provided me with encouragement and suggestions. Thanks here go especially to Jeff Sobal, Bill Whit, Jan Poppendieck, Donna Maurer, Ann Murcott, David Kallen, Dorthy Blair, Paul Thompson, Bill Friedland, Larry Busch, Bill Lacy, Janet Solis-Long, Audrey Maretski, Anne Hertzler, Jo Marie Powers, Jackie Newman, Mia More-Armitage, Ann Tinsley, and many others.

I also owe much to Peggy Shifflett, for the grant proposal funding I received from USDA to study the elderly's food habits came because of the proposal she wrote (as a student, she was not eligible for this funding, so her proposal was submitted under my name). This collaboration resulted in a number of articles and inspired the proposal I wrote for the National Institute on Aging (NIA). I have gained immensely in working on these various data sets with students like Betty Kucera, Jenna Anding, Amy Tram, Annie Godwin, Cheryl Usery, Connie Chitwood, and others, all of whom have written theses or dissertations that extended sociological perspectives to nutrition.

I also wish to recognize the tolerance, support, and occasional prods I have received from many faculty members and administrators at Texas A&M, especially Jim Copp, Mary Zey, Pat Guseman, Jane Sell, Steve Murdock, Dudley Poston,

Jon Alston, Letitia Alston, Bill Kuvlesky, Howard Kaplan, Jim Burk, Ben Aguirre, Ed Murguia, David Sciulli, Arnie Vedlitz, Pat Bramwell, and Ben Crouch.

Thanks, too, to Texas A&M and Cornell University for the development leave I spent in Ithaca. In addition, my colleagues and I gratefully received numerous small grants from the College of Liberal Arts and the Texas Agricultural Experiment Station to conduct a number of pilot studies. I would also like to thank the National Institute on Aging (R01-AGO-04043) and the United States Department of Agriculture (Competitive Grant No. 5901–0410–0126–0) (Peggy Shifflett's dissertation funding) for the grants I received. Thanks are also owed to the Department of Rural Sociology for purchasing the World Bank data and to Darrel Fannin's efforts in converting what were essentially data tables into an SAS data file. Without the help of Cynthia Cready, Robin Bateman, and Jackie Burns, much of the analyses of these data would not have been available for presentation here.

I would also like to acknowledge my reading group, the "NAR" (so called because there is nothing "semi" about this seminar) for its contribution (or lack thereof) to my intellectual development. The group is multi-disciplinary and thus our readings encompass the far and wide. I have learned enormously from my fellow "Narophites," as we like to characterize ourselves. This education has included not only subject matter to which I otherwise would not have had exposure but also a deeper understanding of how to read books critically. Any mischaracterization or superficial interpretation of literature I discuss in this book are, of course, the fault of these colleagues!

Lynn Jenson, Linda McIntosh, and Winnie Brower are owed much of the credit for the readability of the manuscript. They edited and proofread countless times. Thank you one and all. Linda deserves special mention, because without her efforts this book might never have seen the light of day. I'm also indebted to Jackie Sandles, Carolyn Green, Ginny Davis, Barbara Becvar, Winnie Brower, and Janet Fleitman of the Department of Sociology as well as Rick Weidmann of the Department of Rural Sociology for the many drafts that they have done and redone without complaint and for their encouragement.

We owe our parents much and I cannot begin to express enough thanks to them for their patience and encouragement. Finally, my wife and children have always been sources of joy and inspiration, and I thank them for their tolerance and support during our years together.

CONTENTS

1

INTRODUCTION

While it has long been accepted that eating is more than a biological act, most sociologists have shown little interest in the sociology of food. In fact, food is frequently taken for granted as an element in a variety of sociological theory, as demonstrated by such diverse works as those of George Herbert Mead, Karl Marx, Talcott Parsons, Walter Wallace, Gerhard Lenski, Charles Tilly, Anthony Giddens, and Immanuel Wallerstein. All of these theorists have either alluded to or made explicit reference to the human need for food and the social activities that attempt to meet that need. The majority of these associations concern the production rather than the consumption of food. Of the theorists, only Simmel [1915] (see Symons, 1994) and, more recently, Bourdieu (1984) have paid explicit attention to food consumption. Symons's (1994) translation of Simmel's analysis of the social functions of the meal makes it available in English for the first time.

As a consequence of this lack of interest, the sociology of food consumption has languished until recently. However, in the past decade sociologists not only have made promising beginnings but have called for the development of a sociology of food and nutrition (Mennell, Murcott, & van Otterloo, 1992; Sobal, 1992; Whit, 1995). During this same period, rural sociologists have renewed their interest in production agriculture (Albrecht & Murdock, 1990; Buttel, Larson, & Gillespie, 1990). In the meantime, the fields of anthropology, economics, and psychology have forged far ahead in food studies and in the development of areas of graduate specialization. The lack of sociological attention to food has meant that most of the current work on food by social scientists takes either highly individualistic or highly cultural approaches.

Psychologists attempt to explain variations in individual behavior through differences in individual biological and psychological traits. The psychology of food has thus focused on such topics as eating disorders (anorexia, bulimia), obesity, the acquirement of individual food preferences and aversions, and the physiological mechanisms involved in taste and smell. For instance, studies in this field have attempted to explain obesity as a reaction to stress, arguing that this disorder results from an individual either eating to relieve anxiety produced by stress or confusing the internal stimuli caused by anxiety with those caused by hunger (Mehrabian, 1987). Preferences and aversions are partially determined by genetic makeup, personality factors such as "sensation seeking," and the food item's reputation in terms of its healthfulness and taste (Boakes, Popplewell, & Burton, 1987). Regarding taste, psychologists have identified locations on the tongue at which specific receptors detect one of the four taste primaries, that is, sweet, sour, bitter, and salty (Logue, 1991).

At the other end of the spectrum lies the anthropological approach, which deals principally with societal-wide behavior governed by culture (Sahlins, 1976). Levi-Strausian structuralists argue, for instance, that material aspects of culture, such as food and clothing, reflect a universal psychological-behavioral code that originates in the human brain. Other anthropologists suggest that food and clothing characteristic of a given society represent a specific linguistic system with semiotic and communicative properties (Barthes, 1972a, 1972b). An exception to this general macroapproach consists of those anthropologists who focus on variations in the possession of material items in a society, noting their use in demarcating and legitimating differences in status, ethnic identification, and religious background (Goody, 1982; Rizvi, 1991). Goody (1982) has referred to his approach as "sociological."

Some anthropologists are more interested in the nutritional consequences of culture (Harris & Ross, 1987). Generally, their concern lies with what are ordinarily considered irrational food beliefs and practices. One school of thought argues that this aspect of culture is dysfunctional for human survival (see Meigs, 1984). For example, Wendell Berry (1990) has claimed that modern societies have lost touch with the roots of their food supply and thus pursue diets that will eventually lead to irreversible environmental degradation. Studies of protein restrictions, with their resulting negative consequences for infant birth weight and infant mortality, provide a prominent example. Another group, however, suggests that while the effects of such irrationality may be negative for individuals, the latent effect of protein restrictions, for example, is the reduction of population pressure through increased infant mortality (see Harris, 1979).

Somewhere in the region between psychological and anthropological studies of food and nutrition lies the work of economists on these topics. Much of this work involves linking the effects of income with the sale of food. Income has proved highly successful as a predictor of food purchases, often explaining 80 to 90 percent of the variance in such expenditures. Many of these economists have had a great deal of influence on the making of national food policies as well as in the collection of national-level food consumption data. For example, economists have written a major proportion of the questions asked in the decennial Nationwide Food Consumption Survey, which provides valuable information regarding trends in food purchases.

Another approach taken by economists focuses on the results of food consumption in terms of nutrient intake. In this case, income is used to predict intake of various nutrients. Recent studies by Oral Capps (Nayga & Capps, 1994a, 1994b) and Barry Popkin (Popkin, Haines, & Reidy, 1989; Popkin, Haines, & Paterson, 1992) are indicative of these efforts. This kind of work again emphasizes individual economic circumstance and individual purchase and intake. However, economists such as Correa (1963, 1969) and Correa and Cummins (1970) have linked aggregate-level food consumption and nutritional status to economic growth, arguing that interventions such as supplemental feeding programs or reductions of certain nutritional deficiency diseases can make major contributions to the growth and development of society.

Despite the informative value of the psychological, economic, and cultural approaches, they neglect the social nature of food. Many relationships between individuals are created and maintained by food; under some circumstances, food is associated with their destruction. So food is bound up in the fundamental social processes of integration and conflict. For example, persons use meals as a setting in which to forge stronger relationships. Families maintain existing relationships through daily contact at the table. At the same time, spousal relationships may founder over meal scheduling or dishes served (Murcott, 1983a, 1983b); relationships between neighbors become hostile in conflicts over the ownership of farmland (Paige, 1975).

The nonsociological approaches to food and nutrition provide us with ideas from extreme viewpoints. We must study the food behavior either of separate individuals or of whole cultures. Similarly, we must view food either as a material object or as a symbol, but not both. Yet we know that some human behavior cannot be explained by reliance either on culture, economics, or personality. Humans form relationships and establish networks and groups. Organizational life is a part of modern reality. Similarly, it is unwise to view things as either largely symbolic or largely material. Just as we have discovered the importance of reuniting the mind and body, so should the symbolic and physical attributes be rejoined. In our case, it is important to remember that food is both material and symbolic and has both material and symbolic consequences for people.

I have written this book with the intent of demonstrating that sociological approaches to food and nutrition have tremendous potential for the explanation and understanding of food production and purchase as well as nutrient intake and its consequences. Further, I contend that such studies will not only make sociology more relevant but ultimately contribute to the growth of sociological theory. However, a single book cannot hope to examine all of the ways in which food and nutrition are suitable for sociological study. What I try to do in this book is provide the beginnings of sociological approaches to these topics, attempting to show that not only can sociology add much to our understanding of food and nutrition, but also the study of these topics will contribute to sociological theory. I have opted for theoretical pluralism rather than theoretical closure to demonstrate the potential that sociological studies of food and nutrition have to offer not only to the food and nutrition sciences but also to sociology itself. A result of this approach is reflected in the book's title, *Sociologies of Food and Nutrition*. This wording is selected to suggest the many theoretical avenues open to the study of these subjects. However, when I wish to refer to this area as an organized field, I will rely on the more familiar rubric "Sociology of Food and Nutrition."

Like many books, this one is incomplete. It would entail the writing of several more volumes to fully link sociology with food and nutrition studies. This book reflects both my own interests as well as my blind spots. Much of the book focuses on the macrolevel, with the state, social change, class systems, and the world system discussed in terms of countries and societies. However, some chapters deal with mesolevel ethnic differences and processes within families and other organizations. Perhaps the most glaring omission is the microlevel, represented by social psychology. Phenomenology and symbolic interactionism *are* utilized to discuss food and the body. But aside from this exception, social psychological studies of food and nutrition are given only brief mention. The reason for this disregard lies chiefly in the fact that social psychologists have already made a number of contributions to food and nutrition studies. My aim in this book is to encourage sociologists to break new ground by applying non-social psychological theories to food and nutrition.

Because the book is written to interest other sociologists in participating in what I think will become an emerging field, I have purposely avoided bringing closure to many of the questions I raise and the issues I illuminate. Determination of the interrelationships between culture, the state, social organization, social stratification, and social change and food and nutrition has only just commenced. I view this book as a first step in my own efforts to explain these phenomena.

The book begins with the problem of defining and justifying a new subfield within the discipline of sociology. I accomplish this through a comparison of the new subfield with those of rural and medical sociology, two related yet different subfields within sociology. Both fields have made contributions to sociological theory, yet preserved somewhat separate identities. I believe that a sociology of food and nutrition has similar potential. Chapter 2 focuses on the nature of the sociology of food and nutrition and makes a case for it as a new area by comparing it with the related areas of medical and rural sociology. While food and nutrition have clear relationships to food production and health, they are more than either of these. People eat food, not nutrients. That is, they generally see the substances they ingest through the lens of culture and social relationships. In addition, food represents a lifestyle. Thus, models drawn from rural and medical sociology tell us a great deal about choices in production practices or reasons for seeking health care but very little about food purchase and consumption. At the same time, research by medical sociologists on the health care profession suggests a number of fruitful extensions to studies of dietitians and nutritionists.

The third chapter attempts to expand the cultural analysis of food beyond both the symbolic and materialist approaches employed by anthropologists. This is accomplished by examining food habit change from the perspectives of modernization, postmodernism, consumerism, and ethnic studies. Chapter 4 considers the integrating and dividing aspects of food as parts of both the gender division of labor and power structure within families. In particular, women and men's roles in families, on family farms, and in the restaurant industry are examined in terms of food production, food preparation, and food consumption.

Agricultural economists have long studied food production and purchase, using the standard supply and demand models at both micro- and macrolevels of analysis. While this work has explained a great deal about food behavior, it has paid little attention to the behavioral differences predicted by theories of social class. Recently, rural sociologists have begun to apply Marx and Weber to food production (Friedland, Barton, & Thomas, 1981; Friedmann, 1978a, 1978b; Heffernan, 1972; Mann, 1990; McIntosh, Thomas, & Albrecht, 1990). Following the lead of Bourdieu (1984) and Lamont (1992), class analyses of food habits offer great insights into understanding differing lifestyles. Chapter 5 attempts to extend the rather rudimentary attempts by non–social scientists to go beyond standard economic treatments of class to food and nutrition. At a more macrolevel, sociologists have very recently begun to test hypotheses drawn from world systems and dependency theories to examine consequences for human health and nutritional status. The remainder of this chapter attempts to further develop the application of these theories to the history of food exchange and the development of deficiency diseases, including speculation regarding the extension of core country culture to the remainder of the world.

A number of hypotheses are suggested in Chapter 5 as well as subsequent chapters. I attempt to test these using data provided by the World Bank as well as various organizations of the United Nations. The number of countries used to test particular hypotheses varies with the amount of data available for particular variables by country. This results in samples sizes that range from 50 to 121, depending on the analysis in question. Furthermore, the organizations providing these data series often provide little or no documentation regarding the data's reliability or its coverage of a country's population. I suspect that a number of cases are based on regional or local studies and then extrapolated for the entire country. I discuss the validity of these data relative to the concepts they are thought to represent at an appropriate point in each chapter.

Diane Farshow of the University of California, San Diego, once told me that a sociology of nutrition without a consideration of the body was severely incomplete; in recent years, Turner (1992) has made the same argument. Chapter 6 discusses the part the body plays in the production process and the implications of resulting body alienation for food and alcohol consumption. In addition, the body self is an important aspect of self-image. Using both symbolic interactionism and phenomenology, the implications for body self are discussed in terms of the commodification and objectification of bodies and body parts.

The phenomenon famine plays an important role in 19th-century theories of social change. In this century, it has become largely the subject matter of historians, but more recently it has drawn the attention of economists, geographers, climatologists, and anthropologists. Sociologists are among the latest group of scientists to take famine seriously as a subject matter. Sociologists not only want to understand the role social factors might play in inducing famine, but have developed a renewed interest in famine as a cause of social change. Chapter 7 briefly discusses a number of causes of famine proposed by a variety of scientists and examines evidence for these arguments, paying particular attention to those that claim that famines result from social actions. A discussion of the social consequences of famine follows, drawing on case studies provided by anthropologists and economists. Suggestions are made regarding contributions sociological perspectives could make to this burgeoning area of study. Finally, I observe that the anthropology of famine has focused on the household level of response to famine, yet histories of famine in China indicate that both the state and local governments play a role in dealing with famine. Sociological studies of community and governmental efforts that deal with the consequences of famine are needed.

Theories of social change have made the most consistent use of food production as an avenue of technological change and resource generation. Evolutionary theories have paid the most attention to the importance of agricultural development for societal change, but even the equilibrium and conflict theories have included agriculture in their discussions. I examine the role that food plays in both early and contemporary evolutionary theories; as in these theories, so-called equilibrium or social ecology models of social change find that food is a major causal force. Similarly, conflict theories of change such as the Marxian, as well as non-Marxist theories of revolution, refer to food and food deprivation as implicit factors in societal change. Chapter 8 discusses all these theories and how the role of food might be made more explicit in their further development.

States are built on food. During the early years of state development, resources have to be generated and concentrated to support a rudimentary bureaucracy and military. Food is one of the few resources available for achieving such goals. States continue to play a part in food, affecting agricultural and food policies, intervening to provide food to the needy with an eye to social stability, and intervening in eating habits to promote a healthy labor force and the combat potential of the armed forces. Chapter 9 reviews the role of food in the rise of the state, the development of state responsibilities for insuring a steady food supply, and the political economy of food and nutrition policy.

Food and nutrition are associated with a multitude of social problems including obesity, eating disorders, unhealthy foods, unsafe foods, and vegetarianism. These problems are discussed from both objectivist and social constructionist perspectives, with an emphasis on the latter. Here the discussion focuses on the role of the mass media, official statistics, and pictures in persuading members of the public that a problem exists. Chapter 10 is devoted to this approach. The final chapter was added at the advice of the series editor, Gary T. Marx. It conducts a "sociology" of the sociology of food and nutrition. This is accomplished in several ways. First, the theoretical trends in the sociology of food and nutrition are discussed and assessed. Future trends are given some attention as well. Next, I discuss the organizational basis for the sociology of food and nutrition and assess the future growth and development of such organizations. This is followed by the results of a study of those sociologists most heavily identified with the sociology of food and nutrition. A discussion of the future of this emerging field completes the chapter.

2

AN OVERVIEW OF SOCIOLOGICAL APPROACHES TO FOOD AND NUTRITION

INTRODUCTION

This chapter argues in support of the emerging field, the sociology of food and nutrition. A skeptic may well ask why sociology needs yet another field, particularly one that has several apparent shortcomings. The first fault is the obvious overlap that such a field would have with rural sociology and medical sociology, and the second is the atheoretical, applied-appearing nature of such a field. I will argue that while the sociology of food and nutrition shares some of the same subject matter as rural sociology and medical sociology, it also encompasses topics left untouched by these two fields.

I will also argue that the sociology of food and nutrition has already begun to make theoretical contributions to many areas of sociology such as social change, the state, culture, social organization, social stratification, and social problems, to name just a few. Critics will likely judge this new field as they have rural and medical sociology, as one more application of sociological theory and method to a new set of social problems with little chance of providing new theoretical insights. Thus, the new field would make little contribution to the development of sociology as a scientific discipline. I suggest that the characterization of rural sociology and medical sociology as having had no impact on the discipline is untrue and that the sociology of food and nutrition will make similar contributions to sociology.

This chapter accomplishes these goals by discussing the subject matter of the fields of rural sociology and medical sociology in terms of (1) the degree to which they overlap with the proposed field of the sociology of food and nutrition and (2) the contributions they have made to sociological advancement. I will suggest that food and nutrition encompass subject matter beyond what generally is considered either rural or medical sociology and that by incorporating this new subject matter into the new subfield, substantial contributions to sociological theory are possible.

MEDICAL SOCIOLOGY/NUTRITIONAL SOCIOLOGY

The Sociology *of* and *in* Medicine[1]

Medical sociology has struggled with an identity problem since the 1950s. Straus (1957) attempted to alleviate the problem by separating a sociology *of* medicine from a sociology *in* medicine. The sociology *in* medicine focuses on the social causes of health; the sociology *of* medicine examines social relations within both formal and informal health care settings.

Much of the sociology *in* medicine involves the application of sociological theories, concepts, and research methods toward elucidating the distribution of morbidity and mortality across groups of persons and the group attributes that cause this morbidity and mortality. These efforts are classified as "social epidemiology." Emile Durkheim's (1951) [1897] work on suicide is frequently cited by both sociologist and nonsociologist medical researchers as one of the classic works of social epidemiology. Many of the nonsociologists who work in social epidemiology borrow heavily from the social sciences, particularly sociology (Berkman & Syme, 1979; Cassel, 1976).

The sociology *in* medicine (nowadays referred to as the sociology *of* health) examines the effects of status characteristics such as class, gender, and race and then argues that these produce differences in health (Angel, 1989; Marmot & Theorell, 1994; Syme & Berkman, 1976; Verbrugge, 1989; Woolhandler, Himmelstein, Silber, Bader, Harnly, & Jones, 1989). Each status position carries with it both resources and constraints. For example, status permits differential access to occupations that pay well and whose conditions are less stressful. Those with more education or who are male or white are at an advantage in this regard. Status differences also affect the kind of medical treatment an individual receives (Jones, 1989; Riessmann, 1994). In addition, role characteristics produce differing levels of stress. Multiple conflicting roles, role overload, and role-specific strains such as nonreciprocity or inadequate role performance resulting in depersonalization, lack of control, constriction of self, and inadequacy of rewards may affect both physical and mental health (Kandel, Davies, & Raveis, 1985; H. B. Kaplan, 1986).

---

[1] Jeff Sobal has also developed the parallel between the sociology *of* and *in* health and a sociology *of* and *in* nutrition, which he discussed at the first annual meeting of the Association for the Study of Food and Society, Aquinas College, Grand Rapids, Michigan, June 1987.

The sociology *of* health focuses on social relationships that result from either real or anticipated changes in health status. Here the emphasis lies in either formal (e.g., doctor-patient) or informal (e.g., spousal) relationships that arise out of a change in health (e.g., a person becomes ill) or an anticipated change (e.g., a person is exposed to a virus or has grown older). If the content of what constitutes sociological subject matter involves both social antecedents and social consequences, then neither the sociology *of* health nor the sociology *in* health are sociological when taken alone. Taken together, however, a configuration arises in which a social antecedent produces health consequences, which then produce social consequences. Thus social antecedents have social consequences through physical and mental mechanisms.

Furthermore, many argue that health constitutes both a social as well as a biological state (Herzlich & Pierret, 1987 [1984]; Gerhardt, 1989). Persons suffering from an acute condition such as a cold virus are said to take on the "sick role," which means that they have permission temporarily to cease to comply with their other obligations until they become well (Parsons, 1951). Taking on the sick role also means that the individual accepts certain responsibility for behaving in a manner that indicates an interest in getting well. Persons suffering from chronic illnesses may not be able to perform at the same level as prior to the illness or to regain roles held at that time. Here the sick role expectations and obligations are less clear; disability may become a deviant status.

The Sociology *of* and *in* Nutrition

As stated previously, the sociology *in* medicine refers to social epidemiology. The sociology *in* nutrition is, in part, a social epidemiology of inadequate diets, stunted growth, obesity, and poor nutritional health. These states result from many of the same status differences that produce ill health: class, gender, and ethnicity (Harriss, 1990). Obesity, for example, occurs more frequently in women, minorities, and the poor (Sobal & Stunkard, 1989). Adverse life events associated with various role behaviors affect nutritional status as well (McIntosh, Kubena, & Landmann, 1994a). Anorexia nervosa, until recently, afflicted young, white, middle-class females (Gordon, 1990). Some medical sociologists assert that health problems have both social antecedents and consequences. For example, a number of class-based lifestyle choices, such as eating diets high in fat, greatly increase the risk of heart disease, and persons who contract heart disease frequently experience changes in social relationships and downward social mobility.

Problems associated with nutrition are affected to an even greater degree by social class, lifestyle, and gender differences than is health. Anorexia nervosa, for example, largely results from both problematic relations between adolescents and parents, the culture of slimness, and various types of social inequality (Brumberg, 1988; Gordon, 1990; Thompson, 1994). Social consequences of nutrition include the impact of obesity on self-image (Allon, 1973) and on marital changes (Sobal, 1984a). Others have linked malnutrition to lessened role competence (Kallen, 1971, 1973; McIntosh, 1975).

The sociology *of* health involves the study of the social activities that characterize both formal and informal medicine. Some of this work begins with Parsons's insights regarding the sick role and its relationship with other roles, such as that of the physician. Others have conducted examinations of actual encounters between patients and health professionals, from either ethnomethodological or power-dependence perspectives (Stimson & Webb, 1989; Waitzkin, 1989). Still others have examined the effects of societal forces such as bureaucratization and political economic interests on the medical care system (Estes, Gerard, Zones, & Swan, 1984; Flood & Scott, 1987; Light, 1989; Turner, 1987). These same forces have implications for both access to health care as well as the quality of that care, and thus their study is important for policy making. At the same time, this research has made contributions to the study of complex organizations and political economy.

The sociology *of* health would involve those social relationships that characterize both formal and informal dietetics, that is, relationships between dietitians and their patients, dietitians and physicians, dietitians and the food industry in general, and dietitians with the public.[2] The latter is illustrated through the use of dietitians as expert sources by the news media and the appearance of food and health newspaper columns written by dietitians. In addition to studies of role conflict and contested legitimacy, the process by which dietetics has undergone professionalization would make an excellent case study.

Many of the same impacts of bureaucratization and political economy likely impact on dietetics, but these impacts have yet to be studied. Of particular interest would be studies of the more mesolevel politics of dietetics and nutrition in universities. Some campuses maintain separate colleges of dietetics or nutrition. Others, however, locate these disciplines within departments such as food science or animal science. Such departments are generally highly dependent on funds from agricultural commodity groups and food industries. Nutrition and dietetics may take lower priority in these settings, and the nature of the research pursued may differ as well.

The sociology *of* nutrition would involve the study of activities that characterize both the formal and informal relations within dietetics and nutrition fields. This could involve a very wide range of studies. Researchers could examine how the working location of dietitians and nutritionists, many of whom either practice or conduct research in multidisciplinary settings, impacts on their status and re-

---

[2] Marjorie DeVault (1995) has already made a contribution in this general direction in her study of role marginality of "nutrition professionals in the health care hierarchy." Regarding dietitians and the food industry, see "Corporate Support" (1995).

search priorities. Many dietitians are employed by hospitals or by other health care organizations; some go into private practice; others are found in various academic departments or institutes (DeVault, 1995). Initial studies might, in fact, focus on the differing role expectations of dietitians working in these various settings. For example, role expectations, professional autonomy, and role strain all likely differ between dietitians who work in hospital settings, those in group practice settings such as HMO's, and those in independent practice. Sociologists would find differences in research priorities between nutritionists who work within colleges of home economics and those within colleges of agriculture, particularly nutritionists found within departments of animal science.

Second, bureaucratization and rationalization have increasingly impinged on all professions, but no one has examined their effects on the delivery of nutrition education and other services. Third, an increasing number of studies of the political economy of medicine have recently appeared, with a focus on the impact of economic and policy changes on the quality and distribution of medical care. With the exception of studies of the political economy of food stamp access (Hirschl & Rank, 1991), little is known about how forces of change have impacted the delivery of nutrition services such as the Supplemental Feeding Program for Women, Infants, and Children (WIC), Expanded Food and Nutrition Education Program (EFNEP), and other nutrition programs. Finally, the impact of industry interests on dietetics and nutrition research remains unknown.

The sociology *of* and *in* health have added to the sociological body of knowledge through an enlarged understanding of labeling and deviance, social control, professionalization, and role performance. Hospitals and associated professions provide societies with a substantial alternative to imprisonment as a form of social control (Foucault, 1973; Goffman, 1961b; Scull, 1993). Abbott (1988) and Halpern (1990) have utilized psychiatry and medical specialties, respectively, to develop and test theories of professionalization. The sociology *of* and *in* nutrition will make similar contributions. Furthermore, the sociology *of* food and nutrition will range well beyond those areas associated with medical sociology, in that adding food to the description broadens the area of study by a substantial amount. Issues of food production, processing, retailing, purchasing, and consumption are thus added to the picture.

Table 2.1 provides a summary of the overlap between sociological approaches to health (or medicine) and sociological approaches to food and nutrition.

RURAL SOCIOLOGY

Rural sociology has met with the same criticism as medical sociology; it is often considered too applied and insufficiently theoretical by some of its own

Table 2.1. The Sociology *of* Health and *in* Health Contrasted with the Sociology *of* Food and Nutrition and *in* Food and Nutrition

Sociology *in* health	Sociology *in* nutrition
A. Ecology and etiology of disease.	A. Ecology and etiology of under- and over-nutrition, hunger.
B. Variations in attitudes and behavior regarding health and illness.	B. Variations in attitudes and behaviors regarding hunger, eating habits, nutritional status.
1. Sociological continuities (e.g., social class differences).	1. Sociological continuities (e.g., social class differences).
2. Reorientation of sociological concerns: deviance, stigma.	2. Reorientation of sociological concerns: deviance (certain forms of vegetarianism, stigma associated with obesity).
Sociology *of* health	Sociology *of* nutrition
A. Recruitment and training of physicians.	A. Recruitment and training of dietitians.
B. Relations of physicians to others in the role set .	B. Relations of consumers (or dietitians) to others in the role set.
C. Effect of the changing political economy on distribution of health care.	C. Effect of changing political economy on access to food and nutrition services.

Note: Adapted from Wolinsky (1980: 41).

practitioners (see Copp, 1972; Falk & Gilbert, 1985; Friedland, 1989). Others criticize rural sociology not for its involvement in applied issues but because of the side it has taken. Friedland (1989) and others believe that rural sociology has followed the lead of the various agricultural sciences in becoming "client oriented," which means doing research that aids the various commodity groups.

Rural sociology began as a "problems" discipline. As evidenced by trends in the subject matter of *Rural Sociology*, the official journal of the Rural Sociological Society, rural sociologists wrote about rural problems and social justice during the formative years of the discipline. Later, the emphasis switched to studies of community life and rural families, demographic change, and the adoption and diffusion of agricultural technology (Buttel et al., 1990; Christenson & Garkovich, 1985). Even this latter work was directed at policymakers in an effort to improve conditions on farms and in rural communities. Falk and Gilbert (1985) have described much of the early work by rural sociologists as atheoretical and applied, although sociologists such as Sorokin, Zimmerman, and Taylor successfully pushed the discipline toward a more basic science position; their success, however, was due less to the persuasiveness of their case than to the political pressures from agricultural interests. Both Copp (1972) and Friedland (1989) have echoed the position that rural sociology has lost its critical edge.

Despite the concerns regarding ideological stance, rural sociologists have made major theoretical contributions during the last 30 years. By examining the work in the sociology of agriculture, adoption-diffusion, and human ecology accomplished by rural sociologists, for example, the field would appear to have made significant contributions to theorizing in sociology. Frisbie and Poston's (1976) development of the sustenance organization concept and operationalization has added significantly to the knowledge of how communities survive and prosper. Friedmann's (1978a, 1978b) extension of the commodity chain perspective to agriculture has greatly broadened the concept of globalization. Despite its applied reputation, the adoption-diffusion perspective developed at Iowa State by Beal, Bollen, and others and extended by Brown (1981) represents one of the few models available that ties together the processes of micro- and macrolevel technological change.

Buttel et al. (1990) have argued recently that rural sociologists have turned their attention to the "structure of agriculture," which has meant that once again rural sociologists have begun to pay attention to rural social problems. However, this renewed concern differs somewhat from the early concerns in that the problems under study have societal if not global implications, and the problems are approached from a theoretical perspective, rather than applied, policy-oriented perspectives. Included here are the concerns of Rodefeld (1978) and Friedland et al. (1981) for the negative effects of technological change in farm labor and family farm viability, Heffernan's (1972, 1984) documentation of trends toward industrialization, and concentration in the U.S. broiler industry (Buttel et al., 1990). Friedmann (1978b) has traced the increased commodification of food as it increasingly becomes part of globalized "commodity chains." Albrecht and Murdock (1990) document the increased interest in the sociology of agriculture, observing that the number of articles fitting this subject matter increased from less than 15 percent in the period from 1939 to 1975 to 23 percent during the period from 1976 to 1985.

More recently, rural sociologists have begun to study consumer issues as well, focusing mainly on consumer fears regarding the healthfulness of agricultural products and the potential health and safety hazards of new agricultural and food processing technology (Hoban, Woodrum, & Czaja, 1992; Jussame & Judson, 1992; Sapp & Harrod, 1989; Zey & McIntosh, 1992). McIntosh, Christenson, and Acuff (1994b) and McIntosh, Acuff, and Christenson (1994c) have examined the effects of the public's knowledge of personal food safety on food safety handling in the home. These studies have utilized social psychological models, in contrast to the political economy approaches taken by those in the sociology of agriculture.

Sociologists working in the new field of the sociology of food and nutrition may experience the same sort of criticism as have both medical and rural sociology. A number of the early studies in the area by sociologists have not relied heavily on sociological theory. Furthermore, much of this effort gives the appearance of a sociological application to problems in dietetics. However, researchers such as Allon (1973) and Sobal, Rauschenbach, and Frongillo (1992) have begun to examine how obesity impacts self-image or hinders chances in the marriage market. Tests of world systems and dependency theories have utilized food purchases, food availability, and nutritional status as outcomes in processes of exploitation and immiseration (Bradshaw, Noonan, Gash, & Sershen, 1993; Burns, McIntosh, & Zey, 1994; Wimberley, 1991a, 1991b). Studies of food riots, such as those published in the Walton and Seddon (1994) collection, contribute greatly to the understanding of conditions that lead to collective behavior and social change. These are just the beginning.

An Independent Role for a Sociology of Food and Nutrition

The discussion thus far demonstrates that sociological work on food and nutrition issues overlaps substantially with work in both medical and rural sociology. If those areas of overlap constituted the full range of sociological work on food and nutrition, a new field would be redundant. However, food and nutrition can contribute to studies of the development of self-image, play a role in cultural studies, constitute a major concept in theories of social change, and serve as a focal point in research on a number of social organizations, including families, factories, and restaurants. Thus, sociological studies of food and nutrition will contribute to theoretical and empirical developments in world systems theory, cultural sociology, social psychology, social organization, and social problems. Studies that involve food and nutrition have already had an impact on theory development in such areas of macrosociology as the development of consumer society (Fine & Leopold, 1993), the rise of the state (Tilly, 1992), the state versus society debate (Gilbert & Howe, 1991; Skocpol & Finegold, 1982), collective behavior (Walton & Seddon, 1994), and world systems theory (Bonnano, 1994; Freidmann, 1988; McMichael, 1994) as well as in the microareas of the phenomenology of the body (Turner, 1992) and social support theory (McIntosh, Kubena, & Landmann, 1989a; McIntosh, Shifflett, & Picou, 1989b).

These areas lie at the very heart of sociology, and thus contributions from a sociology of food and nutrition can avoid the mistakes and attendant problems of both rural and medical sociology by demonstrating the role it can play in the further development of sociological theory. By doing so, it can avoid the stigma associated with the characterizations of "applied" and "atheoretical." This new field remains in a somewhat disorganized formative state, and work on many of the fronts discussed above has just begun. This field thus has a great potential for making significant contributions to sociology yet requires further development as a field to reach its potential. To capture this sense of lack of coherence yet high potential, the term "sociologies of food and nutrition" will serve as the rubric for the sociological studies of food and nutrition. Only when the possibility of a formally organized field is under discussion will I revert to the singular version "sociology of food and nutrition."

3

Culture and Food

INTRODUCTION

The cultural represents one of three predominant approaches used to explain food use and nutritional health, the others being the economic and the psychological. Anthropologists have accounted for the majority of cultural studies of food and nutrition, although sociologists and historians have given some attention to these subjects.

Anthropologically based cultural schemes traditionally have emphasized either cultural materialism or variants of symbolic structuralism. Recently others have created models in which the material and symbolic aspects of food (and other objects) play equal roles. In addition, descriptive studies of food and food practices exist.

While some of these studies have been produced by anthropologists, folklorists and historians have also made major contributions. Sociologists have only recently shown an interest in food as a cultural phenomenon. Much of the work by sociologists (and others) on origins of consumerism and its implications for society have application for the study of food. Furthermore, sociologists have expended a great deal of effort on reexamining and reformulating the concept of culture itself, which may advance the study of food and nutrition.

Mennell et al. (1992), Murcott (1988), and Whit (1995) have reviewed and critiqued the various anthropological approaches to food and nutrition, making it unnecessary to do so here. Anthropologists have tended to focus on either the materialistic or the symbolic aspects of food and nutrition, and the debates among them have centered on which of these ontological positions is correct. The functionalist approach of Malinowski (1944) largely focuses on the cultural and social arrangements that develop in response to the biological needs of human beings. Sociologists have built upon this framework in order to construct sociological approaches to nutrition (McIntosh, 1975; McIntosh, Klongan, & Wilcox, 1977; Sobal, 1991a, 1991b). Evolutionary or developmentalist arguments by both anthropologists (Childe, 1963) and sociologists (Lenski & Lenski, 1987) have pinpointed the importance of agricultural innovations and surpluses in making possible the increases in urbanization and differentiation-specialization associated with societal evolution.

The cultural materialism theory of Marvin Harris and others has shed a great deal of light on overlooked, seemingly "irrational" food behaviors that contribute to long-term societal viability (Harris & Ross, 1987). Harris's famous example concerns the role that "irrational" beliefs against eating animal flesh plays in ensuring that a sufficient number of cows are maintained so that generations of buffalo may be produced. These buffalo serve as the chief means by which Indian farmers cultivate their fields. The farmers justify their behavior in religious terms rather than through their recognition of its contribution to long-term survival.

The French structuralism school and its offshoots found in the work of Mary Douglas, Roland Barthes, and Pierre Bourdieu have had increasing influence as the sociology of culture has experienced a renaissance. They make insightful connections between the symbolic aspects of food, on the one hand, and social relationships, on the other. Both anthropologists and sociologists have thoroughly evaluated and critiqued these approaches (see Goody, 1982; Mennell, 1985; Mennell et al., 1992; Murcott, 1988; Whit, 1995).

The works of Harris (1979, 1985) and Lenski and Lenski (1987) appeared heavily undergirded by functionalism, and thus suffered from many of the problems associated with that ontology. However, Mennell et al. (1992) observed that the perspectives of Harris, Mintz, and Mennell himself were more developmental than functionalist, which meant that food habits changed in response to changing social and ecological conditions. In the case of Harris, in particular, food habits were said to evolve in a "Lamarkian" manner. That is, adaptive food patterns were learned and passed on to successive generations through socialization. This elaboration, while sensible, did not rescue materialism from all the pitfalls associated with functionalism. There remained the problem of the disjuncture between what people understood as the reason for adhering to certain food habits and the apparent "wisdom" of these habits for the long-term survival of the group. Hindi farmers spared their cattle because of religious prohibitions on eating animal flesh, not because they perceived the need to maintain cows as the source of buffalo.

If the requirement that food habits always serve some larger functional purpose is relaxed such that functional and dysfunctional patterns are both recognized as possibilities, then materialism of the sort promoted by Harris is far more useful. Mintz's (1985) materialistic perspective proves more beneficial than Harris's because it ties the development of food habits to the economic interests of the dominant class. This and other developmental or evolutionary perspectives are evaluated in Chapter 8.

Sociologists have found Mary Douglas' (1973, 1991 [1966]) work more practical than either that of Levi-Straus or Barthes because she made no claims regarding universal cultural categories. In addition, her food categories (and other categories) are tied to social categories of groups. She connects distinctions in food to distinctions in hierarchical position, on the one hand, and the dichotomy of food/nonfood to the distinction between in-group versus out-group members, on the other. She also suggests that the strength of categorical distinction increases with the degree of hierarchy and sharpness of intergroup difference.

As will be seen, these arguments have some utility. However, Douglas's (1984) most recent work on food gives a clear indication that the underlying order existing between food categories connects to no similar underlying order with regard to social complexity. This failure, however, should not preclude more systematic searches for links between structural complexity and food habits. Furthermore, hierarchy and strength of intergroup distinction are by no means the only frameworks for distinguishing between groups. Other forms of social differentiation exist, and differences in political, economic, and ideological power lead not only to differential access to foods but also to differential ability to control the definition of what is "good to eat."

Anthropologists have made many contributions to our understanding of the social and cultural bases of food production, distribution, and consumption. Much of their work focuses on historical, prehistoric, and nonmodern cases. Furthermore, their accounts, with only a few exceptions, ignore intrasocietal class and ethnic differences in food habits and nutritional status. These represent some of the areas where sociologists can make major contributions.

SOCIOLOGICAL APPROACHES TO CULTURE

The remainder of this chapter shifts the focus away from anthropological perspectives on food, nutrition, and culture to potential insights that might result from a number of sociological perspectives on culture. Admittedly, some such approaches rely, in part, on anthropologists such as Douglas and Levi-Straus, but many base their work on insights drawn from Durkheim, Weber, Marx, Simmel, Veblen, Elias, the critical theorists, neo-Marxism, and postmodernism.

One line of thought lies in sociological explanations of the processes that brought about modern societies and how such societies differ from traditional ones. Some have focused on processes of differentiation-specialization and rationalization; others, on the process of commodification and the elevation of the exchange of commodified goods above those exchanges that foster social integration. This latter topic constitutes a major theme in the work of critical and postmodern theories. The purchase of goods with exchange value (and ultimately, with sign value) becomes paramount in the lives of members of modern societies. The concerns of these approaches shift attention away from historical and nonmodern cases and onto modern society.

As the above suggests, several approaches to culture, including critical theory, neo-Marxism, and postmodernism, begin with the premise that a modern society contains a capitalist economy. This particular institution manipulates other institutions and culture itself to maximize profits and maintain order in the market place. This approach to the culture of commodities and consumerism has largely dealt with fashion and durable goods, with only recent application to food and nutrition.

A second approach lies in the treatment of culture as a resource by which one class dominates another. Work here draws on Max Weber, Thorstein Veblen, and George Simmel, with Pierre Bourdieu providing the most visible and effective contemporary work. Prominent in Bourdieu's analysis of class competition in France are examples of foods, restaurants, and concerns for nutritional health.

The third approach to culture is more strictly "cultural" than either the neo-Marxist/critical theorist or class dominance perspectives in that it considers culture the outcome of noneconomic processes. Culture in the first two approaches has no independent or causal status of its own: it is an instrument by which profits can be increased, social order maintained, and status preserved. Several recent discussions of the origins and importance of consumerism indicate that cultural, rather than economic, forces lie behind commodities and consumer behavior. D. Miller (1987) and Campbell (1987) reflect recent efforts at developing cultural explanations of modern consumerism. This kind of work has had little application to food and nutrition, but I will attempt to demonstrate its potential utility.

Fourth, sociologists consider the study of ethnicity and, in particular, ethnic group relations to be "bread and butter" issues. Salient topics in these studies are the maintenance of ethnic identity, processes of assimilation, and processes of exclusion for they suggest reasons for differential food habits and lack of access to certain food sources. While sociologists have paid scant attention to the role that food and possibly nutritional status might play regarding these issues (see van den Berghe, 1984, and Alba, 1990, for exceptions), some fruitful ideas can be generated when theories of ethnicity and ethnic relations are brought to bear on food and nutrition.

Finally, both sociology and anthropology have an interest in the adoption and diffusion processes that surround technological and other innovations. Much of the work that exists has dealt with the adoption and diffusion of agricultural technology in both premodern and modern times with some attention paid to innovations in cooking and food choices. Once again, further understanding of changes in food beliefs, food behavior, and nutrition are possible through the extension of these perspectives.

MODERNIZATION THEORY

Modern societies consist of differentiated institutions that themselves are divided into specialized units for purposes of effectiveness and efficiency. The institutions connect through abstract media of exchange such as power, influence, money, and commitment. Principles of rationality operate in most institutional spheres and impinge on institutions such as the family and religion, which have thus far escaped the process. Furthermore, modern culture itself promotes instrumental rationality and, increasingly, value rationality as well.

For many, technological innovation powers the engine of modernization. In increasing the energy extraction from the environment, it increases surplus food and other resources needed to support larger populations at a higher standard of living (Sanderson, 1990).

As the horizontal dimension of society grows in terms of new roles and institutions to achieve greater differentiation and specialization of tasks, the vertical dimension changes as well. A differentiated class structure develops in which the bulk of the societal population has shifted out of the lower classes into the middle categories as achievement replaces ascription as the mechanism of placement (Lenski & Lenski, 1987).

Finally, modern selves change as well. The modern personality holds beliefs in the efficacy of science and technology and in the importance of planning ahead and saving resources for future use (Inkeles & Smith, 1974). Modern selves are rational selves, willing to impose self-restraint and defer gratification, including both eating and drinking practices (Gusefield, 1991; Schwartz, 1986). At the same time, modern selves are said to experience a certain amount of mistrust and uneasiness regarding the benefits of modernity. We begin the discussion of modernization and food with technological changes in agriculture.

Modernization of Agriculture

Until recently, sociological theories of modernization tended to focus on the causes and consequences of industrialization and political and cultural change. When these theories have included agriculture as a factor, they have viewed it as a means to modern ends: the mechanization of agriculture improved productivity to the point that an increasingly large urban population could be supported with inexpensive food. At the same time, this productivity could be achieved with fewer workers, releasing needed labor for urban factories (Braudel, 1979b; Weiss, 1980). In addition, some of the more recent discussions have focused on the improvements the modernization of agriculture have created for increased quantity and quality of the human diet (Floud, Wachter, & Gregory, 1990). Some, however, have disputed the hypothesis that nutrition improved significantly as a result of industrialization (Sagen, 1987; Whit, 1995). Finally, modernization has transformed the storage, transportation, processing, and preparation of food.

Specific Changes and Their Import

The modernization of agriculture involves the substitution of new technology for labor as well as for older technologies. The general result sought is that of increased production, a goal which has often been achieved in a spectacular manner. While too numerous to list in their entirety, certain general areas of technological change are worth noting. In horticulture, the advances have occurred in soil and water management (cultivation, irrigation, fertilization) and in plant breeding; in the world of domesticated animals, breeding and range management stand out.

As Cronon (1991) and others have documented, technological change in the form of transportation and preservation contributed greatly in overcoming temporal and spatial barriers to food distribution. The invention of the railroad, grain and refrigerator cars, grain silos, meat packing plants, and marketing boards all contributed to the ability to transport food stuffs well beyond their point of original production. An additional implication of these innovations was that a greater variety of ecosystems could be tapped and their products marketed (Fischler, 1980). These changes led, for example, to access by American families to a greater diversity and quantity of meats at lower prices (Cronon, 1991).

Modernization in association with capitalism has had yet another effect, one which was largely unintended. The increasing separation of food from its source of production increased the possibility of adulteration by the unscrupulous. In fact, the original motive for establishing the Chicago Board of Trade was to institute quality standards and mechanisms for their enforcement (Cronon, 1991). As the distance from the original site of production and the number of hands through which the product passed increased, customer suspicion grew.

The modernization of cooking processes is said to have lagged behind those in production agriculture (Cowan, 1983). Cooking technology renders foods more edible, digestible, and palatable. As in agriculture production, it can affect the productivity of the activity as well as the labor process. The invention of the stove, for example, has increased the number of items that could be cooked simultaneously and permitted the expansion of types of cooking (Cowan, 1983).

Prior to the stove, Europeans primarily used the hearth, which generally permitted only roasting and fast boiling. Stoves allowed both slow and fast boiling, baking, and broiling, often at the same time. Refrigeration extended the life of products, allowing extensions not only in their marketing but also in their preservation in the home. The latter had the potential for reducing the frequency of trips to the market; the later invention of supermarkets, however, which eliminated neighborhood stores, led to longer distances traveled to obtain food and other supplies (Cowan, 1983; Walsh, 1993).

Social Differentiation and Differentiation of Cuisine

As Goody (1982) argued and Mennell et al. (1992) further developed, cuisine followed social differentiation. Societies with greater social differentiation (or grid, as Mary Douglas referred to it) had a more differentiated cuisine as well. This was principally a hierarchical distinction, the notion of an elite cuisine versus the common meals, dishes, cutlery, and norms regarding deportment of the nonelite.

Control and manipulation of the symbolic aspects of class help maintain class boundaries. Hierarchical societies manage to deny inhabitants of the lower order access not only to goods considered necessities, but also to those goods whose very possession denotes upper-class status. In societies in which hierarchical control is less, as lower-order groups obtain sufficient resources, they are able to command access to these status goods. In order to continue to maintain possessional, and thus, symbolic distance, upper status groups must seek new goods and symbols. We will return to this theme of exclusion at a later point.

Processes of Modernization and Changes in Food

Childe (1963) and others observed that literacy generally developed in hierarchical societies. The ability to read and write not only differentiated one class from another but increased the power of elite classes over an illiterate nonelite. Both Goody (1982) and Symons (1991) argued that dietary distinctions occurred only in those societies whose populations had achieved some level of literacy, some degree of urbanization, and large agricultural surpluses. The importance of these latter characteristics followed closely the evolutionary logic of both Childe (1963) and Lenski and Lenski (1987) and agreed with Giddens's (1984) assessment of the importance of urbanization.

Symons (1991) and Braudel (1979a) round out the picture by suggesting that trade and imperialism were sources of added variety to elite cuisine. Symons (1991) perceptively observed that the ordinary diet–cuisine distinction was insufficient and proposed a further step in the historical process of differentiation: traditional cuisine evolved further into reflexive cuisine as a result of societal rationalization. Under these conditions the kind of elite described by Freeman (1977) began to appear. This elite thought about, discussed, and experimented with food. Its numbers must reach a critical mass to support a cadre of like-minded chefs, a condition fostered by urbanization. In addition, Symons (1991) believed that cuisine reflexivity and literacy were mutually reinforcing.

Symons (1991) argued that in addition to urbanization, literacy, differentiation-specialization, and the development of hierarchical rationalization of the diet contributed to cuisine development. He argued that the long-term evolutionary sequence included increased energy extraction, storage-distribution, and control over the environment through the application of rationalization to agriculture, then food processing, and finally cooking. Rationalization was clearly at work in agriculture, reaching down to the level of the so-called family farm, transforming the distribution and storage processes and, most recently, the processes involved in food preparation both at home and in the commercial sector.

This approach, which emphasized vertical differentiation, is not without its problems. For example, Goody (1982) emphasized that substantial social distances between classes in society led to major distinctions between class diets. However, this observation may not hold universally, as a recent description of the Thai diet suggested. In her comparison of the food eaten by royalty and commoners, Van Esterick (1992) found little distinction. It should be noted that elite speak a different form of Thai and wear very different clothing than do the nonelite (and are much wealthier than the average Thai). The dishes chosen to eat and the ingredients selected by their cooks were quite similar. Perhaps Thai cuisine might have developed greater status differentiation had Thailand began to urbanize at an earlier point in time, or the Thai simply relied on other means of status differentiation.

A similar problem with Goody's approach was observed by Mennell (1985) who found that while the French court developed an elaborate cuisine designed specifically to distinguish it from the bourgeoisie, the pluricentric distribution of power in England resulted in far fewer culinary distinctions. Yet such differentiation remains the order of the day in France, but few such differences are observed in American society (Lamont, 1992), nor are they apparent in English cuisine. Perhaps the former difference results from greater mobility changes in the United States, yet the latter difference cannot be so simply explained: social mobility is relatively low in England.

Finally, while some societies have produced a single "high" cuisine associated with a so-called courtly class, others such as Italy, India, and China produced haute cuisine based largely on ethnic and/or regional traditions (Appadurai, 1988). Mennell et al. (1992) argued that such cases represent multiple rather than unitary societies. For example, China was not a single society, but rather a number of loosely united societies sharing some common elements of culture and social structure (Jones, 1981).

The issue of multiple cultures held together by political, economic, and perhaps some cultural arrangements leads to the consideration of multiethnic societies. Where class and ethnic categories do not neatly coincide, the relationship between social differentiation and culinary distinction is less clear. In fact, dietary variety may displace culinary distinction, depending on the circumstances. Dietary complexity will likely vary with the manner and degree of ethnic group incorporation.

Complete assimilation would mean the disappearance of each group's own cuisine. Complete separation would mean the ghettoization of cuisine. In both cases, cultural complexity is thus low. Under more pluralistic circumstances, while each group maintains many of its customs, the more tolerant atmosphere encourages a greater participation of out groups in an in group's cultural practices. Thus, for example, in a situation of complete assimilation, no "ethnic" restaurants would exist; there would only be restaurants reflecting the dominant group's culinary heritage. Under complete separation, each ethnic group would maintain its own set of restaurants, serving its own cuisine with little patronage by nonmembers. Under greater pluralism, a greater variety of restaurants would be frequented by all.

Ethnicity and Food

Modernization, in theory, brings with it a reduction in ethnocentric beliefs and primordial attachments, replaced by both nationalism and a sense of citizenship (Geertz, 1973). The theory of assimilation, or inclusion, further assumes that as individuals immigrate from other societies, their national and ethnic beliefs and attachments will subside once exposed to the forces of cultural and structural inclusion. These views have been modified greatly since their first advancement in the 1950s. Not only do so-called traditional societies have difficulty in subverting ethnocentrism, but it continues to prevail in even the most advanced of countries. Thus, some modernization theorists embrace a model of "pluralism with equality."

At any rate, ethnic identification remains strong in the United States among Anglos, Hispanics, blacks, and Asians. Within each of these major groupings further diversification exists. The designation Hispanic establishes a convenient label for what constitutes a number of widely differing ethnic groups. Hispanic reflects persons from such diverse origins as Mexico, Cuba, Nicaragua, Columbia, Uruguay, and so on. The category Asian, for example, represents Japanese, Chinese, Filipino, Thai, Lao, Vietnamese, Indian, and so on. Researchers continue to find major differences in language (including slang), beliefs, and customs across these groups. In addition, each group has differing immigration histories that have affected the types of adaptive cultural responses made to living in the United States.

Ethnicity among non-Hispanic whites (often referred to as Anglos, despite the inaccuracy of such a term) remains a meaningful distinction as well. A great deal of structural assimilation has occurred among non-Hispanic whites. Members of such groups participate fully in both the economic and political institutions of society, and high proportions of each white ethnic group have intermarried with members of other white ethnic groups (Alba, 1990; Greely, 1974). Nevertheless, cultural distinctions remain. For the white ethnic, these distinctions are to a certain degree voluntary; individuals can choose to embrace or deny their ancestry. In some senses, the use of ethnic identity in the construction of one's self is the sort of lifestyle choice modern societies permit, as in Giddens's (1991) view.

Alba's (1990) study of self-identified "white ethnics" found that nearly 85 percent could identify their ethnic heritage; 33 percent could identify a single ethnic ancestry; 36 percent, two; 26 percent, three or more. These respondents were then asked to identify ethnic experiences that in their own eyes were central to their ethnic identity. Of the native-born ethnic whites, 26 percent could identify no such experiences, but 23 percent could identify six or more. Three experiences appeared to have the greatest relevance for identity: first, the eating of ethnic foods; second, the utilization of certain words or phrases from the language of their heritage; and third, carrying on customs and traditions. A fourth, participating in ethnic festivals, approached these three in relevance.

Alba (1990) then analyzed the relationship between the importance of ethnic heritage with the tendency to eat foods of the respondent's ethnic origins at least on a monthly basis and found that the greater the importance of heritage, the greater the likelihood of eating such food. In addition, he found that those who both *identified* with a single heritage as well as actually possessed such a heritage were more likely than others to eat ethnic foods at home and on special occasions. While no significant differences were found regarding the propensity to use special ingredients during cooking, even here such use was greater among those who both subjectively and objectively could be classified as having a single ethnic heritage (Alba, 1990:85–91).

These findings are important, for they give credence to the claims that ethnic heritage remains central for some and that food plays an important role in the maintenance of such heritage. Pierre van den Berghe (1984), in fact, claimed that ethnicity is primordial as well as situational and that ethnic cuisine represents the ethnic group's long history of reciprocal relations between kinsmen and members of the same community. This sense of long-term interdependence provides basic resources for survival, including food. Because of the close association of food with ethnicity, on the one hand, and ethnicity with self-identity, on the other, cuisine remains strongly rooted even after language and other customs disappear during inclusion processes.

Certain structural factors may facilitate cuisine retention. For example, the city of Alhambra, California, the majority of whose population is Chinese, 200 restaurants serving such cuisine exist (Davis, 1992). In fact, urbanization, while normally associated with the breakdown of ethnic cultures, also leads to the concentration of members of various ethnic groups. As a result, increases in the economies of scale may occur to a sufficient degree so as to allow ethnics to maintain their cultures (Kalcik, 1984).

When assimilation occurs, it carries with it certain costs. Some writers have observed the pain that cultural assimilation causes several generations later when the very success of assimilation leads to estrangement with one's heritage. One writes: "I feel torn between desiring for my children's acceptance within what we call a multicultural society and wishing they had a stronger identification with their Japanese, Chinese, and Filipino heritages. I also recognize that at this time in their lives they could do little more than clothe themselves in their grandparents' culture; for because they have been raised almost solely on McDonald's and Sesame Street, their cultural search would make them just another set of ethnic tourists" (Kaneko, 1993:184). Agueros (1993:227) described his experience of returning home and eating the bread of his country again: "Ah, Bread, you make me realize that it is hard and wasteful to be purely ethnic in America—definitely wasteful to be fully assimilated."

The process of intermarriage further encouraged the loss of ethnic identity, as heritage becomes diluted. Alba's (1990) data clearly demonstrated that the importance of ethnic identification declined fairly steadily by generation and that this process was exacerbated by the number of ethnic groups in the person's background. Positive responses to the inquiries regarding the eating of ethnic foods declined as ethnic identity lessened. Furthermore, Alba's (1990) subjects reported that while previous generations successfully passed on food traditions, their authenticity decreased with each successive generation.

Anderson (1988) found that cuisine assimilation occurs more rapidly in families that experience both peer and institutional pressures to conform to local food norms, as when children are exposed to school lunch programs. While some school lunch programs have attempted to provide meals that reflect the cultural backgrounds of their students (Biagi, 1992; "Mexican Food," 1994), such efforts appear neither widespread nor sufficient to accomplish anything more than the retarding of assimilation's momentum. Food consumption researchers in the United States have found that the regional differences in cuisine that once characterized American foodways are in rapid decline; class and age are now better predictors of such habits (Guseman & Sapp, 1984, 1986).

Camp (1989) and Pillsbury (1990) described extensive regional differences that lasted well into this century, reflecting the initial as well as later immigrant settlement patterns described so well by Meneig (1986). However, Pillsbury's (1990) attempt to demonstrate empirically that regional differences in cuisine remain strong is not convincing. An examination of his tables indicates that while each region was characterized by the type of restaurants available, the percentage differences across regions were not particularly great. Furthermore, the national chains that continue to sweep the nation, leaving only the less populated places untouched, have made only half-hearted efforts at developing their own versions of regional cuisine. Pillsbury (1990) reported that the chains do better business in some regions compared to others, but these would appear to be only temporary setbacks.

Others have reported a renewed interest in ethnic cuisine in the United States (Levenstein, 1993), but much of this interest is faddish—one cuisine will become popular, only to be replaced by another. Thai food has begun to supersede the once highly popular Chinese food in some areas of the country; in others, Chinese restaurants remain the more numerous.

Ethnic food products have also found a major market niche in the United States; the *Houston Chronicle* (Boisseau, 1992) has reported on the growth in sales of La Minita's Mexican Food Products, which produces 1.6 million tortillas per day. Nationwide, tortillas now outsell bagels, English muffins, and pita bread. The article further reports that Mexican food was the country's fastest growing ethnic food, with sales of more than $2.2 billion in 1992. As others have observed, however, the popularity of ethnic foods waxes and wanes.

It is currently unclear whether the renewed interest in ethnic foods is a genuine move toward cultural pluralism or is faddism driven by the forces discussed earlier. Furthermore, the degree to which these ethnic food products achieve authenticity is also in question. Much of the demand for tortillas, for example, derives from the fast food industry's attempt to expand their repertoire, rather than maintain tradition. Groups, many of whose members are recent immigrants, create market niches. Many Hispanics, for example, preferred high-fat milk and have increased their consumption of it while consumption by other groups has declined (Senauer, Asp, & Kinsey, 1991).

It is also important to note that modernization has broken down many regional differences not only through the spread of fast-food restaurants but also through the spread of producers of national and regional food goods and by supermarket chains. This process is made possible by innovations in food preservation and packaging. These moves toward a more national cuisine are found elsewhere as well. In Japan, both international tourism and the mass media have turned "regionally unique dishes" into national fare (Ashkenazi, 1991:296). The forces at work here are those of massification, rationalization, and capitalism.

Remarks regarding culinary differentiation must be tempered as well. Members of modern societies belong to numerous groups whose boundaries do not neatly coincide. Members of the same ethnic group may also belong to the same religious group but are far less likely to have the same occupation, live in the same neighborhood or region of the country, or belong to the same kinds of voluntary organizations. These cross-cutting social ties insure less rigidity of group boundaries. Furthermore, these ties increase the likelihood of exposure to a greater variety of cultural conventions as well as the likelihood of a greater willingness to experience them firsthand.

Horizontal Differentiation

Modernization theorists, unlike many evolutionists, have tended to focus less on vertical and more on horizontal differentiation. Thus, another way of looking at modernization is to determine whether diets become more complex (i.e., contain greater variety) with increasing role and occupational differentiation. In modern societies, horizontal differentiation is high and is based principally on occupation. There is some evidence that occupational cultures develop that spill over into the private lives of members. The effects of occupational differentiation are discussed in Chapter 5.

More complex societies tend to differentiate activities and goods produced, and they also tend to have greater trade involvements. However, these same societies may make far less use of the potential food items available to them, while less modern societies make extensive use of the plants and animals available in their environments. A complex society such as the United States makes culinary use of only a fraction of the mammalian species available for consumption and makes no use of its abundant insect population. At the same time, while the food stores in complex societies seem to abound with differing products, one could argue that many of these products differ more in terms of labels than ingredients.

Much of the preceding discussion rests on a great deal of speculation. More systematic attention needs to be paid to the complex interrelationships between food and its symbolic relevance, on the one hand, and the changing nature of class systems, on the other, including their degree of openness, increases in horizontal differentiation, and the cultural and structural relevance of ethnicity. In particular, the effects of the degree of social integration and cross-cutting ties on cuisine exclusion and dietary complexity require direct examination. This calls for original research because existing data sets such as the National Food Consumption Survey and the National Health and Nutrition Examination Survey lack a complete inventory of status roles.

Modernization as Destruction

A neglected theme in the modernization literature concerns the destruction of the past. Modernism displaces and destroys tradition (Behrman, 1988), replacing it with what is considered new and modern. Modernization represents a process; however, as what was new and modern yesterday becomes outmoded, it too is replaced. Modernization has the potential to destroy the spiritual connection culture has with its food.

A number of traditional cultures developed a close association with a particular food. Some European societies were once associated with the bread they both produced and consumed. This appears less the case today, largely due to modernization. At the same time, traditional symbols may be reasserted as a means of moderating the destruction of traditional culture.

Ohnuki-Tierney (1993) argued that rice has consistently played a pivotal role in Japan's "myth-histories." It represented a metaphor for the Japanese collectively in that it connoted commonality among human beings and between human beings and spirits. It reflected the difference between organized society and the wilderness, and it set boundaries of "imagined space, seasonality, and Japanese history" (Ohnuki-Tierney, 1993). Of interest, however, was that rice became a central symbol during the "Early Modern period" and most especially during the Second World War. It stood for the symbol of the "purity of the Japanese self" in response to threatened encroachment from the West, and, in reaction to the current invasion of American fast foods, the popularity of Japanese cuisine has actually increased (Ohnuki-Tierney, 1993).

At the same time, however, modernization creates greater fluidity in the creation and destruction of symbols. For example, Lewis (1989) has argued that the lobster has come to symbolize Maine. This is not the result of some deep structural process, but rather a conscious attempt to further develop a tourist industry. Lobster became a desirable regional cuisine and a means to symbolize one having visited the Northeast through the possession of lobster images on tee shirts and as jewelry. As Lewis (1989) has observed, the symbols extend both the spatial and temporal range of the highly perishable original.

The arguments made by those who support the view that the symbolic aspects of food play a deterministic role in a society need careful scrutiny. It is clear from Lewis's (1989) analysis that both status and financial interests motivated the elevation of lobster to its current symbolic prominence. The situation described by Ohnuki-Tierney (1993) provided a number of political reasons why rice has been raised to its position of prominence. From Mann's (1993) perspective, such symbols are a source of power developed and wielded by those who wish to achieve tangible social goals.

Modernization frees people from the constraints of tradition, which is often based on rigid ethnic and status differences. People can now access what they are able to afford, regardless of their background (Fischler, 1980). Cuisine is open to all. At the same time the forces that once bound people to one another are loosened. Fischler (1980) has boldly argued that the delinking of people parallels the delinking of food from the greater, meaning-providing symbolic order, creating a situation of gastromie, the food equivalent of anomic social relations.

Modernization involves a belief system that includes an emphasis on progress. Transformations of nature become matters of routine application of technology. Faith in the efficacy of this technology is present. The ability of technology to produce intended results buoys up this faith. Granted, technological change results in numerous unintended consequences, but their connection to the originating technology is often obscure.

Technological innovation and social differentiation are not the only destructive forces associated with modernization. Considerable evidence suggests that rationalization and commodification processes may equal or exceed the impact of technology and differentiation.

THEORIES OF ADVANCED MODERNITY

Advanced modern societies reflect many of the same tendencies said to characterize modern societies but carry them to greater extremes. Theorists of advanced modernity argue that in addition to capitalism and strong states, advanced modern institutions include a significant surveillance component. Furthermore, the state practices reflexive monitoring; that is, the state sets goals, pursues them, and alters course when necessary to pursue other goals. Such direction requires the widespread control of human behavior.

The second major feature of modern institutions lies in their disembeddedness: institutions are "lifted out" of their local contexts to operate at national, and sometimes global, levels. This is achieved through the media of exchange or what

Giddens calls abstract systems and expert systems that "bracket time and space through deploying modes of technical knowledge which have validity independent of the practitioners and clients who make use of them" (1991:18). Institutions have the capability of separating time from space constraints: the when and where of conduct are no longer intrinsically linked (Giddens, 1991).

In order for institutions to perform adequately, they must instill a sense of trust. In fact, day-to-day interactions involve trust; humans need to trust in order to obtain what Giddens (1991:19) referred to as ontological security. Trust, however, is not a given. It must be earned by both the institutions and the individuals with which a given actor is connected. A certain amount of distrust, perceptions of risk, and insecurity characterizes modernity, and the scientific method leads to perpetual doubt. Finally, the modern self is said to be reflexive; that is, through continued self-monitoring the self undergoes frequent change: we are what we make of ourselves; what we make of ourselves is based, in part, on how we define and redefine both our past and our potential future; we self-actualize by maintaining control over our personal time and by balancing opportunities and risks; we extend reflectivity to the body itself—the body becomes an action system rather than remaining the passive object of earlier periods of human history (Giddens, 1991:75–79).

Theorists of late capitalism echo some of these sentiments but view the modern self as having much less individual autonomy. This is partially due to the importance they place on the institutions of capitalism and the state. Capitalism is essentially exploitive, and the state is a mechanism that not only enhances exploitation but maintains stability in the face of potential disruption caused by protests and complaints over exploitation. Culture itself has become not only a commodity but, through the cultural media, a mechanism of exploitation as well. Finally, late capitalism has generated contradictions and crises that have led to the unraveling of the welfare state (Habermas, 1976; Offe, 1985). Society is characterized by corporate takeovers, vertical integration, and downsizing of factories and farms; decline of blue collar industrial positions and their replacement with low-skilled white collar jobs; globalization of markets; and colonization of the lifeworld (the commodification of heretofore primary relations) (Crook, Pakulski, & Waters, 1992). However, it is the relentless spread of rationalization into every area of life that has received the most attention in the food related literature.

Advanced Modernity and McDonaldization

Commentaries on agriculture in advanced modern societies have focused on the industrialization of agriculture, or what some have called "factory farming" (Goodman & Redclift, 1991; Johnson, 1991). While some types of animal agriculture and certainly some segments of dairying have industrialized, as Goodman and Redclift (1991) observed, much of agricultural production itself remains craftlike.

Beyond the farm gate, however, value-added processing is highly industrialized and becoming more so with time. This aspect of agriculture is Fordist in nature, creating industrial products that have a long shelf life and are convenient for the consumer to prepare by using interchangeable inputs similar to the manufacturing of durable goods.

George Ritzer's *The McDonaldization of Society* (1993) used the principle developed by the McDonald's Corporation and other modern organizations to illustrate the observation Weber made regarding the processes and consequences of rationalization. Ritzer noted that the rationalization process involved the institution of procedures that insure predictability of operation, calculability of actions to access their costs, control of the labor process by substituting machines for workers, and greatly standardizing the routines of the employees who remain to further insure a predictable product. One unintended outcome, however, was irrationality. The very steps taken by McDonald's and its mimickers, while insuring instrumental rationality, led to dehumanized working conditions and value rationality. That is, valued noneconomic pursuits became commodities.

Ritzer (1993) noted that McDonald's and Club Med represented rationalized forms of leisure, negating the very meaning of leisure. Recreation was meant to be an escape from the "iron cage," not simply another version of it. As Ritzer also observed, alternatives to McDonald's-like cages existed, pointing to Marvelous Market and Ben & Jerry's Ice Cream as alternatives. Blue Bell Ice Cream of Brenham, Texas, also attempted to create an image of a less rationalized, less bureaucratized food company, in part by producing small batches of high-quality ice cream. In such examples, we find that substantive rather than instrumental rationality are the primary driving forces: taste and quality served as the purpose for doing business, not simply efficiency, predictability, or calculability.

Ritzer (1993) ended his treatise by arguing that we can escape the iron cage by never entering it: avoiding establishments such as McDonald's and frequenting places such as Marvelous Market. While this may be good advice generally, it presupposed first the availability of such alternatives and second the wherewithal for each of us to take advantage of these more expensive alternatives. Furthermore, there was some suggestion that alternative food producers such as Ben & Jerry's cannot avoid the standardization that resulted from changes in scale and so increasingly rationalize as their markets expand.

CRITICAL THEORY AND POSTMODERNISM

Critical theory represents an attempt to tie important insights from Weber and Freud to Marx's critical view of capitalism. Weber's insistence that the modern world reflects the outcome of a long period of rationalization and bureaucratization in Western societies and Freud's observation that civilization leads to certain regressive tendencies among people are thought to be necessary additions to Marx. Over several decades critical theory has moved away from Freud, using other works such as Kohlburg's developmental personality perspectives to fill the gap. Critical theory permits the study of the state in the context of exploitive capitalism, develops the means by which the various crises of the late twentieth century may be explained, and again makes central the perception that late capitalism exploits not only labor but, more importantly, consumers. Consumers become objectified and reified through the same mechanisms as labor (Goldman, 1992). Furthermore, the so-called lifeworld, or that private arena exempt from market transactions (family, community, friendship, religion), is increasingly "colonized" by the market, turning nurture and support into purchasable products. Baudrillard's (1981, 1988) work is in some senses the most recent rendition of critical theory, although he carried his vision to a point where he accused Marx of bourgeoisie social constructionism. Marx accepted the bourgeoisie notion that production represents the fundamental force in society. According to Baudrillard, the force is exchange. However, exchanges in the market are distortions of the primitive gift exchanges that Baudrillard (1981) believed to represent undistorted social relations. In addition, Baudrillard incorporates ideas from poststructuralism. He is thus not only associated with the poststructuralist camp but also with postmodernism—an association he claims to detest.

Culture as Domination

Essentially, culture serves as a mechanism of domination over those without control of the means of production by those with such control. The thrust of the culture-as-domination approach is to consider culture as a means of social control and manipulation of consumption. Culture, from this point of view, is thus robbed of its civilizing as well as humanizing functions. Critical theorists and neo-Marxists have particularly pushed this theme, arguing that a "culture industry" exists in capitalistic societies. This industry makes individuals willing accomplices in their exploitation (Marcuse, 1964), leading to conformity in behavior and a loss of a conscious understanding of their circumstances (Adorno, 1975).

This manipulation serves to eliminate dissent and questioning or at least channels it into nonthreatening directions. As important as culture is as a stabilizing mechanism, it plays a central role in capitalistic expansion. As the existing market becomes saturated, new markets must be created through the creation of new goods. Through marketing, advertising, and mass media influences, images are manipulated to create a desire for commodities not yet possessed. Certain clothing, cars, and foods become associated with lifestyles expressed by actors on television and in movies (Bell, 1976).

This trend has recently accelerated through the prominent display of brand names in the scenery of films or in the dialogue of actors. Similar (and earlier) trends in novels are described by Harris (1990). This process has appeared to take yet another step with the announcement that the Kellogg name and its cereal products would soon appear with the NBC logo prior to programming on this television network. Shows would be brought to the public by Kellogg and NBC. In exchange, NBC's logos and the names of the stars of six current NBC shows would appear on various Kellogg's cereal boxes (Sloane, 1993). Thus far, no such exchange has occurred.

Such manipulation and its driving motivation were even clearer in advertising. Ads involved the manipulation of symbolic imagery in such a way as to associate a desirable persona or lifestyle with a particular product. Early in this century the image manipulation potential of the commercial was recognized. Prior to this time ads for products simply identified the product and relied on endorsements and half-truths about the product. Attractive packaging and claims such as health properties began to be routinely used to improve sales. For example, promoters of yeast, salt, and chocolate all made unsubstantiated claims about the vitamin content and health-inducing qualities of their products (Levenstein, 1988). Food packaging and advertisements continued to promote their products in this way.

In the 1920s the idea of consumer engineering was born. It began with the idea that the product had to be beautiful, and its imagery had to tap deep-rooted desires in consumers. Furthermore, it was thought that an emphasis on beauty would undermine the practical aspects of the good, permitting compulsive consumption (Ewen, 1988). Manipulation of imagery, in fact, could create new desires, partially through linking them to dreams and daydreams (Campbell, 1987; Williams, 1982).

Cultural domination began with the dominant class as it accepted and manipulated cultural objects to influence the tastes and desires of other classes. Mintz (1985), for example, analyzed the development of a culture of sugar among the elite in England, the incorporation of sugar into mass production, and the ultimate spread of this good down the class ladder, propelled by lower prices and drawn by desires to emulate the upper classes.

Following Gramsci's (1971) lead, Gvion-Rosenberg (1988, 1989) argued that the culture of the hegemonic class is used to dominate the taste and consumption of other classes. From this point of view cultural pluralism is merely a dodge; tolerance of differences actively entails assimilation of differing cultural elements into a single cultural system.

Gvion-Rosenberg (1988, 1989) provided interesting evidence for the processes of hegemony through her analysis of American cookbooks published since 1945. In her first analysis, she showed that culinary pluralism, represented by the incorporation of ethnic dishes into the American diet, was actually culinary hegemony in that ethnic dishes are transformed or Americanized either by (1) incorporating the dish and presenting it as American (e.g., macaroni and cheese, apple pie), (2) replacing foreign ingredients with local ones, or (3) inventing "ethnic dishes which are granted a culinary affiliation not known in their supposed country of origins" (Gvion-Rosenberg, 1988:11–12).

This view of a hegemonic melting pot in which goods, robbed of their original cultural significance, simply may reflect broad processes of cultural change that has occurred in all societies rather than only capitalist systems. For example, Klopfer (1993) described the development of Padang restaurants in urban areas of Indonesia. These restaurants seeked an image that reflected a specific ethnic and regional origin, but, in fact, the cuisine and customs represented had been emptied of "culture as knowledge and practice." Instead, ethnicity was isolated as a performance of a few colorful customs. In terms of the social nature of Minangkahaw cuisine, this meant loss of "context for masculine and feminine roles and for the social significance of eating daily food and ceremonial food" (Klopfer, 1993:303). Thai versions of Chinese restaurants produced Chinese dishes using unmistakably Thai spices. Ashkenazi (1991) observed that the Japanese have historically adopted foods from other Asian and Western societies, often redefining them as Japanese.

Postmodernism

Postmodernism picks up much of the critical stance of the "late capitalism" school but carries the critique further into the realm of culture. Postmodern societies, according to postmodern theorists, no longer liberate but subjugate. They engage in hyperindustrialization and hyperdifferentiation. A postmodern society represents the domination of commodified relationships in noneconomic contexts and the continued differentiation regardless of functional consequences. Hyperrationalization and hypercommodification exist, in which consumption, freed from taste, becomes a dominant concern. The state's functions are now surveillance and external defense; citizen's rights have eroded; the distinction between high and low culture has disappeared; the aesthetics substitute for function in products as well as art. Ultimately, both meaning and self are fragmented (Crook et al., 1992; Rosenau, 1992).

Both critical theorists and Baudrillard find that Marx's notion of "fetishism" is a particularly insightful concept when it comes to the study of commodity consumption. When a commodity becomes the bearer of value, it is fetishized. The fetish represents exchange value rather than the more "natural" use value and becomes part of the exploitive nature of social relationships under capitalism. Critical theorists have carried this idea forward to argue that objects take on an exchange value that comes to represent an image of the type of person (and thus the type of social relationships in which such a person engages) who most likely uses such a good. Baudrillard (1981) carries the notion of fetish even further by arguing that people in advanced capitalism do not exchange goods, but rather signs. The signs themselves have become vast fictions of what the good is worth and what it represents.

Many students of consumerism draw equally on critical theorists such as Benjamin, on poststructuralists such as Barthes, and on postmodernists such as Lyotard. The thrust of their studies deals with music, food, and literature as commodities that can be marketed. More importantly, however, are the perceptions that things that enter the market become commodified signs. That is, they are bought and sold on the basis of the image they reflect, not on the basis of their use value.

According to Crook et al. (1992:37), postculture contains no fixed boundaries between "art" and "popular art" or "commodified art." "Postculture does, indeed, exhibit a semiotic promiscuity and preference for pastiche and parody which commentators widely associate with postmodernism...a television commercial sells cat food by setting the sales pitch to the music of a Mozart aria" (Crook et al., 1992:37).

In this view, packaging was a means by which producers communicated with consumers, using eye-catching illustrations, color selections, and brief messages relating to the product's "importance." For example, the package may claim that a product was "new," "high fiber," and/or "fat-free." Strasser (1989) argued that as food production underwent industrialization, companies sought methods to distinguish their products from others in order to sell in larger quantities to increase profitability and to be able to claim an adulteration-free good. Packaged products served these purposes. Susan Willis (1991) carried this argument further, asserting that in the postmodern world packaging is fundamental to the creation of the product's sign value or image, however disconnected from use value.

Advertising

Advertising represented a cultural form, unique at least in its origins, in modern societies. Advertising developed in the United States, according to Strasser (1989), to increase demand in the face of rapidly increasing supplies of products created by mass production. As new products and brand names were created to increase the consumption of a particular company's goods, advertising provided a particularly suitable vehicle for this purpose.

Ads do affect purchasing behavior. Using aggregate data on spending on advertising and food purchases, Forker and Ward (1993) demonstrated that expenditures on both generic and brand name commercials substantially increased sales of food commodities such as beef, milk, cheese, eggs, and various vegetables. McIntosh, Kubena, and Peterson (1993b) showed that exposure to specific ads and newspaper stories that link health outcomes to diet affect food consumption.

Modernists, perhaps best represented by economists, generally argued that ads do not manipulate, they inform. Consumers already know what they want and used ads as sources of information about alternative products. Schudson (1986) argued similarly that ads helped consumers rank a product relative to other products along a status continuum.

Other social scientists generally evaluate advertising more critically. A conservative version, offered by Bell (1976), suggests that advertising has helped create the consumer ethic at the expense of the work ethic. Marxist and critical school theorists have regarded advertising as a method of capitalistic manipulation, creating wants and needs that heretofore did not exist (Baudrillard, 1981; Goldman, 1992). Postmodernists share many of the same ideas held by the critical theorists regarding advertisements. Many thus view ads as essentially manipulative, with Baudrillard holding the position that advertisements have become "obscenities." "Certainly the new level of advertising marks a distinct break in the degree of directness....The technique...is one of 'perverse provocation', as if the bank were saying, in Baudrillard's words, your arse interests me, give me your arse and buttocks and I will bugger you and you will enjoy it" (Gane, 1991:87).

Goldman (1992) and others relied on Baudrillard's notion that advanced capitalism maintains a political economy of signs, one in which signs, increasingly divorced from both use and exchange value, are exchanged. In such an economy, advertising becomes important in creating and transmitting symbols.

A product such as beer is given a particular name, say "Micheleob." The beer has certain properties and functions that its maker hopes will appeal to consumers. These may have to do with taste, caloric value, price, and so on. Ads for Micheleob, however, rarely focus on either taste or calories, but upon particular experiences that hold particular meanings. Weekends have come to mean leisure, relaxation, extended time in the private or life world. Thus the ad proclaims: "Weekends were made for Micheleob." Over time the valued event becomes symbolized by the product so that when confronted with Micheleob, the consumer associates it with the pleasures of weekends, with relaxing. Beer ads represent a particularly good source of attempts at portraying products as signs for desired experiences and events. "Old Milwaukee" and special times in the great outdoors are spent with friends, usually brought together around some valued event such as grilling steaks or recently caught fish or boiling lobster on the beach. "It doesn't get any better than this," claims the ad. "Heineken" becomes, if the ads are any indication, synonymous with success; "Coors" ads portray "Silver Bullet" (Coors Light) consumers as both young and desirable men and women. The ads place these persons in settings that foster promising interaction: bars with dancing and mixed gender volleyball games at the beach. In this environment, shyness disappears; meeting attractive strangers lacks the usual discomfort and fallibility.

Jhally (1987) argued, similarly to Goldman, that ads empty products of their real (use value) meanings and create new meanings for particular audiences. Thus the producers of products are said to buy specific groups of people or audiences when they buy commercial time during a particular time of day. He set out to demonstrate not only "fetishization" but also audience differentiation by examining a sample of 1,000 prime-time and sports-time commercials, arguing that products discriminate between female and male users. Thus, television stations aired ads for males during those times at which the largest audience of males were likely to watch television programs, such as sports programs.

Ads for female viewers aired during prime time when they were most likely to watch (Jhally, 1987). Ads for females linked families, family activities, and romantic relationships with beauty aids, house cleaning products, and foods. Food ads constituted 23 percent of all prime-time ads, but only 3 percent of ads shown during sports programming. These figures reversed when the product was alcohol—only 3 percent of prime-time ads were for beer, but 23 percent of the sports-programming ads promoted this product (Jhally, 1987).

As groups such as women are further segmented, the orientation of the ads changed. Monk-Turner's (1990) comparison of advertising themes in two American magazines (*Glamour* and *Cosmopolitan*) with those in two British magazines (*Options* and *Woman's Journal*) indicated that the American magazines contained a much higher percentage of ads with beauty or science themes while the British magazine ads were more likely to emphasize taste and efficiency. Had she selected *Good Housekeeping* or *Women's Circle*, the ads would have focused on other themes, as these magazines likely have an audience that differs from that of *Glamour* and *Cosmopolitan*.

True postmodern ads, however, go beyond simple attempts to make a product something more than it isn't: something that reflects a totality of desirable experiences. A true postmodern ad would reflect a simulacrum; that is, it would represent a reality that isn't a reality at all but rather only an image of reality. Recent Marlboro cigarette ads demonstrate this well. The ads attempt to make smoking look both natural and healthy by depicting smokers as active individuals in the great outdoors, but, at the same time, they have the mandatory Surgeon General's health warning placed at the boundary of the ad (Kellner, 1991). In the realm of food advertising, perhaps the term "lite" serves as the best example. Lite products are sometimes low in calories, other times not; sometimes low in fat, other times not. Lite beer ads, furthermore, suggest their product "won't slow you down."

A second way that such postmodern ads achieved their purpose lies in those that scramble meaning, scramble "signifieds and signifiers," and blur the art of high culture with that of mass culture. Goldman (1992) provided excellent examples of such advertisements. None dealt with food; a canonical case was a recent Reebok ad that combined a number of images taken out of context to create a convoluted image. The ad consciously attempted to portray itself as "not an ad," suggesting that the consumer was too hip to be fooled by advertising.

Postmodern advertising may bury the brand name in a welter of imagery (Goldman, 1992) or ignore it altogether:

> Where raisins from California were once marketed according to specific brand-name identities such as "SunMaid," they are now promoted as the "California Raisins" and embodied in a band of wrinkly-faced black "dudes" with skinny arms and legs, who chant "I heard it through the Grapevine" while soaking up the California sun. "California Raisins" do not represent a return to the pre-brand-name generic commodity, but rather a hyper-commodity whose connection to rock music and black culture heroes precipitates a vast array of spin-off products, from grotesque dolls to beach towels emblazoned with "Raisins" (Willis, 1991:2)

The commodified relationships Goldman (1992) detected in recent McDonald's ads may also reflect hypercommodification as well. He claimed that corporations have recently attempted to cash in on the current angst over the decline of the family. Campaigns for products such as Coke, McDonald's, and Taster's Choice served as examples of efforts to connect private emotions with products portrayed to represent idealized families and family relations. McDonald's ads began by presenting an idealized family in an idealized setting; at the end of the ad, McDonald's is linked to these idealizations. Like the idealized family in an otherwise chaotic world, "McDonald's depicts itself as a 'haven in a heartless world'" (Goldman, 1992:99). McDonald's seized on anxieties stimulated by separation and isolation and implied these can be neutralized and conquered through consumption of McDonald's as a commodity sign. McDonald's becomes a community of friendship and kinship (Goldman, 1992:100). At the same time that companies reaffirm the importance of the private world, they undermine it through commercialization.

Most commercials for food, however, have shied away from such extremes. Instead, while advertisers have tied food items to many of the same lifestyles as products such as shoes, they can also link food with convenience and good health. Advertisers may view direct rather than obscure approaches as the most effective means to promote food products.[1]

---

[1] I have looked and challenged others to do so. Only Gaye Seidman of the Department of Sociology, University of Wisconsin–Madison, (personal communication) produced a plausible candidate. She explained that the Taco Bell ads that involved the piano player and chorus in the back of an old pickup truck contained enough confusing pastiche to qualify as postmodern. Bishop-Tramm (1995) observed that series of bizarre ads for milk that involved full-page, color photos of sports and media starts. These icons were well dressed and well kept save for a slim "mustache" of milk on their upper lips. Text was practically nonexistent and stated little about the value of milk. Instead, the ads implied that the rich and famous drank milk and were not ashamed to leave its lingering residue as a badge of honor. An ad showing milk spilled on one's front would defeat the intent to show that one can be cool and sophisticated while at the same time sloppy.

Malls and Fast-Food Restaurants

Postmodernists have singled out malls and fast-food establishments as characteristic of postmodern economy and culture. Both have encouraged hypercommodification, use bizarre combinations of imagery involving the new and the old, and create images of unreality. Langman (1991:217) described malls as opportunities for "self-production of recognition seeking spectacles," a self-hood that is both lonely and voyeuristic.

Mestrovic (1992) argued, however, that postmodernists and critical theorists too quickly condemn malls and fast-food restaurants. He quite correctly observed that these sites of consumption, for all their glitter, glitziness, and emphasis on commercial transactions, also provided individuals with "all of the functions of the old-fashioned town square. Senior citizens can participate in walking or jogging groups. Primary groups form around the video arcades, coffee shops, and indoor restaurant plazas...the mall protects the individual from the small-town gossip and surveillance that were always present in archaic societies" (Mestrovic, 1992:134). This suggested that malls represent a continuity with past changes in social arrangements of eating and drinking in public.

The earliest restaurants and boarding houses provided men who were separated from their families with meals and informal social contacts. Only later did restaurants become oriented toward serving families (Pillsbury, 1990). Bars in the nineteenth century, while considered coarse and corrupting, became a place where young, unmarried immigrants could find friendship, information, meals, and women (Powers, 1991). In fact, bars selling ale were actually encouraged in nineteenth-century England in an attempt to discourage the working class from drinking harder spirits (Gofton, 1986). Today, many find the bar a place for friends to meet, a place to make contacts with unmarried women, and as an escape from the harsh demands of an unrelenting work ethic (Alasuutari, 1992).

Postmodern Foods

Postmodernist food examples have been more prominent in the form of isolated cases. Barthes (1973, 1982) described the Japanese meal, with its lack of a central dish, as fundamentally postmodern. He described this as a "crisis of the sign, elimination of the critical distance, de-centering of authority, conflation of production and consumption." A Japanese owner of a Euro-Japanese restaurant in Hawaii traveled to France to learn French-style Japanese cooking. So-called Japonais cooking involved little that is actually Japanese in origin but, rather, is Chinese. The intent of Japonais cuisine was to create a particular image by appropriating widely from a variety of Oriental food cultures (Tobin, 1992). A final example came from Diane Barthel (1989), who described the cultural modernist disdain for chocolate boxes as their belief that Victorian artifacts are both outmoded and in bad taste. Yet chocolate has remained a food of luxury and fantasy, and it is considered postmodern. The design of chocolates rendered "the simulacrum an art form" and chocolate combined images of self-pleasure with obscenity, lack of self-control, and overindulgence in a weight-conscious world.

Health Magazines

Health magazines have proliferated along with those oriented toward the outer features of the body such as *Shape*. Some of these publications reflect modernist values, but others contain messages of suspicion of modern institutions such as medicine and the pharmaceutical industry. *Eating Well* takes a unique position among such magazines. It manages to combine health, the aesthetics of food dishes, and taste in its presentations. In print since 1990, every cover of this monthly publication presents a stunning photograph of a food dish. On the cover of the January/February 1993 issue (vol. III, no.15), an attractive slice of banana cream pie seems to rise from the page toward the reader. The colors of objects around the pie are earth-tone brown, yellows, and greens. The caption reads "Luscious Low-Fat Banana Cream Pie." Standard columns in the magazine include: "The Healthy Skeptic," "RX for Recipes," "The Rush Hour," "Dinning Well," "Nutrition," and "Market Place." The remainder of each issue is devoted to recipes, all of which contain beautiful photographs of the end result, all the while recognizing them as low-fat, nutritious, unique, and tasteful.

Povlsen's (1991) study of changes in pictures of food in women's magazines suggested that aesthetics only recently have displaced more utilitarian portrayals of food. From the 1950s to the 1980s, pictures were used to help communicate how to prepare a dish by showing how the results should actually look.

The Health Food Movement

The health food movement has many attributes that would make it appear postmodern in nature. Health food ideology involves a mix of science and spiritualism, along with a nostalgia for the "natural" and for nature. Adherents believe that through individualistic self-control over their own behavior they can perfect and purify their bodies. Relying on expert advice from various health movement leaders, these individuals argue that a healthy life is obtainable through the reunion of mind, body, and spirit (Goldstein, 1992; Kandel & Pelto, 1980; Murcott, 1986). This mix of seemingly contradictory ideas from science and nonscience, the nostalgic view of what circumstances foster health, and the drawing from a great diversity of sources of wisdom are among the characteristics that make this movement appear postmodern. In addition, many in the movement believe that society is a corrupting influence; however, as society can't be changed, the only viable means available for achieving good health is through their own individualistic efforts (Whit, 1995). Finally, despite the emphasis on health as an individual problem solvable through personal efforts, a number of the organizations associated with the movement emphasize group solutions (Goldstein, 1992). For example, Overeaters Anonymous uses the same 12-step approach as Alcoholics Anonymous. Overeaters Anonymous emphasizes the need to remain a practicing member for the remainder of one's life in order to stay slim or, as in the case of AA, to remain sober.

However, comparisons of the current health food movement with the health food movement of the nineteenth century suggest great similarities, making the current movement's postmodern status suspect. As in the current movement, health foodists of the last century emphasized spiritualism, science, and pseudoscience, and both movements emphasize the untrustworthiness of modern institutions (Gusefield, 1992). Thus, both have perceived modern medicine as a source of health problems rather than their solution. It might be added that both have suspected that the food industry willingly compromises the healthfulness of their products in the pursuit of profits.

One difference between the health movements of the two centuries, though, may lie in perceptions of governmental culpability. During the nineteenth century, the consumer could not expect protection by government from business; now consumers do. However, many currently appear to have grown disillusioned over the ability and willingness of the U.S. Department of Agriculture (USDA) and Food and Drug Administration (FDA) to regulate agriculture and the food industry.

SOCIOLOGY OF RISK AND DIET, NUTRIENTS, AND HEALTH

Several sociologists have argued that societies in the stage of advanced or high modernity exhibit risk as a characteristic (Beck, 1992; Freudenburg, 1993; Freudenburg & Pastor, 1992; Giddens, 1991). Their intention is not to claim that life is far more risky than before; in fact, the opposite appears to be the case. People live longer than ever before as societies devote more resources to the improvement of health and welfare. Specific medical, social, and engineering innovations have produced these improvements. Rather, risk constitutes a cultural outlook (Beck, 1992; Giddens, 1991).

The very improvements that have enhanced life chances have increased our understanding of what puts us at risk, and as our knowledge increases, so does our ability to make predictions about harmful outcomes. This very ability increases awareness and fears of these outcomes. In addition, institutions such as the economy, government, and science/technology increasingly take actions that have unintended consequences. At the same time these institutions contribute to delocalization. That is, actions that have harmful effects on local areas are taken by those whose connections to those local areas have greatly lessened.

Finally, a number of consequences created by such institutions were far more global and final than earlier actions. Nuclear and global warming suggested apocalyptic endings never before possible. Freudenburg (1993) argued that the public has come to recognize a certain "recreancy" on the part of progress-generating institutions, that is, a perception that institutions that supposedly shield us from the negative consequences of technology frequently failed to do so. These breakdowns may occur, in the public's view, because of (1) technological incompetence, (2) dishonesty, or (3) inability of the system to cope with unanticipated problems.

Both Giddens (1991) and Freudenburg (1993) focused on global or community-level risks ranging from nuclear holocausts to leaks of radioactive waste into the local water supply from a nearby waste deposit. Global warming and local environmental and sustainable agricultural concerns were examples as well. However, I have claimed that, in addition, current concerns over irradiated foods, growth hormones in meat, and the lack of sufficient nutrient content in food were all part of a recent loss of public faith in public institutions to protect us from risks.

The historical evidence of mistrust in the food industry tempers this strong assertion somewhat. As stated earlier mistrust appears to increase with increasing distance between consumer and producer. The latest evidence of mistrust in food science may reflect the even greater separation created by innovations in food technology, rather than a recent break with modernism.

Critics suggest that food companies have effectively captured the regulatory mechanisms of both the USDA and the FDA, arguing that neither the food supply nor its regulation for safety and quality deserve our trust. In addition, while defenders of food advertising claim that ads provide an important source of information that consumers would otherwise lack in attempting to make informed purchases, critics charge that these efforts are neither truthful in content nor sufficient in amount to serve as useful sources (Gussow, 1990).

As the amount of information and its inconsistencies increases, fear and mistrust also increase. Apparent inconsistencies, such as the disagreement among scientists over the role of dietary fat in coronary heart disease and whether margarine is truly safer to eat than butter, have led some to give up their quest for better health and have led others to seek alternative ("new wave") authorities who share the same concern and mistrust. Trust has shifted from the food industry and food scientists to local purveyors of natural foods (Giddens, 1991:23).

The ecology movement, in general, and the sustainable agriculture movement, in particular, reflect reactions to the disembeddedness of agribusiness and agricultural science and technology whose interventions have resulted in local as well as global concerns for environmental quality and long-term sustainability of human life (Allen, 1993; Buttel, 1995). Radical solutions proposed by the sustainable agriculture movement include conducting agricultural research within local settings in which the results will be applied and involving both local producers and their knowledge of sustainable practices (Victor & Cralle, 1992). Thus, agricultural research becomes decentralized and participatory.

These arguments recall the optimism of the late 1950s and early 1960s in which many of the NGOs (nongovernmental organizations involved in technical assistance to Third World countries) practiced local solutions for local problems and principles of self-help. Those were days in which such policies were prompted by visions of the elimination of poverty and the modernization of society with all of the seemingly desirable characteristics of modernity. The renewed interest in local solutions and self-help derived not from an optimistic but from a pessimistic vision: Changes must be made not to improve lives, but merely to sustain them over the long haul.

Perceptions of risk lead to mistrust not only of what modern institutions produce but what "expert systems" express about those products. Such experts have long defended r-BST and food irradiation, but instead of persuading the public of the merits of these, the motives and the abilities of the defenders have come under suspicion.

The extent of the gap between consumers and experts is evident from a number of studies that have shown that while experts rank food-borne pathogens as the greatest food safety risk to consumers, these dangers are ranked last by consumers themselves, who instead feel that they are at greatest risk from "additives" of various sorts including pesticides, food coloring materials, heavy metals, and growth hormones (Groth, 1991; Lee, 1989). Such differences exist in Europe as well, although the experts there are more concerned about salt, fat, and sugar than bacteria (Sellerberg, 1991).

As previously mentioned, the experts themselves frequently disagree, and over time many change their position with regard to a particular finding. From newspaper accounts of dietary fat and heart disease research, it is quite evident that not all medical researchers agree that such risks exist or that the public can engage in behavior changes that would substantially lower their risk of heart disease. It is perhaps less evident that within dietetics and nutrition similar disagreements have occurred regarding what advice should be given to the public with regard to dietary fat and as to whether or not the food industry ought to be criticized. Some argue that the food industry merely provides what people want; it gives them choices by which they can make informed selections, depending on their need for convenience or health. Others argue that the choices are illusionary in that a number of the options are not real alternatives, based on real differences, at all. In addition, they charge that product labels differ from what the product actually contains or mislead in terms of their meaning. "Lite" until recently has had no standardized meaning; 97 percent fat free implies a fat-free and therefore "safe" food to eat for those wishing to restrict their fat intake, but the more important information, the percentage of calories from fat, which is usually much higher than 3 percent, is missing. Regulations are currently forcing changes in such practices.

If our culture and society may now be described in terms of risk, how widespread has the perception and concern for risk become? Empirical studies, in fact, indirectly point to widespread concern, although these results provide insufficient evidence to support the notion of a culture wholly consumed by fears of the future. Indeed, concerns for risks are not uniformly held across class structure or gender (Hoban & Kendall, 1993).

However, Giddens (1991) observed that as society refines its ability to calculate and communicate risks, the perception of risk grows. The new nutrition labels for foods, which begin with fat content, and the forthcoming safety labels on fresh meat products may result in the unintended consequence of a heightened fear of food.

Finally, the idea of "risk society" developed in the context of a perceived likely nuclear holocaust and global environmental destruction. While the demise of the Cold War has reduced the likelihood of the first form of mass destruction, the latter potentially still hangs over humankind. When drawing a contrast with the Middle Ages, however, it is clear that for inhabitants of Europe during that period, the possibility of the destruction of the world as they knew it appeared highly likely. As Camporesi (1989) has suggested, these fears and obsessions resulted not only from real conditions of scarcity but also from hallucinatory states caused by hunger, the conscious use of poppy and hemp seeds in the preparation of bread, and in the use of moldy flour in bread making. Matossian (1989) provided statistical evidence of widespread presence of these mycotoxins in bread, using data from the seventeenth to nineteenth centuries. Claims regarding today's world include aspects of the environment that are said to make people ill, not hallucinate. Furthermore, the Europeans feared what are today regarded as natural calamities, while present-day fears draw on images of human-caused calamities. The contrast may appear less compelling. The point, however, is that Europeans of earlier, less globally connected times held fears similar to those of current Europeans.

NEW SOCIAL MOVEMENTS AND RISK SOCIETY

Perhaps because of the new risks and the changing nature of social relationships in postmodern societies, new kinds of social movements have appeared. As indicated, groups have rallied around the issues of food safety, environmentalism, animal rights, and saving the family farm. In a number of respects, such issues are hardly new. Conservationism began in the nineteenth century; issues of food safety drove public and governmental concern at the turn of the century. New social movements, however, differ from the old in several ways (Crook et al., 1992; Galtung, 1990; Rosenau, 1992).

First, more so than social movements of the past, the new movements are value driven. Giddens (1991) has argued that the very appeal of the new social movements is in their ability to connect members of advanced societies with moral and existential questions long repressed by institutions. Their goals—clean environment, sustainable agriculture, and safe food—are not means to some more ultimate end such as greater equity in the class structure but instead are ends in themselves. The intended contrast is the labor union, which is modernist; its goals of higher wages, better benefits, and better working conditions are the means by which labor seeks to equalize its working conditions with other classes.

A second difference lies in the relationship of the new movements to traditional political parties. Unlike modern movements such as organized labor, which aligns itself with and often has become subordinate to traditional political parties, the new movements attempt to maintain organizational autonomy and distance from traditional politics in an effort to avoid compromising their goals.

Third, new social movements more likely practice democratic principles internally and have thus far avoided bureaucratization and oligarchization characteristics of labor unions and political parties. Finally, the new social movements have aligned themselves with the culture industry, arguing the importance of speaking for individualistic rights in the realms of creativity, freedom of choice, and liberation (Touraine, 1995).

The new social movements tended to be highly issue oriented. This may involve temporary coalitions with other groups to pursue a particular goal for often very different reasons. Rosenau (1992:148) illustrated this contention with the opposition to the opening of a Carl's Jr. hamburger franchise on the University of California at Irvine campus. Boycotts and picketing were organized by "consumer and animal rights groups who were joined by Japanese Americans, lesbians, gays, and people with disabilities."

Discussions of the new social movements have not carefully examined interrelations and potential disharmonies among the movements that may, in fact, be quite widespread. For instance, many who support the idea of an extremely low fat diet may support public efforts to lower fat in the diet, elect to eat such a diet, and recommend it to others. They may support legislation promoting such diets and criticize the food industry for making only cosmetic changes toward the production of a low-fat diet. Some may adhere to low fat diets because the stand they have taken in opposition to the exploitation of animals for food and research purposes. However, not all of those who believe a low fat diet is healthier necessarily find fault with industry, and those who choose to criticize industry may, at the same time, have no quarrel with the use of animals for either sustenance or research. For example, the Physicians Committee for Responsible Medicine (1990) has strongly promoted vegetarian diets, arguing that, unlike the Prudent Diet promoted by the American Heart Association, vegetarian fare not only lessens the intake of fats but eliminates animal protein and cow's milk. Such a diet, its proponents claim, actually reverses heart disease, lowers blood pressure, and lessens the risk of diabetes, gallstones, kidney stones, osteoporosis, and asthma. This group promotes what it calls the new four food groups, which consist of whole grains, legumes, vegetables, and fruits.

In 1990 a number of nutritionists questioned the credibility of the Physician's Committee, noting that one of its most prominent members was also connected to animal rights activism. His motives for recommending such a radical change in the human diet were thus considered suspect relative to his known commitment to animal welfare.

STATUS-STRIVING, CONSPICUOUS CONSUMPTION

Weber (1968) distinguished between life chances and lifestyles. Position in the social stratification system bears on both. One's position in the hierarchy of resource access determined, to a great extent, how long one lived and what level of health one enjoyed. These were a person's life chances.

Thus, we are speaking of access to a quantity and quality of food that renders a diet healthy, an environment less contaminated, and formal health care. Weber (1968) also described resource distributions associated with lifestyles. These distributions map out social differentiation among groups of persons.

Lifestyle resources were not used to extend life or make it more comfortable but instead to achieve distinction from others. In some societies simply having food on a predictable basis may serve exceedingly well as a means to distinguish one's self from others. Certainly during the Middle Ages, a time of periodic food shortages and famine, having enough was "having it all." As Camporesi (1989) eloquently described, during much of the Middle Ages, Europeans were consumed by fears of disease, hunger, and the night and were obsessed with getting enough food, the availability of bread, and concerns that undeserving others (e.g., monks) might have gotten too much. It was a time during which a "fair price for bread" symbolized the right to live (Thompson, 1971). Furthermore, persons from all class levels were obsessed not only with obtaining food but also with food's effects on their bodies. They worried about eating enough bread so as to have sufficiently frequent bowel movements. Thus, during medieval times, lifestyle differentiation, at least with regard to food, was minimal.

As sufficient agricultural surpluses eliminated famine over time, however, reducing with it the fears and obsessions associated with insufficient food, more attention was paid to differences among classes. Differences in quantities consumed by various classes was superseded by concern over the quality of the food consumed. Thus, cuisine was born (Mennell, 1985). The changing nature of food and the manners associated with its eating arise largely from the so-called civilizing process described by Elias in *The History of Manners* (1978) [1939]. Mennell supplemented Elias's material regarding cuisine but, more importantly, extended the Elias perspective to status mobility as the dynamic element in the continued change in taste, manners, and cuisine.

A number of writers since Veblen's *Theory of the Leisure Class* (1953) [1899] have argued that the consumption of goods in modern Western societies is driven less by basic human needs than by socially defined needs. Further, these wants frequently consist of what other persons of higher status already possess. This point of view has received various support by sociologists such as Mukerji (1983), McCracken (1988), and Bell (1976) and has been described as "conspicuous consumption" or the "consumption ethic." Some of these writers claim that the consumption ethic was a precursor to capitalist production (Murkerji, 1983); others argue it is the result of the breakdown of the very Protestant ethic that led to capitalist production (Bell, 1976).

The desire to appear of higher status implies that lower income groups will attempt to consume beyond their immediate means. The role of the installment plan (Bell, 1976) and the recent development of near instant credit in the form of credit cards means that, even if momentarily, a person can rise above his or her status. A common mechanism of momentary status change is the restaurant. A person does not have to belong to an exclusive club to dine on high cuisine, only have the means (cash or credit) to do so. Many exclusive restaurants restrict access, thus increasing their desirability by limiting the number of patrons they serve. Others do so by simply elevating their prices. The diner gains both the cuisine and the elegant circumstances thought to characterize the everyday lives of those with higher social status. Finklestein's (1989) classification of restaurants aptly demonstrates that their owners realize that dining out is for public display and thus that image may be more important than the taste of the food served.

Bourdieu (1984) has continued Veblen's rather vicious descriptions of conspicuous consumption and class competition. Despite Gartman's (1991) claim that Bourdieu is no more than an extension of Veblen, Bourdieu's work is, in fact, difficult to categorize neatly. Bourdieu has attempted to blend French structuralism's emphasis on unconscious linguistic structure with Marxist materialism (Garnham & Williams, 1980) by refusing to separate object and subject, intention and cause, and materiality and symbolic representation (Wacquant, 1992:5).

Systems of symbols serve not only to demark one class from another but also to "maximize" the reproductive interests of one class relative to others. Symbolic violence is the "preferred mode" of dominance in societies in which material resources are few. Even in countries where resources are more plentiful, reducing class mobility by limiting access to cultural practices remains an important weapon.

Bourdieu (1984) attempted to disentangle the class system in France through the analysis of taste. Taste represented internalized ideas regarding where the person fits in social structure, what her or his relationship is to others, and those orienting practices that range from the "most automatic gesture or the apparently most insignificant techniques of the body-ways of walking or blowing one's nose, ways of eating or talking...to the most fundamental principles of construction and evaluation of the social world" (Bourdieu, 1984:466).

Taste permits individuals ways of distinguishing their own class membership from that of others, and this taste becomes a social weapon used to maintain class boundaries. Part of taste is acquired within the family, but much is obtained from the educational system. The educational system produces cultural capital in that it provides individuals with a sense of what matters most in life and how those things ought to be viewed and discussed. To produce such taste differentiation, the educational system itself must be stratified.

Food played a major part in the Bourdieu scheme. He described food as the "archetype of all taste" for it "reflects directly back to the oldest and deepest experiences" (Bourdieu, 1984:79). Furthermore, practices and goods associated with different classes were organized in accordance with the structures of opportunity. The main opposition relative to food consisted of income. However, true differences were in the "opposition between the tastes of luxury (or freedom) and the tastes of necessity" (Bourdieu, 1984:174).

Those with the "taste of necessity" were considered the "people who don't know how to live; who sacrifice most to material foods and to the heaviest, grossest, and most fattening of them, bread, potatoes, fats, and the most vulgar, such as wine" (Bourdieu, 1984:179). In the face of the new ethic of sobriety for the sake of slimness, peasants and especially industrial workers maintained an ethic of "convivial indulgence." Tastes in food related to "a whole conception of the domestic economy and division of labor between the sexes" (Bourdieu, 1984:185). Tastes in food also depended on the idea each class has of the body and of the effects of food on the body, that is, on its strength, health, and beauty (Bourdieu, 1984:190).

Recent work indicates that distinctions, symbolic violence, and class competition may differ both in nature and in degree in other societies. In fact, a recent study indicates the relative absence of such competitiveness in the United States. Michele Lamont's *Money, Morals, and Manners* (1992:3) contrasted the upper middle-class cultures of France and the United States, finding that "cultivated dispositions and the ability to display an adequate command of high culture" was far less important in the United States than to French members of the dominant class. More than their American counterparts, the French drew boundaries on the basis of sophistication: "there are rules for everything: when should one use *vous* instead of *tu*? Does one know at a glance the difference between a fish knife and a cheese knife?" (Lamont, 1992:103). Americans who *did* make these kind of distinctions do so on the basis of what is considered cosmopolitan: an interest in the cultures of others expressed through travel, language learning, and experiencing differing culinary traditions (Lamont, 1992:107).

Domination and Resistance

A recent study of food and domination among the Zumbagua Indians in Ecuador showed how useful this approach, especially when integrated with others, can be. Weismantel (1988) produced an analysis much like Bourdieu's (1984) in that food was the fundamental vocabulary in the discourse of domination. Food topics frequently appeared during interactions, and particular foods were used to denote class and ethnic distinctions. For example, reference to particular food items could serve as the expression of wishes, rebukes, insults, or snubs (Weismantel, 1988).

Such references, in turn, served to connect Zumbaguans to the wider world of social and political forces that "created their position" relative to other Ecuadorians. Zumbaguan cuisine spoke loudly of subsistence and backwardness relative to the modern, market-based diets of other Ecuadorians.

Finally, Weismantel (1988) emphasized the material nature of food, which structuralists and Bourdieu tended to take less seriously. Precisely because food may be manipulated by social practices, the structure of cuisine lost its fixity. The intergenerational and gender struggles that occurred in Zimbaguan households, many due to differential exposure to and acceptance of wider Ecuadorian society, led to struggles over what will be served and how it will be cooked.

The Return of Veblen

A number of observers have upheld Veblen's perspective regarding the barbaric nature of conspicuous consumption and of status striving. The gentlest description comes from work by Charles Derber (1984) on the pursuit of attention. Modern life has stripped individuals of opportunities for drawing attention to themselves. However, expenditures for goods and services consumed in public redress this loss. Part of the enjoyment of eating meals in restaurants derives from its very public nature: one not only obtains the attention of the host, but of waiters/waitresses, cooks/chefs, and other personnel. Furthermore, the bulk of this attentiveness is enjoyed surrounded by witnessing others. Finklestein (1989:26) has made this point more forcefully, arguing that the very public nature of such service is ultimately decivilizing.

Finally, several observers have alluded to so-called foodies (MacClancy, 1992; Simmonds, 1990). Epicureans, an educated minority, have been replaced by the entire middle class, who, as foodies, are compelled to possess knowledge of food and an aesthetic appreciation of it; to name drop restaurants and to seek out "novel or strange edibles" (MacClancy, 1992:23). Eating out at restaurants is the central activity of foodyism. But unlike the consumers described by Finklestein (1989), whose motivation appears to be self-image building, foodies go for the food itself; even seduction and entertainment take on a lesser role. In fact, foodies are considered self-absorbed hedonists by critics (Simmonds, 1990). This view carries us back to the postmodern image of uncontrolled desires.

CULTURAL EXPLANATIONS OF CONSUMERISM

Few writers have challenged the status striving and conspicuous consumption views of consumerism. One notable exception, however, was Campbell (1987), who argued that Romanticism, an ideological force that played a similar role as Puritanism in the economy, was not consciously developed to encourage consumerism. The Romanticist legacy as it evolved, however, emphasized empathy, dreams, and fantasy. These qualities eventually became a major motivating orientation in dealing with the world of produced goods. Williams (1982), while accepting the view that much of consumption was due to status striving, also argued that dreams and fantasy act as an important motivator in consumption. She and others noted the conscious linking by the market of dreams and goods. Thus, McCracken (1988) stated that consumer goods serve as bridges, especially prior to ownership, between an individual's actual circumstances and an "idealized life." As obtaining an object eliminated the bridge, desire for newer objects occurred.

Producers draw the consumer's attention by using fantasy to entertain while, at the same time, they make a connection between the fantasy worlds the consumer finds desirable and their goods. Thus, vacations, beers, and the like potentially connect the consumer with places filled with happy, young, beautiful people. Buying the product brings that fantasy world to the consumer. Perhaps the most blatant use of fantasy exists in the area of food and exercise products associated with weight loss. Not only are miraculous changes in weight said to be possible, also entire changes in the self and in others' perceptions of the self are promised. Advertisements first depict unhappy, extremely overweight persons, wearing no makeup or attractive clothing, and who are generally portrayed as being isolated and alone in the "before" the product image. The "after"-the-product-is-consumed picture shows slim, happy, attractively dressed and made-up persons now surrounded by smiling, approving friends and family.

Gronow (1991:49), relying on Campbell, argued that food consumers can change their preferences dramatically and within short periods of time, e.g., "from fear of additives to fear of cholesterol." But Campbell (1987) focused on dissatisfaction generated by the differential between the product's promise and the actual experience of the product. Campbell's (1987) model would appear to apply well to the automobile industry, whose ads played on the emotional experiences one expects to enjoy upon purchasing the product. Again, dieting aids provided the clearest example of Campbell's approach to food. Women long to appear similar to the young, slim, attractive models depicted in the ad's "after" pictures. Discovery that the product failed to deliver on its promises apparently neither extinguished the longing nor the belief that the "right" product at some point will come to their rescue.

Levenstein (1993) provided more usable examples in this regard. He described the rise of attraction of French cuisine and its rapid decline in popularity once it became "too common place." Consumers shifted toward Northern Italian, Chinese, and Japanese cuisine. The current rage has been Thai. These shifts are encouraged by cultural entrepreneurs such as Julia Child, Michael Clayborne, Thomas Greene, and Jane and Micheal Stern.

CULTURE AND AGENCY

Many of the cultural perspectives in sociology are realist in nature, emphasizing cause and action at the macrolevel, and arguing that individual behavior results from these macroevents. Others, particularly the social action theorists and structuralists such as Giddens, have attempted to create a perspective in which individuals operate with a certain degree of autonomy. This perspective operates within the constraints generated by culture, institutions, and class. The difficulty of such approaches lies in identifying the amount and nature of such autonomy.

John Fiske (1989, 1991) has described culture in terms of its production and consumption aspects. For instance, he has argued that adolescents purposely attempt to control their own lives through the subversion of conventional culture. Malls serve as sites for such activities, increasing the necessity for greater surveillance and control. Additional guards and cameras generally are insufficient control devices. Clothing styles—the all black look of the 1980s, the pierced ears of males—were all attempts both to separate the youth from the adult culture and to mock the conventions of controlling adults. Fiske is well aware that while parents and other so-called conventional others experience the intended bewilderment and anger, the economy simply looks at such efforts as new marketing opportunity. If the style is all black, manufacture all black; if it is the "grunge" look, manufacture new clothes that appear to have come from a "Good Will" outlet. If body rings are worn because earrings no longer shock and older adult males already wear them, manufacture body rings. Manufacturers have found a market for rings that fit noses, navels, and other body parts. Fiske, as does D. Miller (1987) and Willis (1991), recognized that once a purchaser gets the goods home, the power of the product's sign greatly diminishes. When products are worn, new cultural meanings may develop that may contradict those intended by the manufacturer. Furthermore, the poor may lack the wherewithal financially to immerse themselves in the "social and cultural fluidity" implied in packaged, labeled goods (Fiske, 1991:63).

However, DeVault (1991) has described the entire process of home food accumulation, storage, and preparation into specific meals as involving a great deal more conscious planning, even in lower-class households, than observers might first imagine. This parallels DeVault's (1991) description of women shopping for groceries, which shows active purposive, consumers who strive to achieve the goals they have set for this particular kind of shopping excursion. To do so they cut through the ads, packaging, and other hype used to attract customers.

The struggle over control of the concept of "natural" reflects this point—counterpoint view of culture. As part of the risk orientation that has developed in advanced societies, some consumers have adopted the notion that natural substances are by definition preferable to manufactured products. They are said to be less toxic, more healthful, "what nature intended." As described by Belasco (1993:203), "A predominant theme in both the counterculture and the mass media, nostalgia revealed itself in food marketing surveys as a growing demand for roots, nature, tradition, family warmth and togetherness, local color, and craftsmanship." The challenge for the food industry, in response, has been to meet the demands for nostalgia along with the expectation that food products would be increasingly *more* convenient than before. Some, however, apparently are willing to sacrifice convenience in exchange for natural products, even though the concept of natural may in fact be vague, wooly, and mystical, according to MacClancy (1992). In fact, consumers appear to rank convenience much lower than nutritional value or taste (McKenzie, 1986).

Not all presentations of modern consumerism are so negative. D. Miller (1987) has rejected the view that modern consumption estranges and alienates. Instead, he has argued that the act of consumption—the actual using or using up of the good—"often subjugates these abstractions in a process of human becoming" (D. Miller, 1987:192). Thus the use of the good is potentially liberating. Similar to Giddens's (1991) suggestions that individuals self-reflexively draw on commodities to build desired selves, goods are used in particular ways and in particular contexts to develop images for oneself and for others. Arguing that consumption is a form of creative work, D. Miller (1987:191) has used beer drinking in a pub to illustrate his point. Beer drinkers tend to frequent the same pub, ordering the same beer. These choices not only link the drinker with persons of a particular gender, ethnicity, class, and region but also generate "possibilities of sociability and cognitive order, as well as engendering ideas of morality, ideal worlds and other abstractions and principles. Although, for some, the age of the pub and the authentic nature of 'real ale' may be important, others may perceive an atmosphere of plastic facades, parodied images and find the products of international breweries as more proper, unpretentious and tasteful" (D. Miller, 1987:191).

CULTURAL CHANGE AND FOOD

Theories of modernization assume that innovations eventually spread and eventually replace all old habits and products. Postmodernist and consumer theories have also assumed the relative inability of consumers to resist new products. Few have examined the differential adoption of innovations over time. As with other changes in culture, these result from a variety of forces. In many ways, changes in food consumption are similar to changes studied using adoption-diffusion models in sociology and anthropology. In other ways, changes in consumption may differ from conventional cultural change. Some, as Rozin (1987) has done, argue that food's basic connection to survival increases the stability of food habits. Others might well argue that rapid political and economic changes have forced basic changes even in this area.

William F. Ogburn (1964) some years ago described the obstacles facing the introduction of any new idea. Many dismissed Ogburn as an out-of-date, misguided functionalist, but his description of the factors that either hinder or facilitate adoption captured well contemporary thinking on the topic. He noted that barriers included vested interests and cultural compatibility at the macroend and habit and economic resources at the microend. The introduction of foods from other societies may be blocked by those whose livelihood depend on continued consumption of traditional foods. For example, Japanese rice farmers have resisted successfully the importation of rice grown in the United States and elsewhere and have received support from consumer groups who feared that an open market for rice would increase food insecurity (Yamaji & Ito, 1993). Governments may resist imports because they fear becoming politically weakened by overdependence on nondomestic food supplies. Thus, Britain's reluctance to become a full partner in the Economic Community of Europe arose from its traditional concern for British vulnerability during wartime because the country can be easily blockaded. At the same time, under different circumstances, both political and economic interests have often been served by encouraging the importation of foods from elsewhere.

Barriers at the individual level involve a host of factors including habit (or what Giddens describes as practical consciousness), strong cultural incompatibilities, or lack of resources (Ilmonen, 1991). Food habits are a part of practical consciousness, that part of individuals' everyday repertoire that cannot even be easily recognized and discussed, as DeVault (1991) found in her study of shopping, cooking, and other food habits. Part of the difficulty in making changes lies in the ease with which an individual can rely on habit versus the additional effort that must be undertaken if one chooses change. Routines may involve, for example, not only a narrow range of choices for what one eats for breakfast, but also how many meals are eaten, where they are eaten, and with whom they are eaten as well. Parents spend a great deal of time attempting to influence children's eating habits

(Birch, 1990). Commentators have claimed the meager fruits of success in these efforts appear during adolescence (although no real evidence for adolescent food rebellion exists, unless, anorexics are considered stormers of the food barricade). As a person ages food habits supposedly become entrenched, although research by Peggy Shifflett (Shifflett & McIntosh, 1986–87) found that elderly persons frequently made both adaptive and nonadaptive changes in their food repertoires (see also McIntosh, Fletcher, Kubena, & Landmann, 1995).

Income and education also affect the adoption of new habits; generally those who have more of both of these resources are more willing and able to experiment with new crops, new cooking techniques, and new foods. Frequently, individuals have good reasons for nonadoption. One of these includes the risk involved in changing from familiar to unfamiliar ways of behaving. For example, the switch from a traditional variety to a "miracle" seed involves, for many, the use of herbicides, insecticides, and more precise spacing among seedlings when planted. New varieties are often more difficult to harvest because they mature at lower heights. Finally, the new variety may require not only a change in the way it is prepared for eating but also a change in taste.

At the same time, however, evidence exists that demonstrates the adoption of either single foods or of major reorganizations of foodways by numerous cultures. Historians and anthropologists have done much of this work, but sociologists have contributed by way of studies of the spread of innovative agricultural techniques.

One discussion used concepts drawn from both Rogers (1983) and Hagerstrand (1976) and observed that adoption and diffusion processes involving food were often slow. The fuel for the engine of change appeared to be economic change: either an increase in prosperity or its decrease (Wieglemann, 1974). For example, the importation and use of goods such as sugar, coffee, and tea, all considered luxuries, depended on an upper class positioned to take advantage of these goods. With continued prosperity and an increased supply to the degree that such goods became more reasonably priced, the middle and eventually the lower classes became consumers as well (Mintz, 1985; Schivelbusch, 1992; Wiegelmann, 1974).

During less prosperous times, "famine foods"—substances associated with poverty and desperation, such as grasses—became widespread in use. There existed insufficient evidence to predict whether poverty or prosperity was the more effective fuel for the engine of change in food consumption. Even under conditions of necessity, agricultural and other innovations were adopted at a fairly slow pace (Lenski & Lenski, 1987). For example, the plow was said to have spread at a rate of approximately 1 mile per year; China thus received this innovation approximately 3,000 years after it spread outward from Mesopotamia. Of course, the plow lacked a twentieth-century mass media and advertising campaign to aid its diffusion.

Wiegelmann (1974) also observed that not all food innovations successfully diffused across all classes or across all societies. Part of the problem may lie in the incompatibility of the food with the existing constellation of foods. More fundamentally, there may be a moral barrier to the adoption of certain foods. Coffee spread slowly in the Middle East, not only because of concerns over "coffee euphoria" or intoxication but because of the conditions under which it was drunk, namely, in coffee houses, thought to be places in which immoral and treacherous conversations took place (Hattox, 1985). In Sweden, by contrast, coffee spread widely despite beliefs that coffee drinking was both unhealthy and led to immorality, specifically to a refusal to work (Nelson & Svanberg, 1993)! A culture may simply find, in addition, the potential new food was not viewed as a food at all within its boundaries. Thus, only a few restaurant patrons in the United States have found raw squid—with its particular property of sliminess—attractive.

Current research suggests that innovations in food consumption in the modern world appear to be driven principally by necessity. Both Goodman and Redclift (1991) and Ilmonen (1991) have observed that changes in labor force composition have led to the acceptance of convenience foods in Britain and Finland. In both cases, the entry of females into the labor force, an economic necessity, led to the use of these products. Goodman and Redclift (1991) observed that in order for women to accept convenience foods, a fundamental redefinition in sex roles had to occur. But as Hochschild (1989) and Ilmonen (1991) asserted, sex role changes have occurred insufficiently in terms of male participation in household labor. Women may embrace those innovations in foods and appliances that they perceive will save them time. This issue is explored in chapter 4. As stated earlier, Ogburn (1964) has identified vested interests as an impediment to change. Others have argued that the link between diffusers of an innovation and its potential adopters is embedded in a host of institutional arrangements that include organizations that provide credit (McIntosh & Zey-Ferrell, 1986; Zey-Ferrell & McIntosh, 1987). Households may require credit in order to purchase major appliances, and most farmers rely on credit in advance to purchase farm machinery.

Walsh (1991, 1993) provided ample evidence that innovations in food processing potentially affect packers, transporters, wholesalers, and retailers. He found that the successful spread of an innovation thus seemed to depend on the size, power, and coalition-forming abilities of those groups that either oppose or favor the innovation.

There has been little systematic investigation of individual innovative behavior, such as in the area of cooking. McIntosh and Shifflett (1993) found that recipe innovators had more contact with members of their social networks, participated more in religious activities and in voluntary organizations, had higher incomes, and were able to pay for necessities. In contrast, traditionalists were less involved in voluntary organizations and had denser network relationships. In other words, innovators had the wherewithal and were less subject to the greater demands for conformity associated with dense social ties.

Finally, the rapid changes in the U.S. diet since 1910 have resulted, in part, from traditional supply and demand factors. The role of the mass media behind such trends as the rise in soft drink use and decline in milk intake has yet to be investigated.

CONCLUSION

Sociological theories of culture complement those offered by anthropology. Anthropological theory provides us with functionalist-developmentalist views of the significance of food for human adaptation to material circumstances. It also causes us to consider the deeply symbolic importance of food. Sociological theories of culture complement these efforts by further examining the interrelationships between food habits and symbols and social structure. These theories lead to an examination of how the forces of capitalist expansion weaken the links between social structure and culture in order to mobilize symbols in the effort to increase profits.

Modernization Theory

Modernization theory deals with issues similar to those raised by Levi-Straus, Goody, and Douglas. That is, modernization theory connects changing food habits and symbols to increases in rationalization, massification, and differentiation. However, this work has not uncovered universalistic relationships between social and dietary complexity. Symons's work has taken steps in this direction, but, clearly, more could be done by pursuing these relationships further.

Modernization theory describes processes of social differentiation that proceed along vertical and horizontal lines. Furthermore, modernization means rationalization and homogenization through massification and assimilation. The first set of forces should increase the diversity of foods and food symbols available to members of society, but the second set lead to a reduction of diversity. This suggests that current trends in foodways and food symbols are the outcome of these competing forces. However, this is largely speculation. Studies are needed to link changing food habits and symbols with the various processes of modernization. These studies will not only help understand current and predict future trends of modernization but will also aid in determining which of these processes have the greatest effect on culture.

Of particular interest is the role that food might play as a device in maintaining group boundaries. Thus, Alba's (1990) recognition of the importance of food habits in determining ethnic identity is a welcome addition. Clearly, a great deal more can be done, using both the survey research methodology employed by Alba as well as the qualitative efforts of Goode, Curtis, and Theophano (1984), who has found that adherence to traditional food patterns among Italian Americans varies by day of the week and by the scheduling of work inside as well as outside the home. More importantly, the analysis of ethnic identity should examine the use of food as an exclusionary versus an inclusionary mechanism. If van den Berghe (1984) is right, then food serves not only to integrate an ethnic group but also as a mechanism for excluding nonmembers. At the same time, Goode et al. (1984) have described the difficulties in maintaining a distinct cuisine within a dominant culture that places a great premium on time. These groups not only have to defend their children from the homogenous school lunchroom diet but must also contend with the processes of rationalization and commodification that destroy authenticity and meaning.

Class Culture

Theorists such as Bourdieu have forced us to return to the insights of Veblen regarding the qualitative differences in the consumption choices and what the choices symbolize to the various segments of the class structure. Bourdieu's is not talking simply about differentiation but rather class-based means for maintaining class differences and boundaries. These differences and boundaries vary across societies in their intensity, but his approach suggests an entire new line of research on foodways and other items of material culture.

Critical Theory, Postmodernism, and Agency Theory

Critical theory and postmodernism theory suggest that the trends of food habits and symbols are the result of manipulation by the forces of capitalism. There is certainly no argument that advertising attempts to alter habits of all sorts and to link culturally important symbols to products. These efforts may have effects powerful enough to overcome those associated with modernization. Here too we have nothing but speculative arguments, for little work has been done that demonstrates that advertising has its intended effects on consumers.

Existing studies have not linked exposure to particular ads or to the use of particular foods as props with changes in beliefs, attitudes, or behavior. These studies have also not focused on the consequences of ambiguous or misleading implications of ads and food as props.

With the exception of changes in sexual mores and the acceptability of violence, social scientists have paid little attention to the effects of the mass media on culture. We know little about whether ads and other depictions of drinking, for instance, increase the number of persons who drink or the amount they drink.

Studies of food advertising should examine the ad's effects on "meal culture" or expectations regarding what constitutes a meal. Both Mary Douglas (1971) and Ann Murcott (1983b, 1993a) have found that people have a clear notion of what constitutes a "proper meal." Similar studies should be conducted in the United States to develop some baseline notions regarding what people in general and those who prepare food expect of their meals. Research could then begin regarding whether print advertising, prime time television, or movies present differing ideas and behavior.

We know little as well about the relationship between advertisements and definitions of the self. One approach to studies in this area would begin with the connection between consumption and unrequited dreams depicted by Campbell (1987) and Williams (1982). Slenderness ranks as one of the most powerful of unfulfilled wishes. Many women have developed highly unrealistic images of how they should and could look if they only found the right diet, form of exercise, or device. Products exploit this desire with highly deceptive ads that make either explicit or implicit promises to fulfill these dreams. Such ads appear to have had great success, given the level of expenditure for such products.

Furthermore, as Fiske has argued, consumers remake the symbolic importance of purchased goods. Adoption-diffusion research tells us that new products are not automatically accepted or purchased. This line of research categorizes nonadopters as "laggards," under the assumption that the "new" is worthy of adoption. Turning this view on its head might lead us to classify such individuals as "resistors."

Food and nutrition studies may thus also play a part in efforts by sociologists to further develop agency theory (see Ahrne, 1990, for example). Not all consumers are passive receptacles. They make food choice changes in response to new information regarding the linkage between food and health and boycott products they believe unsafe or the result of labor exploitation. Despite the content of ads and programming, they resist.

4

THE SOCIAL ORGANIZATION OF FOOD ACTIVITIES AND NUTRITIONAL STATUS

INTRODUCTION

Insight into the effectiveness and interconnectedness of food production, acquisition, processing, preparation, and consumption activities requires an understanding of social organizations. These include organizations such as families, farms, commodity associations, restaurants, food companies, transnational conglomerates that own and control food companies, voluntary organizations that aid the hungry and those with eating disorders, universities where food and nutrition research takes place, and the state that sets agricultural and food policies (see Chapter 9). A second reason for a focus on social organizations such as these is because forces of rationality, commodification, and concentration occur not in individuals but rather in groups. These forces have a significant and increasing impact on agriculture, the kinds of foods available to people, and eating habits. More significantly, these force have collided with social institutions that serve as cultural icons in many Western societies: the family and the family farm. The latter are thought by some to be the last outposts of those expressive relationships considered necessary for both individual well-being and for social order itself.

Both liberal and conservative thinkers have expressed concern for the family's survival and have mainly disagreed over how best to preserve families. Similarly, observers across the political spectrum have worried about the future of the family farm, either because this mode of living reflects one more instance of independent individuals endangered by the forces of capitalism or because it serves as a continued source of renewal in democratic systems (Browne, Skees, Swanson, Thompson, & Unnevehr, 1992). These same forces are producing changes in the food-processing and food-retailing industries as well that have implications for health and well-being (see Chapters 5–8).

Third, the groups involved in food activities generally include prominent roles for women. Often, however, these roles are either overlooked or are taken for granted. Such roles and the social forces that affect their performance represent important topics for research by themselves, but their importance grows when it is observed that the forces of rationality, commodification, and concentration bear heavily on these roles in terms of changes in the expectations of and resources available to incumbents of such roles. Because of the importance of social organizations and the roles that women play within them, this chapter examines families, farms, social networks, voluntary organizations, and complex organizations of various sorts (e.g., restaurants, universities, transnational corporations) in an effort to describe both the social nature of food activities and what factors affect their successful conclusion.

The chapter reviews various perspectives on organizations attempting to demonstrate, on the one hand, the contribution they make to the study of food and nutrition and, on the other hand, the insights that actual studies of the social organization of food production, preparation, and consumption make to sociology. Particular attention is paid to women's roles in these perspectives.

FAMILY THEORIES AND THEIR APPLICATION

Primary versus Secondary Groups

Over 80 years ago Charles Horton Cooley (1962) [1909] made observations of the socialization process in children. His interest lay in how children internalized culture. He argued that children emerge at birth empty of culture and thus must learn language, beliefs, norms, and values. Such socialization occurs not in school but in groups into which children are immediately thrust and on which the children depend for survival. Cooley (1962) [1909] designated such groups "primary," for they were said to be "first in time, first in intimacy, and first in influence."

Briefly, primary groups tend toward small size, last for a significant period of time, function largely through face-to-face interactions, generate member loyalty, and meet member needs. At the same time members are expected to engage in self-sacrifice for the good of the group. Secondary groups tend to be the opposite; they are larger, do not depend on face-to-face contact, generate less loyalty, judge members on the basis of what they do not who they are, and can expect less self-sacrifice. Many of the differences are absolute, but most are of degrees. While many have long eschewed the terminology of "primary group," the assumptions regarding the nature of such groups continue to characterize discussion of family and friendship groups. The ideas associated with primary groups were blended into structural-functionalist versions of the family by Kingsley Davis (1958);

much of today's work continues this tradition and is referred to as the institutional approach.

The Institutional Approach

The family is one of the oldest and most basic of social institutions; its effectiveness lies in its use of primary relationships in directing human activities. It is the major source of physical and social nurturance for most individuals. Society itself could not exist without the presence of families or some functional substitute.

The individual has the need for love and affection, companionship, and acceptance as a total human being. Such needs are usually met within primary relationships, which are based on intimacy, trust, and loyalty. Family and friendship groups constitute socially legitimated opportunities for these kinds of relationships. The family provides these as well as the context for the provision of physical needs such as food, shelter, sex, and material comforts (Malinowski, 1944). In many parts of the world, the family roles are organized around specific aspects of food acquisition and production activities. Where families principally obtain their food from the market, their roles coalesce around food purchasing, storage, preparation, and consumption. As will be discussed in greater detail, the institutional perspective on families places great importance on the wife-mother role for the provision of the finished goods (such as meals) and services that meet basic human needs. These important activities were described by DeVault (1991) as "caring work."

Families remain principal mechanisms of socialization and social control. Children, for example, enter the world unable to provide themselves with food or protection from an often noxious environment. Because children cannot fend for themselves, the necessity of having needs filled by others, as well as communicating these needs, renders children open to socialization. Much of what passes for knowledge of food (what constitutes edible substances, what doesn't; what constitutes food for us ["good" food] versus food for others; etc.), food and table norms (manners, etiquette), and beliefs regarding the linkages between food and health come to individuals via families.

Based on this brief discussion, the importance of the family in acquiring foods, transforming "raw" foods into finished meals, and organizing their distribution among family members should be clear. At the same time, a functionalist analysis of certain family–food activities provides valuable insights into the family institution in that more detailed descriptions of family roles and role interdependencies are made possible.

The Social Functions of Meals

Parsons developed a social system schema that identified the functions that institutionalized social practices play in preserving both the institutional practices themselves and also the society from which they derive. The function of the family in Parsons's scheme had to do with creating and sustaining the motivational energies necessary to participate in family and other institutional status-roles. Families achieved this by creating a sense of solidarity among its members.

The maintenance and strength of family solidarity results from the participation by family members in familial, religious, and community rituals (Bossard & Boll, 1950). Others have argued that in a modern society the affection and support the family provides its members through family caring activities serve as the source of family solidarity (Caplow, Bahr, & Chadwick, 1982; DeVault, 1991). Family rituals include activities in which caring takes place. A central family ritual is the family meal. "The performance of specific routines at meal time in which the family unites as a whole, gives the family a feeling of solidarity" (Bossard & Boll, 1950:26). Several times a year families reinforce these daily activities through major meal events such as those that occur in conjunction with important religious or community events (e.g., Thanksgiving dinner) (Whit, 1995).

DeVault (1991) argued persuasively that the reason women made such an effort to "construct the family meal" was in their perception that this work is what "constructs the family itself." Accomplishment of family depended on how well she performed this. This suggested, however, that despite the primary group perspective's emphasis on ascription, successful families required achievement.

A second function of the family to which meals contribute has to do with socialization (see Lewis & Feiring, 1982). Even in a modern society in which a school system begins the formal process of socialization relatively early in life, families are still required to provide their children with the basic social and personal skills needed to function away from home. These include certain linguistic abilities, the capability of responding to authority, and how to feed and relieve oneself of bodily wastes. Families provide more than boot camp skills in preparation for the educational system. Families expose their members to values, norms, beliefs, and skills essential for entry into societal roles that schools lack either sufficient time or legitimacy to offer. Some of this socialization will reflect societal culture, while other aspects will involve ethnic and class culture. Such learning includes the norms and skills involved in table manners and the identity of items considered as real food, as good food. In addition, family members learn what items constitute nonfood.

Rozin (1988) argued that through interaction with family members and others, individuals learned various food-related emotions, the most profound of which was disgust. This emotional reaction is defined by Rozin and Fallon (1987:23) "as revulsion at the prospect of oral incorporation of offensive objects." Children obtained these kinds of distinctions and others through interaction with others, particularly parents. It seems reasonable to hypothesize that food-related emotions develop from meal interaction.

Meals serve additional functions for the family as a system. In order to survive, families must maintain a system of status differentiation and a division of labor (Parsons & Bales, 1955). The allocation of food portions in terms of their size and quality reflects both the status hierarchy and division of labor. These involve differentiations by age, sex, and economic responsibilities (Delphy, 1979). Distributional differences are greatest in agricultural societies and remain evident in farm families in industrial settings. As men are responsible for many of the family's agricultural tasks, they frequently are permitted to eat first and best. But even in those African societies in which women perform most of the agricultural labor, men's needs continue to receive highest priority (McIntosh & Evers, 1982). In modern societies, while the entire family eats together and there is concern that all family members receive sufficient food, men's food preferences continue to dominate (Charles & Kerr, 1988; DeVault, 1991; McIntosh & Zey, 1989; Schafer & Bohlen, 1977; Zey & McIntosh, 1992).

Mealtime also provides a routinized context for social interaction, permitting the coordination of family activities, the sharing of information, and the shaping of selves (DeGarine, 1972). Finally, family members who wish to sanction the behavior of another member may utilize the mealtime in order to make an example for other members. In the United States, a popular punishment for deviant family members is to be kept from the family table or to be sent from the table before finishing the meal.

For society the family produces human beings from what were once asocial beings. Through socialization and social sanctions, families teach their members the ability to communicate with other human beings, a sense of acceptable values, and a sense of acceptable means by which those values may be pursued. With these skills and knowledge, the child is sufficiently prepared to enter school and, ultimately, the workplace and marriage. The dinner table serves as a ready forum for such socialization.

These discussions imply that families that function well according to societal expectations, in fact, produce the family meal outcomes described previously as well as well-nourished family members. Studies of interaction patterns among family members at mealtime indicate some families perform better than others. In some the family meal becomes an opportunity to play out long-standing disagreements and for family factions to engage in struggles for influence and control (Douglas, 1968). Analyses of dinnertime conversations found that discipline was the second most frequent topic of conversation (Dryer & Dryer, 1973). Many reported furthermore, that their childhood memories of family meals were quite unpleasant (Hinton, Eppright, Chadderdon, & Wolins, 1963). Finally, the findings of researchers such as Charles and Kerr (1988) suggest that lower-class family fathers see little value in interaction among family members during meals and use their power to discourage it. Likewise, the presence of a television set likely reduces interaction.

Other Food-Related Food Exchanges

David Cheal (1988) has undertaken extensive work on the family. He criticized the functional approach, yet a number of his findings appear consistent with functionalism. He described "gift ceremonies" as a system of "redundant transactions within the moral economy, which makes possible extended reproduction of social relations" (Cheal, 1988:19). He argued further that the moral economy of the family involved a "deep structure" of stable relations that individuals work to maintain.

Cheal (1988) examined the kinds of gifts exchanged for such occasions as birthdays, wedding anniversaries, Christmas, and others. He found that gifts possess either instrumental or expressive properties and are given in response to the underlying principle of the occasion. Purely instrumental occasions included weddings and purely expressive occasions included going-away parties and Valentine's Day. Mixed types, involving both dimensions, were anniversaries, Mother's Day, Christmas, and reunions (Cheal, 1988). The occasion type dictated the nature of what was considered an appropriate gift. Instrumental gifts, for example, involved items that the recipient could use to accomplish everyday goals such as food preparation. Thus, weddings and pre-wedding parties involved a high frequency of giving food and drink as well as food preparation equipment. Events that called for expressive displays utilized gifts of only food or drink items rather than the means by which food or drink might be prepared. The nature of many of the instrumental gifts given at a transitional point such as marriage served to reinforce the importance of the family setting for food work and the responsibility of the wife-mother role incumbent for such work.

In sum, the activities of acquisition, preparation, and organization of family meals are more than just the means by which organized social life meets participants' biological needs. Accomplishing these sustains the family as a social unit and contributes to societal maintenance as well. In this context gift giving serves similar purposes.

Family Systems

Researchers have developed perspectives that incorporate ideas drawn from the institutional approach, treating these as variables rather than constants. One of these efforts is referred to as the family systems perspective (Hook & Paolucci, 1970). In particular, the family is viewed as an important influence on the lives of its members due to the physical and social nurturance it provides (Sims, Paolucci, & Morris, 1972). While much of this work has focused predominantly on the beneficial aspects of the family system, work by Rudolf Moos (1974) indicates negative aspects of family life are important as well.

Family systems that are cohesive permit the expression of feelings, permit independent actions by its members, and encourage participation *as a group* in various recreational and sporting activities are to be viewed as positive, having functional or desirable outcomes for its members. Alcoholism and delinquency are more likely to occur in families lacking these attributes. Dysfunctional or undesirable behavior has been associated with high levels of conflict, rigid behavioral expectations, control, and *extreme* cohesiveness (Kintner, Boss, & Johnson, 1978:635). The few studies of nutritional status that apply the family systems perspective have used marital instability, poor parenting skills, frequent family conflict, alcoholism, and unemployment as indicators of systems' instability and found that many of these variables predict failure to thrive (Chase & Martin, 1970).

A study by Kintner et al. (1978) focused on how the family system affects the dietary adequacy of husbands and wives. Numerous, moderate-sized correlations were found between nutritional adequacy ratio variables and scores on the various dimensions of the family environment. These results would appear to provide further confirmation of the Moos theory as well as demonstrate its utility for the study of food behavior.

In a related study by Pollitt and Leibel (1980), family environment variables were examined for their impact on growth failure in children. Failure to thrive occurred most frequently in families within which little physical contact or verbal interaction took place between mother and children and where mothers received little help in caring for these children.

These and other studies show that when families function well and when relationships are harmonious and intimate, the individual emerges in a healthy state. When normal family patterns are disrupted, individual members suffer the consequences. In a recent study, husbands and wives whose families ate at least one meal per day as a group reported higher levels of family satisfaction, cohesion, and demonstration of affection (Coppock & McIntosh, 1991).

These are useful studies for they distinguish between healthy and nonhealthy environments. Determinants of dis-health, however, are frequently sought in the biographies of family members: is the individual a drunk, an addict, or simply a role incompetent. These studies overlook compositional or organizational features of the family structure and environment that might explain not only the family dysfunction but the individual pathology itself.

Social Networks, Social Support, and Food

Families operate within a wider array of relationships, commonly referred to as social networks. An individual's social network consists of immediate family as well as kin living outside the household, neighbors, friends, coworkers, coreligionists, and coorganizational members. The strength and nature of such ties vary, as do their consequences. Ties to others often involve the exchange of resources that can include instrumental as well as expressive goods, services, and information.

Such ties alert researchers to potential sources of help from which families obtain resources from the outside. Dual-parent, dual-working households may reduce time pressures on caring work by drawing on resources available from kin and friends. Stack's (1974) description of the social networks of ghetto residents demonstrates the important part they play in survival of families receiving their resources. Furthermore, the extension of network ties beyond the family creates otherwise unavailable sources of aid.

Much of the aid involved in such exchanges is food related. The social networks of the elderly, for example, provide transportation to the grocery store, help with cooking, advice about food, and mealtime companionship (McIntosh et al., 1989a, 1989b). For elderly with disabilities these sorts of help may allow them to remain independent of more formalized living arrangements, such as those associated with retirement centers and nursing homes.

As with the institutional approach, the social network perspective has tended to focus on the helpful aspects of social relationships rather than deleterious ones. In this regard, their similarity with primary group characteristics and consequences is emphasized. The findings thus far have been promising.

Results of Recent Social Network Research

Several studies of elderly subjects confirm the utility of applying social network approaches to nutritional status.

The Virginia Study

Shifflett and McIntosh conducted a study of the "Future Time Perspectives and the Food Habits of the Aged" (McIntosh & Shifflett, 1984a, 1984b). While the data set contained only a few social network measures, sufficient data were available to examine the effects of marital status, the number of close friendships, attachments to relatives, friendship density, mealtime companionship, and religious social support. Many of these variables were found to be positively associated with the elderly's nutrient intake adequacy. Furthermore, the study showed that while stressors such as poor financial condition reduced appetite (which, in turn, reduced nutrient intake adequacy), social support variables buffered this negative effect (McIntosh & Shifflett, 1984a, 1984b; McIntosh et al., 1989a).

The Houston Study

Seven years after the Virginia study, the project "Social Support, Stress, and the Aged's Diet and Nutrition" was conducted. Using insights from the Virginia experience, McIntosh, Kubena, and Landmann collected data concerning social network structure (size, density, homogeneity) and receipt of expressive (emotional) and instrumental (goods and services) support from network members such as help with cooking, companionship, mealtime companionship, advice about diets, and encouragement to make dietary changes. A stressful event index as well as disability indices were also used to generate information about those events or conditions that might negatively affect dietary intake and nutritional status.

Structural features of the elderly's social networks affect diet and nutrition. For example, elderly whose networks are more heterogeneous in terms of gender and religious participation have higher mean nutrient adequacy ratios (MARS), more fiber-dense diets, less body fat, and higher blood levels of thiamin (McIntosh et al., 1989b). The provision of emotional aid in the form of general companionship and meal time companionship was associated with more regular meal patterns, good appetite, higher mean nutrient adequacy ratios, greater mid-arm muscle mass, and elevated hematocrit levels. Mealtime companionship increased as network size, connections to neighbors, and church membership homogeneity increase (Torres, McIntosh, & Kubena, 1992).

Preliminary results indicated that among the elderly an accumulation of stressful life events and the presence of physical disabilities lessen meal regularity, increase body fat, and decrease muscle mass. However, the more companionship the elderly got from their support network, the less life events and disabilities lower meal regularity (McIntosh et al., 1989b).

Constraints on Family's Production of Nutritional Status

The organizational characteristics of the family include its division of labor and degree of centralized decision making, both of which impact food related activities. In turn, the labor force participation patterns of the heads of household, the absence of heads of household, and the family's size affect family structure. Many of the structural characteristics of the family, as well as the labor force participation of various family members, interfere with food related activities such as cooking and meal supervision.

This examination will take as a point of departure the role of the wife-mother in the United States and Great Britain. This is done because societal norms designate this position as that with the primary responsibility for shopping, cooking, and meal oversight, but also because the extant literature features this role. This perspective, however, is not meant to eliminate alternatives to this normatively prescribed division of labor. The impact of the father-husband role will also be shown to be of importance and the possibility of its change will be entertained.

The Wife-Mother Role

Most consumption and leisure activities take place within the family or other primary group context (Allan, 1985). The base for many of these activities is the household, with that person filling the wife-mother position in charge of household production and maintenance, much of which is caring work (Slocum & Nye, 1976). These include such food-related activities as shopping, gardening, storing, preserving, cooking, and serving.

DeVault (1991) described the work of the wife-mother as "caring" activities. Like Smith (1987), she argued that caring work is largely invisible. Thus, this work was perceived by those who do it, as well as those who receive its benefits, as easy and uncomplicated—work that required little effort or planning. The efforts to plan and accomplish shopping for food, cooking, and scheduling meals, however, was considerable (DeVault, 1991). The motivation for much of the work of caring was in the extrinsic reward of providing for others. Caring, however, was less rewarding in other ways. The invisible, taken-for-granted quality of this role perhaps explained its relatively low level of prestige when compared to other occupations (Bose, 1980). Caring work has changed greatly as household technology has altered the nature of some tasks and as commodification has eliminated others altogether, like the home manufacturing of candles, soap, and most clothing (Cowan, 1983; Strasser, 1982).

Goodman and Redclift (1991) take a similar approach but link changes in the work of caring to the process of commodification endemic to advanced capitalism. Having penetrated the household with processed foods and "white goods" or household appliances, much of women's household labor has shifted to the food processing industry much in the same way that the cottage industry in textiles moved from the home to the factory. The work of preparing food and maintaining a clean household was said to both be easier and more quickly done, although considerable controversy exists regarding that claim. Cooking, for instance, involved for many opening up a preprepared package of food and placing it into an oven or microwave. Thus a combination of white goods and prefabricated foods have radically altered the process of making a meal, as have the increased availability and use of take-out foods (Senauer et al., 1991).

The costs of the increasing number of white goods considered necessities has contributed to the requirement that women take employment outside the home. As women increasingly participate in the labor force, the food and durable goods industries created still more products marketed as products that ease the burden of working women.

The commodification of food and household labor is not complete, for this would result in making housework paid employment. Housework remains, products or not, the ultimate responsibility of women as caretakers of families. Even ads aimed at working women make sure to remind them of their responsibility regarding care for their families (Goodman & Redclift, 1991).

Because of the functional importance of the family and the primary responsibilities that wife-mother role incumbents have in family functioning, this so-called expressive role is considered vital by many functionalists. Even some who criticize the inequalities created by patriarchy argue that societies need to place the appropriate value on caring activities rather than turn them over to the market or some other institutional arrangement, as others have suggested (Johnson, 1989).

Feminist and Marxist perspectives argue that the family and women's work of caring enable either patriarchal or capitalistic institutions to obtain uncompensated resources, namely, men/laborers prepared to govern/work. Exploitation thus explains the low-status, low-pay nature of caring. Such conditions will continue as long as patriarchy/capitalism controls society. Women thus are seen as servants of men's interests or capitalist's interests. These accounts focus on the nature of the unpaid work and social reproduction. This involves bearing children, meeting their needs, and teaching them what it means to be a member of a family, community, and culture. Other aspects of social reproduction involve providing their husbands—the workers of society—with an environment that enables them to continue in the labor force as productive employees. For all family members the work of caring means prepared meals, clean clothes, and other amenities. Whatever perspective taken, the wife-mother role is clearly quite salient.

Role Performance

The institutional literature also makes the assumption that with proper socialization, women who fill the wife-mother status-role and adhere to its norms perform well. Other research, however, suggests that resource constraints of time, money, energy, health, and power may interfere with performance in this position (McIntosh, 1975; McIntosh & Evers, 1982).

In addition, role performance likely varies with differences in family structure. There are several types of family structures, those headed by a single parent and those by dual parents. Some families have no children, others have one or more children. In addition, in some families, children were born at close intervals; in others, they are farther apart. Within each of these types of family structures, labor may be divided in a number of ways, involving parents, children, and/or sources of outside help.

Family Structure as a Time Constraint

Family size and birth order have long been implicated in children's development (e.g., intelligence, physical development). Family theorists have argued for "dilution" models to explain why family size and birth order have such crucial consequences.

This model argues: "The more children, the more the resources are divided (even taking into account economies of scale) and hence, the lower the quality of the output" (Blake, 1981:421). "Quality" here refers not to the inherent "worth" of an individual but rather to some qualitative indicator of "human capital" such as educational or occupational achievement or, as relevant here, nutritional status (Blake, 1981:421).

The dilution model suggests deleterious consequences occur in children from families in which the resources of money, time, and parental energy are diluted by too many demands. Resource dilution occurs in families where there are a large number of children and/or in which the children are closely spaced. Some have found that in addition to spacing, birth order affects outcomes as well (Lewis & Feiring, 1982).

Family size adversely affects the purchasing and consumption of food, particularly among low income households (Cook, Altman, Moore, Topp, Holland, & Elliott, 1973; Sanjur, 1982). In studies of nutritional status, stunting occured in children from large families (Terhune, 1974; Wray, 1971). Last born children, especially the third and fourth child, were at greatest risk of stunting and wasting (Grant, 1964). Finally, the amount of time spent interacting with each child at the dinner table decreased as the number of children involved increases (Lewis & Feiring, 1982).

Kucera (1986) developed hypotheses based on Blake's (1981) dilution theory, arguing that the larger the family, the poorer the dietary intake of its children. She also hypothesized that the youngest children in a family would eat more poorly than their older peers, suggesting a birth-order effect. Kucera (1986) found significantly poorer intakes of various vitamins and minerals in children from larger families and in children of "late" birth order. Further analysis involving the prediction of whether those children from larger families experienced mean nutritional adequacy ratios of less than 67 percent of the Recommended Daily Allowances confirmed the family-size hypothesis (Kucera & McIntosh, 1991).

A structural constraint related to family size was the size of the eating area. Charles and Kerr (1988) found that while middle-class families have sufficient room to eat meals together, many lower class families had to spread themselves across several rooms to accomplish a meal. Such a constraint likely reduced both the effectiveness of socialization and supervision of children.

Finally, the absence of a parent increased the workload of the remaining parent. This too had negative consequences for children's food habits and nutritional status (Chase & Martin, 1970; Johnson, 1983).

Employment

The amount of time, energy, and effort spent at work will influence the time, energy, and effort an individual has to spend on work inside the home (Fox &

Nichols, 1983). Thus those who work long hours at an exhausting job similar to that involved in food purchasing, preparation, and serving, may less likely desire to return home to perform the same or similar kinds of activities.

However, those working part-time (selected hours per day or selected days per week) may have more time to spend on housework including meal preparation. In addition, the nature of the work will affect the time, energy, and effort one has to spend on the household. If one has to bring office work home to complete in the evenings, must work overtime, or do shift work, it may be difficult to participate in food purchasing, meal preparation, service, and cleanup (Zey, Finlay, & McIntosh, 1986). Some may resort to simple meals; others to a greater reliance on restaurants (Kinsey, 1983). This, in turn, may affect the nutritional quality of the meals produced. Other factors, such as parental income, education, and interest in nutrition may mediate the effects on labor force participation of housework.

Unfortunately, few investigators have examined these potentially complex interrelationships and their impact on dietary quality and adequacy. Mothersbaugh, Hermann, and Warland (1993) have demonstrated that meal preparers who feel pressured for time tend to follow less closely the recommended dietary guidelines promulgated by the National Research Council and the American Cancer Society. However, those with the highest nutritional knowledge were less hindered by time shortages.

Existing studies have investigated segments of these interrelationships. To begin with, much debate has centered on the impact of women's labor force participation on both household decision-making power and the division of labor. Goldscheider and Waite's (1991) interpretation of recent research as well as their own findings, based on the National Longitudinal Surveys of Labor Market Experience, indicated that men have begun to increase their participation in various household tasks including grocery shopping and cooking. This task sharing increased with greater levels of the husband's education and "modern" family attitudes.

At the same time, the longer hours the husband worked the less time he contributed to household chores. Hours worked by wives had an even greater impact on husband's contributions at home. The longer she was away at work, the more help he provided (Goldscheider & Waite, 1991:132).

However, others reviewing the research in this area draw very different conclusions, leading some to claim that men, in the past, never made a substantial contribution to household work. This situation remains unchanged today, despite changes in women's labor force participation, men's education, or changing attitudes (Epstein, 1988; West & Fenstermaker, 1993). DeVault's (1991) in-depth interviews of the couples in her sample revealed differences in men's participation in cooking and shopping, but these do not seem to vary substantially by class or employment status. Instead, they appeared to be based on what husbands decide they wish to do around the household. This reflects men's continued dominance in many households (McIntosh & Zey, 1989).

Finally, Keith and Schafer (1991) examined the division of labor and power issues, focusing on who makes food purchasing decisions, decides how much money should be spent on food, normally buys the groceries, and cooks. In their sample of Iowa couples, Keith and Schafer (1991) found that "food-related activities clearly remain the domain of women". The only exception they identified occurred among couples of retirement age. Here, husbands tended to share some of the cooking duties with their wives. In addition, Keith and Schafer (1991) demonstrated that husbands made few changes in their contribution to the household even when their wives participated in the labor force.

Household Technology

Producers of new household technology have consistently promoted their product's ability to save both time and effort. Evidence for such claims supports only half of these contentions. While appliances such as vacuum cleaners and washing machines, powered by electrical current, certainly have reduced effort, they ironically have, by some accounts, increased time spent (Robinson, 1980). The microwave oven has demonstrated its ability to save time, but it grants its user, on average, less than ten extra minutes per day (Robinson, 1980; see also Senauer et al., 1991). Similar claims have been made for convenience and take-out foods, although little evidence is available. A skeptic might argue that after travel is taken into account, the time saved by these products may be less than claimed.

In the meantime the increase in use of highly processed foods, convenience foods, take-out meals, and restaurants extends the process of commodification into the family. These trends may result in alterations in allocation of responsibility of family tasks.

Who Controls Food?

Related to role responsibility and performance is control over what the family eats. Many have argued that in a nuclear family the wife-mother has this authority. If this were the case, control over this important resource might lead to concessions on the part of others regarding the provision of cooking-related help. Women, however, do not appear to treat food in such a manner. Some might argue that a woman's socialization prevents her from taking advantage of this power. Others, however, have argued that women are responsible for food, yet do not control it (McIntosh & Zey, 1989).

Until recently this issue received little attention. Lewin (1943) developed the "gatekeeper" concept, based on findings from Iowa families that indicated women held the power to make these decisions. Studies of decision-making power in other American families have reinforced this image. Other research indicated that husbands or boyfriends exercise considerable power over these decisions. McIntosh and Zey (1989) argued that having the responsibility for cooking and grocery shopping was not equivalent to controlling purchase and recipe choices. Schafer and Bohlen's (1977) study of Iowa couples demonstrated that husbands exercise effective veto power over dishes served. Work by Zey and McIntosh (1992), DeVault (1991), and Charles and Kerr (1988) strongly suggested that wives gave husbands' and children's preferences highest priority, regardless of either her own preferences or beliefs about the healthfulness of particular foods. Finally, when men helped their wives by handling the grocery shopping, it was sometimes done in order to maintain control over the family's budget.

McIntosh and Zey (1989) and Blumberg (1988) hypothesized that women's control over food decisions increases when her income and status, as measured by education and occupational prestige, equaled or exceeded her husband's. Work on household status production indicates that women control the purchase of status goods including foods and alcoholic beverages (Collins, 1994; Coser, 1987). Such consumption appeared only in upper-middle- and upper-class households.

Nutritional and Other Consequences of Women in the Labor Force

Several perspectives on family acquisition and consumption of food have been discussed. An additional question of interest is: What are the effects of family power and division of labor and changes in these for food and its nutritional consequences? Very little research has paid attention to these issues. DeVault (1991) represents one of the few social scientists to examine food acquisition, preparation, and consumption activities under varying class, household structure, and employment conditions. She never intended it as a study of nutritional consequences. Research that seeks to uncover the impact of a variety of family characteristics on nutritional health remains rare, although Keith and Schafer's (1991) study represents what one would hope as the beginning of an extended examination of these issues by others. What difference does it make whether women have greater control over the actual foods purchased and consumed? Does the participation of husbands/older children in food purchasing/food preparation negatively impact on family members' health or make no difference?

Keith and Schafer (1991) dealt with the relationship between wives' working status and the nutrient density scores of the husbands and wives (derived from food frequency data). They did not, however, examine the effects of household division of labor or decision-making power on nutrient density. Their study contained data from 78 single-headed households but did not report on the nutrient densities of these individuals nor on their work status and its possible consequences. The meals eaten per day, time spent preparing food, percentage positive dietary changes made, and percentage overweight or obese were compared across household types. Single heads of household ate the fewest meals, spent slightly less time in meal preparation, but were most likely to report positive dietary changes than members of dual-headed households. The highest percentage of obesity was found among the single heads.

Work by others, including nonsocial scientists, has dealt with only a small part of these issues. Some observers have expressed concern over the impact that work outside the home has on caring responsibilities. In Third World settings, as women's responsibilities for income have increased with no relaxation of caring responsibilities, the nutritional status of children is placed at risk (McIntosh & Evers, 1982). As a result of such concerns a number of studies were launched in order to detect such consequences. Thus far, the evidence is not compelling. Granted, studies in Iran and the Philippines showed a decline in children's health when mothers worked outside the home (Popkin & Solon, 1976; Rabiee & Geissler, 1992). Others have found that, instead of a decline in well-being, children whose mothers brought home additional income that was devoted to food purchases experienced better health (Touliatos, Linholm, Weinberg, & Melbagene, 1984; Tripp, 1982; Tucker & Sanjur, 1988; Wandel & Holmboe-Otterson, 1992).

Most studies in the United States have failed to find significant differences in the diets of children whose mothers work either full- or part-time outside the home from those whose mothers do not. For example, Johnson, Smiciklas-Wright, Croutier, and Willits (1992) utilized the Nationwide Food Consumption Survey to compare the adequacy of intake of nutrients of two- to five-year-old children whose mothers were not employed, employed part-time, or employed full-time. No significant differences were found in these comparisons nor were children whose mothers' worked outside the home disadvantaged by "over" nutrition in the form of excessive calories from fat. This lack of difference persisted regardless of race, family income, maternal age, and education. Other studies reported that the families of working women eat at restaurants more frequently than families of women without employment, but again no difference in dietary intake was apparent (Kinsey, 1983). Skinner, Ezell, Salvetti, and Penfield (1985) examined adolescent nutrient intake and nutrient density of that intake and found that adolescents with working mothers had lower iron densities than adolescents with unemployed mothers.

DeVault (1991) considered the impact of work outside the home on the very business of constructing families through meals but found that instead of eliminating the family meal its construction was simply that much harder. Thus, women continued to take seriously their role in constructing families.

Resolving this issue will require a great deal more study, designed to include all those factors that might interfere with the effectiveness of family caring activities. What, for example, are the implications for nutrition in households in which both adult heads are involved in highly absorptive work?[1]

Importance of the Role of Women in Food Production and Processing

Ester Boserup (1970) and others have made a compelling case for the examination of women's agricultural production activities. They note that women from various parts of the world produce the bulk of foodstuffs needed for subsistence and make major contributions to cash crop production. They note that like the case of caring work, women's contributions to production are either undervalued or totally ignored. Thus international programs in agriculture frequently failed for they have focused on male household heads, assuming that males carry out most of the production activities. Barriers to innovative behavior in agriculture often involve more fundamental issues of women's inequality: women's unequal access to resources prevents them from adopting new technologies. Carolyn Sachs (1983) discovered that women owner-operators of farms and ranches in the United States are equally invisible and ignored. Yet studies of the division of labor on farms document that women have responsibility for managerial and other tasks (Rosenfeld, 1985).

Further evidence of women's importance to food production was found when "artisanal" activities such as independent baking are examined. Bertaux (1982) described the phenomenon of the "baker's wife" in France. Much of the bread consumed in France was produced by independent bakers who relied on their wives and bakery workers for the intensive, time-consuming efforts to provide customers with fresh bread daily. While the goal of many bakery workers was to own and manage their own shop, becoming a baker is possible for only a few, for would-be bakers required two things: capital and a wife (Bertaux, 1982). Obtaining a loan was easier than obtaining a wife. A baker's wife was someone who works 12 hours a day, six days a week in the bakery while retaining responsibility for the household. Bertaux (1982) found that those who had successfully become independent bakers did so immediately after marriage, before the young women could develop a full understanding of the consequences of becoming a baker's wife. Those unsuccessful at doing so had waited until some time after getting married to attempt to set up such a business. During the interim, the young wife had the opportunity to discover the costs associated with marriage to a baker and develop a pretext for refusing to participate in the grand scheme.

---

[1] Karen Kubena, Jenna Anding, Barbara O'Brien, and I have recently gathered data on these and other family, work, and nutrition-related issues. Annie Godwin is testing parental work–adolescent nutritional status hypotheses and Amy Bishop-Tramm is testing family relationships–adolescent nutritional status hypotheses with this data.

Changes in Women's Family Farm Roles

Other changes in farm families have organizational consequences in addition to consequences for men and women. In fact, Goodman and Redclift (1991) argued that changes in farm families parallel in some respects those occurring in urban families. These had to do with increased women's labor force participation, which, in turn, resulted from the increase in the commodification of family life.

The commodification of agricultural production has a long history. Current trends in the creation of biotechnological inputs and outputs simply extend this process. As with families in general, capitalistic penetration of farms is less than complete. Farmers continue to treat their operations as family traditions rather than strict business operations. Many financial decisions are made on the basis of maintaining tradition rather than efficiency grounds (McIntosh, Thomas, & Albrecht, 1990). Farmers under capitalism are often depicted as self-exploitive. This means that they willingly work longer and harder to obtain the same production levels and that they willingly incur more debt and give up necessities, such as family health insurance, in order to obtain the same production levels or remain in business. Some take employment off the farm in order to capitalize their operations. This perspective assumes that women also seek work off-farm to subsidize the operation directly or to supplement farm income to pay for both necessities and luxuries (Ollenburger, Grana, & Moore, 1989; Rosenfeld, 1985). Others have found, however, that human capital factors rather than economic need more successfully predicted labor force participation (Buttel & Gillespie, 1984; Goodwin & Marlowe, 1990; Simpson, Wilson, & Young, 1988).

Some find the presence of family constraints more important than education or experience (Bokemeier, Sachs, & Keith, 1983). Finally, the availability of employment also affects farm women's labor participation. This is reflected by the nature of the labor market in the geographic region in which they were likely to seek employment (Tickamayer & Bokemeier, 1988) and the diversity of jobs and non-farm technology in a county's economy (Albrecht & Murdock, 1984).

While researchers have investigated the consequences of Third World women's work off-farm, few have examined the effects of the labor force participation by their U.S. counterparts. The role of the farm wife includes participation in farm tasks such as feeding animals, maintaining financial records, and in farm decisions such as equipment purchases. In addition to a farm role, women also have the responsibility for caring work (see Rosenfeld, 1985). Work off-farm negatively affects the nutritional status of children according to some Third World studies (Popkin & Solon, 1976). Others have found positive effects. In the United States, the focus has settled on how labor force participation affects farm-related tasks. Some contend that the woman's farm and family duties change little despite the additional burden of work away from the farm (Rosenfeld, 1985). Others found that the more time women spend on work away from the farm operation, the less time they devoted to farm chores (Simpson et al., 1988).

WOMEN'S ROLES IN SOCIALLY ORGANIZED FOOD PRODUCTION, PREPARATION, AND CONSUMPTION

Women and work is approached through a number of different perspectives by sociologists. Some, like Miriam Johnson (1989), found that a revitalized Parsonian approach to women and work has certain merit. Others have argued that the ideology of patriarchy gives men control over the very processes of defining gender differences in character, roles, and occupations (West & Fenstermaker, 1993). Patriarchy legitimizes the inequalities that result (Collins, 1975; Smith, 1987). However, power differentials between men and women make patriarchy possible (Collins, 1988; Smith, 1987).

In such a context, women are viewed as submissive, nonaggressive, non-competitive creatures made for self-sacrifice and caring; thus women are only suited for those activities that require nurturing, caring, and sacrifice. These activities are perceived in this gendered world as less important than those that require aggression, competitiveness, and achievement.

Others examine sex segregation and dual labor markets, arguing that women take on lower status jobs, not by choice, but because of constraints they face when attempting to enter the market for higher status jobs (Baron & Beilby, 1985). These sociologists find that men more likely concentrate in the professions while women locate in the service industry. Status, salary, benefits, and opportunities for upward mobility are all much greater in professional than in service jobs. For example, women overwhelmingly occupy nursing. According to the 1990 census, women continue to make up over 90 percent of professional and licensed practicing nurses. Within the medical profession, women are concentrated in the lower-status, less lucrative practices such as family and general medicine and obstetrics-gynecology (American Medical Association, 1992).

Reskin and Hartmann (1986) studied occupational trends for women and found that the 20 fastest growing jobs for women were almost all located in the service sector. For example, nursing, an already highly segregated occupation, was expected to grow by 50 percent by the year 2000. Similarly, accounting/auditing would increase by 33 percent; supervisor of blue collar work by 17 percent. The fastest area by far for growth in women's employment, however, was the projected 69 percent increase in women's employment in food preparation and service and fast food restaurants (Reskin & Hartmann 1986). Waitressing was expected to grow by 35 percent and kitchen help by 39 percent. Many of these garner minimum wages, poor to nonexistent benefits, little opportunity for advancement, and "sexualized work environments" (Giuffre & Williams, 1994).

Furthermore, employers have found that forcing workers to labor more intensely during shorter shifts increases labor efficiency (Reiter, 1991).

Finally, continued sex segregation of occupations and the growth of women's employment in the low-wage and service sectors has occurred, despite the greater than ever number of increasingly well-educated women entering the labor force. Some reported that women lacked the sensibilities and behavioral traits required for success in the wider world of work. Kanter (1977) found, however, that women developed a lack of ambition, divided loyalties, and a noncompetitive mode because of the lack of opportunities for full participation and advancement.

Waitressing

Women's work in restaurants has attracted considerable attention. Waiting tables is considered women's work (Creighton, 1982; Hall, 1993). For decades the census has reported consistent sex segregation in this occupation (90 percent of "wait" personnel are women). The literature consistently notes the low-status, low-benefit nature of this work. Women are concentrated in this aspect of food service work not because of its poor socioeconomic returns, but because it involves paid nurturing or caring (Cobble, 1991:2). Despite the stereotype, however, this occupation was dominated by men before the turn of the century.

Currently, the continued gendered characteristic of food service waiting is found in the distinction between "waitresses" and "waiters" (Hall, 1993). Hall argued that jobs are not gendered, but rather persons who fill these jobs "do" gender, to varying degrees. This depended on the particular context and the gender expectations the occupant brought with him or her. She studied 77 percent of the 117 restaurants in Hartford, Connecticut, and found that waiters were predominant in high-prestige restaurants (where high prestige was determined by average cost of a meal), whereas waitresses were in greater evidence in the low-prestige restaurants. However, the middle-level establishments employed roughly equal proportions of waiters and waitresses. She also found few differences by gender in work assignments, hours, or other structural features of the work. Gender meanings, however, remained in "the language of job titles and dress codes," suggesting that to "wait on tables in a fine dining restaurant is to do waiting and to wait on tables in a coffee shop is to do waitressing, regardless of the sex or gender of the worker" (Hall, 1993:342).

Power and Autonomy of Waitresses

As with women's food-related roles within the home, the power and autonomy of women's food-related roles outside the home are an issue, particularly during a period of organizational change. How has the food industry benefited women employees?

Women utilized waiting work at the turn of the century as one of their first avenues into the male-dominated occupational structure (Cobble, 1991). In doing so they developed group identity and a willingness to utilize collective action to deal with their grievances. Unionization of waitressing remained a prominent feature until the 1950s, after which changing perceptions of both unions and waitressing were among those factors associated with its decline (Cobble, 1991).

Unionization, however, appears to have had little effect on the power, status, or wages of waitresses relative to their restaurant coworkers. Thus, another theme that has run through some of this literature is the lack of autonomy and control over one's work that characterizes waitresses. Some have observed the stressful nature of this work in terms of its competing pressure between managerial and customer demands. Literature on the impact of work on health would predict that the lack of autonomy and control experienced in a restaurant are extremely stressful as well.

The waitress lacks autonomy and control because of close supervision by management and dependence on customers for tips. The degree to which a waitress experiences autonomy and control depends in part on the nature of the restaurant. For example, Butler and Skipper (1983) found that some restaurants maintain greater centralized control, greater formality (more rules), and lower opportunities to develop work group identity and cohesion; such restaurants experienced higher turnover. At the other end of the spectrum lie restaurants in which waitresses establish considerable control and autonomy in relation to both management and customers. One difference in such restaurants is whether the establishment is more traditional or is, instead, a product of advanced modernity as described by Ritzer (1993). In the latter, rational procedures dominate in order to achieve control over the labor process.

Ritzer (1993) and Reiter (1991) depicted the control process in McDonald's and Burger King, respectively. First, fast-food personnel (there are no true waitresses) interacted minimally with customers—they are trained to serve the customer within three minutes of his or her entry into the establishment. The customer came to the counter to be waited on and the workers remained at their stations. Interaction was to be minimal and structured so as to make the customer want to come back. Wait personnel no longer depended on patrons for tips. (At the same time, these workers received no compensation for income lost from the lack of tips associated with this position.) Second, the lack of an enclosed, separate kitchen meant that staff had no place to which they could retreat and express their frustration/anger regarding unpleasant customers. Furthermore, the very openness of the kitchen area to scrutiny by customers implied that staff must constantly be "on performance." At the same time, by remaining rooted to a particular part of a work area that was not particularly large to begin with, the several managers always present provided close and continuous supervision. Reiter (1991) indicated that these workers have had little success in organizing so as to improve their conditions. Without voice, it turned out their only choice was to exit. And many did. Burger King's turnover at both the managerial and worker levels exceeded 100 percent per year. This high turnover added to the difficulty of organizing this work force (Reiter, 1991).

Other research on service work in the fast-food industry also began with the premise that this industry has vested interests in labor control through routinization of activities. Leidner's (1993) study of McDonald's began with a discussion of Braverman's (1974) observations regarding the deskilling and alienation that result from employers' efforts to control labor by means of routinizing their work. She noted the same processes were underway in the service industries but with less resistance by workers. She described certain forms of this work as "interactive service work," meaning that the work involved direct contact with the public or "service recipients." Waitressing and apparel sales were such jobs. Routinizing such work extended beyond simply standardizing use of the cash register or steps in dealing with other job-related equipment, as in manufacturing work, but involved "areas of worker's lives usually considered to be the prerogative of individual decision-making or to comprise aspects of individual character and personality. Employers may try to specify what they say, their demeanors, their gestures, their moods, even their thoughts" (Leidner, 1993:8–9).

Service organizations may not only attempt to program employees so that they engage in more efficient behaviors but may, to the extent possible, attempt to routinize customer behavior as well. Leidner (1993) argued that McDonald's has effectively socialized their customers through advertising and restaurant layout such that customers know that they are to stand in line, place their orders, and pay for them in the same standardized sequence that minimizes their time in line and the efforts of the service worker.

Leidner (1993) documented McDonald's efforts in training and, through supervision, to develop and maintain strict behavioral routine; however, her participant-observation and interview data indicated that not all workers or managers strictly adhered to it. Yet, many found the programmed behavior a relief from taking individual initiative and a shield behind which they could hide when customers complain or become angry (Leidner, 1993).

Paules (1991) described a very different situation in a New Jersey truck stop. While her inspiration came from Katz (1968), her characterization of waitressing in this setting mirrored that of the operatives studied by Burawoy (1979). The latter described a process called "making out" in which individual workers attempted to exceed that level of production at which incentive pay began. These efforts not only were competitive but also involved conflict with auxiliary workers on whose efforts the operatives must depend for their own productivity. The failure of the auxiliary workers to provide the shop floor operators what they needed resulted from managerial rather than auxiliary worker decisions (Burawoy, 1979:65). This, in turn, led to conflict between operators and management. Such conflict, however, never resulted in the perception that the operative's common enemy was the management; the workers were too involved in competition with one another to recognize this.

Waitresses "made out" by developing strategies that moderated the exploitive nature of their work. Waitresses at the truck stop developed voice rather than exited. As with the shop operatives, these waitresses had not developed group solidarity to confront their conditions. Instead, they utilized individual strategies in competition with one another. Paules (1991) detailed these strategies. First, the waitresses learned that they had much to gain and little to lose by placing customer's desires ahead of company policy. This would increase tips but did not entail the risk of being fired. Second, the longer the waitress had worked, the easier she was able to refuse to take on either seating areas or tasks that might reduce her opportunity for tips. Third, she might refuse to serve customers who had a history of poor tipping or who appeared to fit the stereotype of a poor tipper. Because of the individualistic orientation, interest in collective actions was nil.

Some have found that waiters and perhaps waitresses engage in theft, either from customers, management, or fellow wait personnel. Detection generally led to firing rather than involvement by the legal system, so the consequences were not severe. Stealing may represent a form of making out (Hawkins, 1984).

FORMAL ORGANIZATIONS AND FOOD

Organization theorists and others have disagreed over the essence of current trends in organizational structure. Ritzer (1993), as discussed earlier, viewed the trend as the continued expression of rationalization processes. Thus, organizational change and the formation of new types of organizations must be interpreted from the standpoint of increased automation, rules, and supervision to increase efficiency.

Postmodern theorists have emphasized flexible specialization or post-Fordism, especially in regard to product differentiation. According to them, the postmodern economy is a consumer-oriented economy. David Harvey (1989) took this approach, although he argued that such changes represent another step in the capital accumulation process, as opposed to a break with the principles of capitalism. Furthermore, flexibility occurred in the manner in which labor is utilized, leading to greater opportunities for control and exploitation. Clegg (1990) made a similar case but argued in addition that the new flexibility is a requirement of changing environmental and technological contingencies; choices made regarding structure may reflect concerns either for efficiency or for control. However, he argued in addition that trends in organizational structure depended greatly on the cultural context in which they are embedded. For example, he viewed the familistic businesses formed by the Chinese in Hong Kong, Taiwan, and other places as an alternative form of rationality, but one which draws on the importance of the patriarchal family that the Chinese have traditionally emphasized.

Some of the changes outlined by Clegg (1990) appeared to be the modernization of more traditional family businesses, as opposed to the taking up of certain traditional characteristics by otherwise highly modernized firms, as postmodernist theory would predict. After all, similar kinds of changes have occurred in family farming, particularly in the United States, and no one has described these as postmodern in nature. Instead, they represented a traditional organization's response to an ever-modern world (McIntosh et al., 1990).

Others have argued that organizational changes represent forces of capitalist accumulation through the means of concentration and mergers. Food companies have been among the biggest and most profitable in the United States. Based on return to equity and profits per share, for example, food companies were the most profitable of any kind in 1992 (U.S. Department of Commerce, 1994:554). Furthermore, many have changed in ways that conform to those trends described by Ritzer, Harvey, Clegg, and others. These transformations represent excellent case studies for the development of models of organizational change. They also suggest that changes will result in a fundamental alteration of the nature of the food supply and its distribution.

Food production processes involve what many have come to call the food system, which itself includes international, national, regional, and local components. In the discussion that follows, the international and national aspects will serve as the point of departure. The international sectors consist of farms as well as companies involved in the assembling and brokering, manufacturing and wholesaling, and transporting and retailing of foodstuffs (Senauer et al., 1991). The processes involve what is known as value-adding or altering the food item in some ways so as to increase its exchange value. Profits generally increase with increases in value-adding. The companies involved have undergone a great deal of change; some represent modernization, others reflect postmodernization and capitalist accumulation.

Farms as Complex Organizations

An examination of trends in farming finds a continuous downward fall in the number of operating farms. However, this decline is not exhibited equally by farms of all sizes. Middle-sized farms have sustained the majority of the losses, while both large- and small-sized units have actually increased in number (Senauer et al., 1991; Staunton, 1993). Small-sized units involve family operations whose members may hold full-time employment off-farm, maintaining the operation after hours and on weekends. In East Texas, for example, cotton and dairy farms are being replaced by small cattle herds. The rise of the larger scale farming operations reflects changing opportunities and constraints on family farming; thus most of the so-called corporate farms are family corporations rather than food company buyouts, as was once suspected.

Studies of the changing organizational structure of farming in the United States have followed either a Weberian or an neo-Marxian perspective (Friedland, 1991; Heffernan, 1972; Rodefeld, 1978). These perspectives have a great deal in common, but, in general, the Weberian account seems most credible, largely because the risks associated with farming are apparently too high for capitalists. Thus, family farms remain family businesses rather than become nonfamily corporations. At the same time, as research demonstrates, farms have taken on certain characteristics held by other small- and medium-sized businesses. These involve attempts to increasingly rationalize the operation.

Modern organizations are thought to best embody the rationalism Weber described. "Capitalist practices render production more calculable through accounting methods, the application of technology, and the exercise of greater control over the production process. To facilitate calculability and control, ownership, management and labor are separated, and administration is made more formal and efficient with legitimacy based on expertise" (McIntosh et al., 1990).

Several studies of farms demonstrated the usefulness of this approach. Dolch and Heffernan (1978) described the large-scale production of poultry from this perspective, utilizing Aiken and Hage's (1968, 1971) variables. They found that such farms have separated production from consumption, clearly differentiating the organization of farm business from the organization of farm family activities. These farms relied on hired management and labor, selected on the basis of experience and skills. The study also discovered that formalized work rules, a division of labor based on skills, and centralized authority characterized many of these farms and that these features tended to be highly correlated with one another. Poultry farms of the sort studied by Dolch and Heffernan (1978) have been described by others as factory farms, which operate as large-batch, assembly line–like industries. These farms, like the industrial farms described by Rodefeld (1978), remain rare, although changes in the dairy industry indicate that it too has begun to develop factorylike qualities. Most modern farms continue as a combination of traditional family and modern organizational characteristics.

Such farms formed the basis for the McIntosh et al. (1990) study, which began with Weber's distinction between "value rationality" versus "instrumental rationality." Farms displayed varying degrees of both orientations; those that possess modern-rational characteristics placed greater emphasis on instrumental rationality while more traditional family farms emphasized value rationality.

A modern-rational farm is one that is large in size (as measured by acreage farmed and gross farm sales), diverse in its products, complex in its division of labor, and rational in its managerial strategies. Furthermore, such organizations make less use of family labor and owned land, preferring employees hired for their skill and the use of rented property. Value rationality reflects efforts to remain true to certain ultimate values. This means, among other things, attempts to preserve the family farm, regardless of the cost.

Instrumental rationality concerns the selection of means that increase efficiency and effectiveness. Certain technologies may increase efficiency and effectiveness, while others may preserve resources for long-term survival. Soil conservation technologies, for example, embody both instrumental and value rational characteristics but vary in terms of which of the two is better served (McIntosh et al., 1990).

The McIntosh et al. (1990) study found that farms that employed rational managerial techniques, a division of labor based on skills, and decentralized decision making utilized a greater number of soil conservation practices that reflected an instrumental-rational approach. Farms practicing the less profitable, but more long-term soil conserving technologies had some of the same characteristics but, in addition, made greater use of family labor and land that was owned rather than rented or leased.

Not all studies in this area have produced consistent findings. Simpson, Wilson, and Jackson (1992) argued and supported with their evidence that farm productivity, a measure of organizational effectiveness, was associated with task dispersion rather than specialization, particularly on medium sized farms. McIntosh et al. (1990) found the reverse to be true, regardless of farm size.

Food Processing

Forty-seven kinds of food processors currently operate in the United States; while they differed in many respects, they have all recently experienced the trend toward concentration (Senauer et al., 1991). Heffernan, Constance, and Gronski (1993) provided specific examples. In the beef and sheep slaughter industries and in corn and flour milling, the concentration of market control maintained by the top four companies averaged about 50 percent in 1987. By 1993, the concentration of market control had increased to over 70 percent in each of these commodity processing industries (Heffernan et al., 1993).

Economists who have examined concentration in the processing of specific commodities have suggested that the effects include distorted prices for finished products, which negatively affect the welfare of both farmers and consumers. For example, pear processing in California exhibited oligopoly and oligopsony (Wann & Sexton, 1992); however, researchers found in the same state a trend toward increased competition among tomato processors (Durham & Sexton, 1992).

Other parts of the food-processing sector have emphasized flexibility in products and manufacturing capabilities (Senauer et al., 1991). The emphases here included market differentiation and re-skilling labor for a more flexible labor force. Market segmentation involved creating new products such as sweeteners and food analogues (e.g., surimi, which is made from inexpensive types of fish, as a replacement for more expensive shellfish) (Senauer et al. 1991).

Mechanization has occurred in sugar processing, for example, which has resulted in labor force reductions. The labor that remained, however, experienced re-skilling by means of multiple tasking (Senauer et al., 1991:126). At the Senator meat processing plant in Stuttgart, Germany, a continuous processing line that involved only one laborer replaced a highly labor intensive set of activities (Jankowiak, 1989).

Food Retailing

Great change has taken place in food retailing, particularly in food marketing. The number of supermarkets declined from 26,321 to 23,722 (a 10 percent decline) from 1980 to 1991 (U.S. Department of Commerce, 1994:299). The large chains have spread beyond their original regional locations, increasing the competitiveness of the environment. This, as well as customer demand for more service, has led to an increase in the average size of the supermarket as well as a diversification of its products. Such stores have begun to routinely include self-service and sit-down deli counters, bakeries, and money machines. Superstores have added postal services, beauty parlors, and greatly enlarged household appliance departments, with the goal of one-stop shopping. Chains show the greatest level of growth, as well as the greatest increase in product diversification (U.S. Department of Commerce, 1994).

Walsh (1993) argued that contingencies created by declining profits, new technology, and changing customers (caused largely by the great increase in women's labor force participation) led to the diversification, decentralization, and re-skilling of some supermarket employees. His study of this industry focused on the meat department. Supermarkets, like other businesses, had sought to control labor costs (Walsh, 1993). In most regards, they have succeeded. However, unionized meat cutters have managed to protect their jobs, both in terms of numbers and status, by resisting those technological changes, such as boxed beef, that would have reduced their importance. Other technological changes that either left untouched or increased the importance of the meat cutters' position, such as the introduction of power saws and meat clerks, were not resisted (Walsh, 1993).

Deli departments were established so that customers could either eat on site or take home preprepared meals (Walsh, 1993). With the development of these and other departments, centralized management became increasingly problematic; decentralization followed, which included departmental control over those decisions about which it had the most expertise. "For example, in the deli department the particular mix of products sold reflected the competence and tastes of the employees and their perceptions of demand at the store level as well as the central office's plans for a marketing strategy" (Walsh, 1993:119). Of final note, Senauer et al. (1991) argued that the shift toward a consumer orientation coupled with scanning technology, knowledge of customer preferences and demographics, plus greater control over what products receive and retain shelf space have given retailers greater power over the food supply relative to processors than ever before.

Restaurants

The restaurant industry has also undergone expansion as more meals are eaten away from home. Some argued that this trend is a direct result of women's labor force participation (Reilly, 1982), while others attribute the change to the increased value placed on this as a leisure activity. The demand for fast foods and ethnic cuisine have led this growth (Staff, 1994), but competition remains sufficiently fierce so as to maintain restaurants' high mortality rate.

William F. Whyte (1948) accomplished one of the first studies of restaurants as social organizations, taking a then-popular human relations approach. He observed that restaurants differ from other businesses in that factories produce goods that are sold by other organizations and retail outlets sell goods produced elsewhere. Thus, factory workers had to deal only with their supervisor; others handled customer relations. In a retail store, on the other hand, the job of labor entailed selling to customers, but without having to produce the goods being sold and thus be supervised for such work. Restaurant workers were involved in both production and sales and had to please two sets of supervisors: on the one hand, the restaurant manager and cooks and, on the other, customers (Whyte, 1948:19). Conflicting expectations may result if the restaurant's management is not both cognizant and accommodating. Whyte (1948) followed this reasoning to the conclusion that the high rate of restaurant failure was due to the inability of the restaurateur to manage these human relations.

Organizational ecologists have found that the death rate among restaurants is sufficiently high to make them useful as a means for developing prediction models of organizational mortality rates.

Freeman and Hannan (1983) used organizational ecology theory to develop models of organizational mortality. They argued that environmental factors rather than features of the organization led to organizational death. Two features of the environment affected organizations. The first, environmental variability, reflected instability in the environment with regard to resources. The second, patterns of environmental variability, indicates whether the variability is evenly spread or clumped. Such environments ranged from fine-grained (evenly spread resources and costs) to coarse-grained (clustering of resources/costs). In the study of restaurant deaths in 18 California communities over a 10-year period, Freeman and Hannan (1983) found that restaurants that specialized their product (i.e., produced fast food, ethnic cuisine, or simply maintained a limited menu) more likely endured in environments that fluctuate greatly (the gross sales of restaurants in the community fluctuate greatly each month). The researchers also found, however, that generalist restaurants were far less likely to perish in unstable, coarse-grained environments. Specialists were twice as likely to survive in environments in which sales varied little from month to month, regardless of the clustering of environmental resources. Perhaps these very environments will foster the anticipated growth in fast-food establishments that specialize in ethnic cuisine.

Others have applied organizational ecology models in the study of founding and mortality of breweries and wineries. Carroll, Preisendoefer, Swaminathan, and Wiedenmeyer (1993) examined the organizational legitimacy/competition aspects of density as these contribute to both founding and mortality. When few organizations of a certain kind existed (for instance, breweries) but were increasing in number, this process was progressively enhanced by legitimacy: as such organizations became more familiar, they became more socially acceptable. After a certain number of these organizations were established, competition became the dominant force. Thus when the number of organizations was small, formation rates were high and mortality rates were low. When the number was large, the opposite was true. Carroll et al. (1993) provided strong evidence for these hypotheses, using data for all brewery establishments/closings in Germany and the United States for the period 1860–1988. Their evidence confirmed the legitimacy/competition hypotheses.

Delacroix, Swaminathan, and Solt (1989) found that the experience of wineries in California lends no evidence to the legitimacy model. Since the beginning of California wineries, a strict "business competition" model seemed to have operated. Rather than going out of business, many sought a neighboring niche to fill or an enlargement of the original niche. The neighboring or new niche became a viable alternative; i.e., import sales for sparkling wines suggested potential markets for such wines. Other wineries found that increasing size was the key to success.

Breweries in the United States have developed new niches as well, though not by encouraging the diversity of beers as the German industry has. Instead, large breweries have bought out smaller regional beer manufacturers, eliminating whatever regional uniqueness those beers offered. Market or niche differentiation has occurred instead through the low-calorie and cold-filtered markets. Similar to Delacroix et al. (1989), Carroll et al. (1993) found that larger-sized breweries remained in business longer than small ones.

Of course, such findings would appear to apply to many organizations. Some of the literature on farm mortality, however, indicates that medium-sized rather than either large or small farms are most likely to survive; other findings suggest the opposite is true. No one has investigated directly the relationship between number of farms and survival, but as farms have increasingly become more productive without a concomitant rise in demand for farm products, farm mortality appears to increase with productivity increases in the industry as a whole. Finally, some have observed that niche specialization in farming increases the risk of going out of business instead of decreasing it.

Voluntary organizations generally are not thought of as competitive; thus researchers have yet to apply the organizational ecology model to such organizations. It appears, however, that the potentially mobilizable portion of the population for a given issue is limited in number, and the amount of resources that any one charity mobilizes declines as the number of competitors grows. In addition, drawing on the organizational ecology model. I predict that as the number and size of charities grow, the higher the mortality rate. However, organizations that focus on new issues may be able to create a niche for themselves. Thus, a hunger relief organization might find it "profitable" to focus on long-term development schemes rather than short-term sustenance. These hypotheses, however, have not yet been applied to charitable organizations.

Transnational Organizations and Food

The world economy is not simply undergoing internationalization but has experienced what Dicken (1992:1) refers to as "globalization." What this means is that countries are no longer merely connected by trade, but also by production processes that take place in multiple firms in two or more countries under the direction of an overarching parent organization. Such a company is referred to as a transnational corporation or TNC. Corporations of this sort often involve many companies spread across a number of countries. Klyveld Mair Goerderier, based in the Netherlands, maintains 498 affiliates in other countries; Citicorp, a U.S. banking firm, has 240 foreign operations (Dicken, 1992:370).

Most of the literature on TNCs has drawn attention to their size and economic power. Some have observed that TNC penetration of the Third World has had a negative effect on those countries' economies (Panic, 1993), but others argue that the results are unclear (del Castillo, 1992). Despite the importance and power of these larger TNCs, recently a number of smaller TNCs have sprung up in what are referred to as the newly industrializing nations of East and South Asia and Latin America. Those TNCs located in Korea, for example, concentrate in the extractive industries and have subsidiaries in North America, Latin America, and Oceania, while Singaporean TNC firms specialize in both heavy manufacturing and food and drink processing.

Sociologists have followed the rise of TNCs with great concern regarding the implications of increasing oligopolistic control over resources and the implication national politics have for citizen control over the direction their nation takes. Harriet Friedmann's (1990) work regarding the rise of a world food order, controlled by a small number of large-scale industries that control food reproduction, processing, and distribution, is one example. Kenney (1986) and Kloppenburg (1988), on the one hand, expressed concern over the implications of limited control over the world's germ plasma, and on the other hand, argued that the university's traditional scientific neutrality is endangered by the desire to reap economic gain from patentable biotechnology invented on campus.

Actual studies of the growth and development of food and beverage related TNCs and their impact on food prices and availability, as well as their implications for health, are limited. In a recent study for the Organization for Economic Cooperation and Development, Rama (1992) presented data on trends in the 1980s. Her analysis clearly showed that food and beverage processing is an area of much TNC activity. Food and beverage TNCs have grown in size (as measured by both numbers of employees and sales), for example, during the 1981 to 1985 period. The average U.S. agro-industrial company grew in sales from 2.7 billion to 4.9 billion dollars with employees numbering nearly 45,000 in 73 affiliates in 17 countries (Rama, 1992:43). Leading U.S. companies included United Brands, Unigate, Campbell Soups, Cargill, ConAgra, Heinz, and Coca Cola. Critics of TNCs have charged that these companies have slowly, inexorably taken hold of food production and consumption in the Third World. Trends in corporate penetration confirmed this prediction in the 1970s. However, the 1980s saw most of the growth and expansion of such activities within industrialized countries (Rama, 1992). With the exception of China and other Asian countries, most of the mergers, acquisitions, and profits have occurred in the United States and Europe. Both Japan and Europe have invested heavily in the United States, for instance, because of a favorable monetary climate. These same companies have withdrawn from the Third World because of the level of debt service with which the countries of this region currently must cope, unfavorable prices for raw materials, and host country food policies that focus on exports for income as opposed to domestic consumption (Rama, 1992). The implications of these changes for improvements in the nutritional status of citizens of these countries is yet unclear. Nor is it clear what the implications of mergers, acquisitions, and a greater extent of oligopolistic control over the supply of raw and processed foods will mean in the future.

However, Rama (1992:109) argued that developing countries may have a great deal of trouble competing with large TNCs as they attempt to develop their food-processing capabilities. As Friedmann (1990) has suggested, many companies have moved away from raw food products obtained from developing countries to artificial products that can be manufactured at plants in the developed world. Others complained that TNC penetration reduced the sovereignty of these nations and increased the destruction of their physical environments (Goodman & Redclift, 1991).

CONCLUSION

A number of other organizations involve themselves with food and food problems. These include voluntary organizations, professional organizations, and universities. Voluntary groups are involved in the establishment and maintenance of emergency food centers in local communities. Formal organizations such as the Food and Research Action Center (FRAC) and the Food and Development Institute were developed by U.S. social activists in the 1960s both to study food shortages and malnutrition at home and abroad and to lobby for their amelioration. The American Dietetic Association has a current membership of over 40,000 registered dietitians. Many university campuses have departments such as animal sciences, food science, dietetics, and nutrition that conduct research, train students, and promote change through extension activities. Few of these organizations have received careful scrutiny from scholars regarding the prominence of women in their ranks, their effectiveness in pursuing goals, their impact on food and nutrition, the types of organizational change they have experienced, or the forces that propel such change. Rural sociologists have developed case studies of departments within colleges of agriculture. Torres (1987), Torres, McIntosh, and Zey (1990), and Torres, Zey, and McIntosh (1991) have examined the relationship between structural features of food pantries and their effectiveness as organizations. We have much to learn about the sociological significance of the institutional setting of food research and training and the environmental constraints on food-aid organizations.

Multiple organizations are involved in the production, processing, distribution, and consumption of food. These organizations vary in size and structure and yet all are subject to the same general societal forces. Families, restaurants, voluntary organizations, and food processors have all been forced to act more rationally in a world in which survival depends on greater efficiency. Voluntary organizations, for example, must increasingly demonstrate that they use their donations wisely. Family members have increasing amounts of obligations outside the home and are under pressure to devote less time to existing family activities. As food has become more profitable through value-adding and through greater commercialization, the number of organizations involved has grown. Dietetics continues to attract an increasing number of students. Food companies have grown larger and have attempted to incorporate an increasing number of food processes under their control. Some argue that such increases occur mainly to take advantages of economies of scale, but others claim that this growth is undertaken to drive smaller competitors out of business (Winson, 1993). Larger companies are able to subsidize price cutting more easily than smaller enterprises.

Left untouched by this chapter are a number of other issues. One that was given brief mention has to do with the biological consequences of social organization and its change. We know that some families develop pathological structures harmful to the nutritional health of its members. Researchers have also argued that fast food diets leave one at risk of lower vitamin and mineral intake and of higher percentages of energy from fat. Whether changing diets prompted by technological change or more sedentary lifestyles are the cause of the rise in obesity levels from 25 to 33 percent of the adult population is an empirical question. We have little in the way of clear evidence as to the nature of potential effects that organizational change may have on the quality of the food supply and thus the quality of the diet. Whit (1995) provides interesting speculations in this regard, but as yet, no research has examined these possibilities.

Second, the role of women in food-related organizations remains important, although in those organizations that possess concentrations of power and wealth, their roles are usually subordinate. Women are given control over those aspects of the food process that are valued least. Furthermore, women are often given responsibilities without control, as in family meal planning and preparation. Waitresses in more traditional but less hierarchical arrangements, as in certain restaurant settings, develop a great deal of autonomy but remain poorly paid. Women remain largely in "waitressing" positions, while men dominate "waitering" and chefs' positions. Low status and low pay thus characterize many of the food roles filled by women. Dietetics and nutrition have high concentrations of females, even at the graduate level. However, men tend to fill the higher status positions, such as nutritional biochemistry. The creation of food technology appears to lie largely in the hands of men as well (Cockburn & Ormrod, 1993). Most cooking technology appears to have been invented by men; while it has perhaps made women's work less difficult, it has not saved them a great deal of time. As women gain greater footholds in a variety of higher-status occupations, perhaps some of these conditions may change. Women are likely concentrated in the creation of new food products, and they may increasingly play important roles in the development of new "white goods."

Third, despite warnings and some evidence, it is apparent that the family meal has not disappeared or lost its importance for family. As discussed earlier, meals represent events in which both hierarchy and integration are present. Overemphasis on the hierarchy or challenges to it, however, represent real threats to integration. Because these threats are real and likely numerous in some families, family members may attempt to intervene in an attempt at reestablishing harmony. Functionalists claimed that all groups develop both task and emotional leaders, and the role of the emotional leader in a family is played by the wife-mother. DeVault's (1991) description of women's work at home as caring would lead us to predict that conciliation during meals is likely performed by the wife-mother. However, the extant conflict may originate in the wife–husband or mother–child relationship. Psychologists have claimed that in dysfunctional families, one or more members may become conciliators, using humor and other attention-drawing efforts to diffuse situations of conflict. Children often take on these responsibilities. Thus, during mealtimes, a child may attempt to bring about a peaceful, if only temporary, resolution to the conflict. However, researchers have given these issues scant attention.

Other sorts of meals have received even less attention. Dating relationships frequently involve eating meals together at restaurants. However, there is some evidence that key aspects of these events have changed. During the 1950s, for example, the male routinely paid the entire check. Meals were often eaten either before or after a movie or dance, usually at a hamburger joint or drive-in restaurant. More expensive meals were eaten at fancier restaurants for more formal occasions such as proms. While perhaps this description holds among couples who consider their relationship "serious," students today report that many of their dates are Dutch treat. The costs are shared. Has the function of such meals changed as well?

There is also some data on how the amount and type of food selected by an individual can affect perceptions of others. For example, women viewed as eating a large meal are considered less feminine than women who eat smaller meals; men who select a salad as their entree are perceived as less masculine than men who order meat as the main dish. The chief interest, however, ought to involve a determination of the role that such meals play in relationships. Perhaps they serve to integrate the individuals further into the relationship. Or perhaps they are at best surface manifestations of change in the exchange relations embodied in dates.

Fourth, technological change has made the food industry more efficient in some respects, and it permits greater consistency across space. Just as technological innovations have led to increases in production and to the reduction in the number of farms as a consequence, such change will also befall the restaurant industry. Of interest is the kind of restaurant at greatest risk of mortality. It is likely that many of those that close will have been family-owned, nonchain enterprises. However, some of those chains in crowded fields such as hamburger or pizza production may go under as new chains move into as-yet-undeveloped ethnic fast foods. Some of these have tried flexible responses to the changing nature of their competition by offering for short periods of time specialty dishes that are ordinarily not found on their menus. The fast food business appears to have great advantage over other sorts of food service establishments; it creates easy take-home meals, and it can venture into foods that are already familiar to the customer. We are already accustomed to Chinese food; having the choice of a fast-food version offers a change within a familiar set of foods.

Fifth, trends in organizations other than the family have involved globalization, increased commodification through value-adding, conglomeration, and specialization. Some parts of the food industry have attempted to increase profits by becoming more efficient, especially with regard to labor. Prime examples can be found in fast-food restaurants and meat-packing plants. Large companies have bought out numerous food companies to increase assets and to gain control of brand names. Some of these companies have begun to sell off some of their acquisitions to pay off accumulated debt. Intense competition among a small number of companies over the breakfast cereal market continues, although this has not led to the introduction of fundamentally different products or lower consumer prices (Winson, 1993).

Sixth, of additional interest is the changing nature of interorganizational relations in the food industry. Farmers are increasingly locked into forward contracts that have consequences for their autonomy and profit making. This trend is particularly ironic in that it appears that the federal government is moving away from its traditional commodity support programs as a budget-cutting measure; one consequence of less funding is less federal control over amounts and types of crops grown, conservation practices, and perhaps wildlife preservation rules. Thus as producers gain freedom relative to government, some of it is lost to the food processing industry.

Another area in which interorganizational relations may continue to change is that involving food processors and food marketers. Food processors tend to be large in size, and many have become subsidiaries of other large companies. Marketers have also grown in size, and some are parts of large conglomerates too. Power once resided in the hands of processors in these interrelationships, but Seneaur et al. (1991) have argued that marketers have achieved sufficient size to challenge processors. This is an empirical question that needs investigation. In addition, the consequences for consumers in terms of food and nutrition that result from a changing locus of power in the food industry are largely unexplored.

Seventh, restaurants face other environmental contingencies as well. For example, older style restaurants attracted customers for their food and ambiance. Part of the latter for most restaurants included a relaxing atmosphere. Thus, while some degree of haste was expected in terms of the service, patrons looked forward to the leisurely enjoyment of their meals. Fast-food restaurants emphasize not only speedy service but speedy ingestion to make room for the next set of customers. For those in a hurry, this must have great appeal. Those looking for convenience and leisurely pace now have the option of buying take-home meals. Specialization of the restaurant's niche has thus occurred, making it more difficult, we would predict, for generalist restaurants to remain in business.

Food safety is an issue that nags at food companies and restaurants. Some fear the consequences of food-poisoning scandals for profits. Others fear increased regulations by Congress, although the new Congress has begun to question benefits of new industry safety proposals recommended by USDA. In the meantime, food companies and others have attempted to shift the responsibility for food safety on to the consumer, arguing that it is currently impossible for meat processors, for example, to eliminate completely the risk of food-borne pathogens. Others have emphasized both consumer responsibility and profitability by explicitly marketing soaps and cleansers containing antibacterial agents. However, the industry may not successfully shift full responsibility for food safety to the consumer. In most states, the state health department is charged with monitoring restaurant and institutional health and safety practices. Because of a lack of sufficient funds, inspections occur with varying degrees of frequency and penalties for infractions generally are light. Because of recent incidents of food poisonings, along with reminders by the mass media of safety problems in restaurants, state regulations and penalties may increase in frequency and severity. This may lead to the elimination of some restaurants and the change in personnel training and supervision in others. Not all restaurants could afford to adopt a Hazardous Analysis Critical Control Point (HACCP) system, for example.

Eighth, the environment faced by farms is changing as well. Trade agreements such as GATT (General Agreement on Trade) and NAFTA (North American Free Trade Agreement) will likely expose farmers to greater competition from commodities produced outside of the United States. Changes in the Farm Bill recently passed by Congress include features that increase farmer flexibility (e.g., removal of the limitations on the number of acres in which a particular crop are planted; elimination of soil conservation requirements) while increasing uncertainty (e.g., elimination of crop price guarantees and substitution of market pricing). Some farmers currently depend on price supports as the means for making a profit. Many of these may go out of business under more competitive conditions. Furthermore, the disappearance of price controls will return agriculture to the boom-and-bust conditions it traditionally faced before the development of environment-stabilizing farm programs. These changes may cause farms to make further adaptations such as diversification of crops and livestock production to avoid being caught with a single commodity the price of which has fallen well below costs of production. Such changes may be difficult for large-scale farmers who purchased a large amount of farm-specialized equipment; similarly, small farms may not have enough land to permit a meaningful level of diversified production. Albrecht and Murdock (1984) found that one response that farms make to more diverse environments is to engage in part-time farming. This adaptation may be insufficient under new conditions.

Farmers have adapted to variations in their environments by adopting various survival strategies. One strategy is to have some family members work off-farm and use the income derived from such work to subsidize the farm operation. Other owner-operators engage in part-time farming. Albrecht and Murdock (1984) found that part-time farming represents an adaptation to a physical environment less amenable to agriculture and a social environment that offers a greater range of off-farm work opportunities. The part-time farmer is more likely in environments in which competitors have not diversified their commodity production (Albrecht & Murdock, 1984).

5

SOCIAL STRATIFICATION
The Distribution of Food and Nutrition

INTRODUCTION

An area of major interest to sociology since its inception is the study of social classes or social stratification. It is also the area of sociology that has had the most influence on the study of food behavior.

Social stratification is defined as unequal access to desired resources (i.e., money, goods, services—education, medical care) or psychic gratifications (e.g., prestige, respect). Access to desired resources is governed by two very different mechanisms: possession of marketable property or possession of marketable skills (Giddens, 1973). The first pertains to capital goods and other forms of wealth; the second, to skills obtained largely through formal training. In advanced societies like the United States, most persons obtain their place in the stratification system through school system attendance, which credentials them for positions in the occupational structure. Even here, however, connections to individuals of higher social status are frequently necessary to obtain employment (Granovetter, 1973). At the same time, social stratification is generally viewed as a system of imperfectlly interrelated elements. However, inequalities in wealth, income, education, prestige, and the like are, in most cases, highly consistent (Lenski & Lenski, 1987). Those who rank low in income typically rank low along other dimensions. Status inconsistencies occur infrequently.

In this chapter, I briefly describe the main theoretical approaches taken by stratification theorists in sociology and discuss how these pertain to food and nutrition. I also examine how certain correlates of social stratification, namely, gender and ethnicity, relate to food and nutrition. Finally, stratification researchers have begun to apply the world systems theory perspective to problems found in the Third World and following the Susser, Watson, and Hopper (1985) and Campbell, Chen, Parpia, Yinsheng, Chumming, and Geissler (1992) lead, I extend this to health and nutrition.

THEORIES OF SOCIAL STRATIFICATION

While various dimensions of social stratification have been used in food and nutrition research, including father's and mother's occupation, education, and income (Baird & Schultz, 1980; Chavas, 1983; Falese & Unnevehr, 1988; Guseman, Bassenyemukasa, & Sapp, 1987; McNaughton, Boyle, & Bryant, 1990; Riecters, Alvin, & Dellenbayer, 1988), the research generally has treated these elements apart from social stratification theory. Sociological approaches to social stratification have generally focused on either the specific lack of access to resources faced by lower class and some middle-class persons or the intergenerational transmission of class advantages. The nutrition literature, perhaps because of its applied nature, has shied away from the structural implications of social inequalities (i.e., the need to reorganize society in some fashion), and when inequities in nutrition status are encountered, the literature generally concludes with a call for more effective education.

The Weberian Approach

The study of social stratification, using a theoretical perspective, has great utility. In some of the earliest writings concerning social class, Max Weber distinguished between groups of persons who are stratified by the way in which they *use* wealth and status and groups of persons who are distinguished by the way in which they *acquire* wealth and status (Gerth & Mills, 1946:180–198). Weber differentiated between the two types of stratifying principles with the terms lifestyles and life chances. Those who acquire greater wealth and status have greater life chances because of associated increases in the healthfulness of their diet, their access to medical care, and their ability to avoid dangerous occupations or circumstances. Giddens (1973) described this differentiation as the result of stratification in production versus stratification of consumption.

Lifestyles are distinct from life chances, for, rather than survival chances, they represent the opportunity to distinguish oneself from others. They provide the mechanism for gaining and maintaining prestige and respect.

A number of authors have noted in some detail that various social classes exhibit distinct differences in food behavior. *What, where, when,* and *how* food is eaten form distinct patterns by social class (Lasswell, 1965). What is eaten is clearly distinct, at least regarding some foods. The lower classes are generally unfamiliar with such upper-class foods as caviar or truffles, while members of the upper class would disdain TV dinners. Dining rooms are more likely a feature in an upper class home than a kitchenette, and fewer members of the upper class find it chic to eat at a lunch counter.

The whole notion of what is called "taste" results from class distinctions. Some have claimed that taste is "peculiarly modern... the hieratic societies of the ancient past and of the Orient did not fret about the finer points of discernment. Even in the European Middle Ages the concept did not exist" (Bayley, 1991:25). Subsistence, not materialistic pleasure, was the order of the day. Taste developed as the middle class sought to distance themselves from the lower classes in a period of relative prosperity. According to this view, taste had to do with "refined sensibilities" rather than innate properties of objects. What was considered "good taste" could be changed to circumvent lower-class capture of the symbols of style and taste. The development of cuisine, in part, owes its existence to status striving through the expression of good taste. While this account may characterize the majority of individuals living in Europe at this time, it disregards the existence of a small but economically powerful and socially distinct upper class that took a great deal of care in maintaining a sharp distinction between its lifestyle and that adhered to by the remainder of society. These distinctions, however, were based more on quantitative, than qualitative differences.

Weberian approaches to social class can thus be highly insightful when it comes to studies of under- and overnutrition, on the one hand, and on the other, of food choices, cooking styles, kitchen equipment, and choice of restaurant.

The Marxian Approach

Marx's view of social class derives from his larger theory of socioeconomic development. In his theory societies advance through the development of their productive forces. Productive forces consist of the means of production (i.e., instruments of production including tools, machinery, and raw materials) and labor power, which includes strength, skills, and knowledge (Cohen, 1978). Particular configurations of these productive forces constitute the various modes of production associated with feudalism, capitalism, and socialism. Development of the productive forces involve substituting instruments of production for direct labor power to achieve a larger output of products, which, in effect, results in labor de-skilling and increased unemployment. Each stage of societal development typically represents an increase in the economic surplus accumulated as a result of both the development of productive forces and the extraction of surplus value from market exchanges.

In capitalism, the process of surplus extraction for capital accumulation has become a manifest part of the economic system. Marx also argues that each stage of development has a characteristic set of relations of production, which have to do with "effective control over persons and productive forces" (Cohen, 1978:63). The main distinction of importance here regards ownership of the means of production and control over labor power. A feudal lord owns most of the means of production and controls most of the serfs' labor power. A capitalist owns all of the means of production, and a laborer controls his or her labor power. An independent producer is someone who controls both her or his labor power and the means of production she or he uses (Cohen, 1978:65).

The two themes from Marxist thought that apply here are the generation of surplus via labor exploitation and the incessant drive by capitalists to increase profits, regardless of the implications for others. The exploitation and de-skilling of labor in food and agriculture is the theme of works such as *Sweetness and Power* by Mintz (1985), *Meatpackers and Beef Barons* by Andreas (1994) and *Manufacturing Green Gold* by Friedland et al. (1981) (see also, McIntosh & Picou, 1985). Other literature has dealt with the possibility of a "capitalist agriculture." Mooney (1986) and others have argued that capitalism has overtaken U.S. agriculture because of increased tenancy, reliance on credit, forward contracting, and hired labor. Each of these involves a loss of control over either the means of production, labor, or both.

Williams (1994) portrayed the rise of coffee agriculture in Central America as an instance of capital seeking high rates of profit. Actual investments were made in those countries where governments removed or reduced obstacles to investment. Mann (1990) argued that the very nature of agriculture precludes its becoming capitalist, observing that farming contradicted Marx's labor theory of value, which stated that the "production of any commodity is based on the socially necessary labor time needed for its production. Socially necessary labor time refers to the prevailing conditions of production existing in a given time and place" (Mann, 1990:33).

Labor time differs, however, from production time, which is the total time required to produce a good. In some production processes, production may continue without labor time expenditure. For example, the biological processes that make up the gestation period of livestock are a fundamental part of production, yet no labor is involved after an initial input (Mann, 1990). The lack of coordination between labor and production time leads to an inefficient use of farm machinery. This feature and the fact that many agriculture commodities are perishable make farming too risky for capitalists.

The capitalistic drive toward profit and greater control over the market is a theme found in discussions of oligopolies in food processing and marketing (Whit, 1995; Zwerdling, 1976) and studies of the globalization of food and agriculture (Friedmann, 1994; Heffernan & Constance, 1994; McMichael, 1994; Reed & Marchant, 1994). The latter literature focuses on the long-term processes of concentration in the food industry. Some of this literature pays attention to the vertical integration of food processing and marketing (Goodman & Redclift, 1991; Whit, 1995); other literature examines the consequences of transnational food corporations (Heffernan & Constance, 1994). The rise of TNCs, according to Heffernan and Constance (1994), has had a deleterious effect in the form of dislocated labor and resulting rural community decline. TNCs have come to determine "what food is grown where, how, and by whom" (Heffernan & Constance, 1994:29). Some have called these far-reaching effects a form of "global proletarianization" of farming through, among other things, the forcing of peasants off their land and turning them into wage workers in either rural or urban areas (Barkin, 1985; Stonich, 1991).

Winson (1993) described the consequences of concentration in the food sector. The breakfast cereal industry in the United States represented one of the most concentrated industries in any sector, with four firms in control of over 90 percent of sales. This degree of concentration exceeded that required for an industry to take full advantage of economies of scale associated with larger-sized entities. Furthermore, prices in the industry resulted not from competition but from "price leadership," leading to excessive costs for consumers (Winson, 1993:123). Further inefficiencies resulted because of this lack of competition: advertising expenditures as a percentage of total costs increase as the market becomes less competitive (Winson, 1993:127).

The Marxists and others use the argument that capitalism eventually proletarianizes the entire labor force as a critique of the movement of agriculture into commercial markets (Friedland et al., 1981; Mooney, 1986). Their concern lies with the notion that commercialization of subsistence farming results in further impoverishment. However, recent longitudinal studies involving substantial samples of both participants and nonparticipants in cash cropping suggests that these fears may be unfounded (Kennedy, 1994; von Braun, 1994).

Social Class as Lifestyle and Life Chances

Older approaches to studies of social class in the United States focused on lifestyle differences. Lloyd Warner's Yankee City studies (Warner, 1963; Warner & Lunt, 1941, 1947) uncovered community social ranking systems based on (1) occupation, (2) source of income, (3) house type, and (4) area of the community in which the house was located.

Recent uses of measures of social class have gravitated toward the measurement of income, education, and occupational prestige. This approach is taken because these are easier to measure than family wealth, political power, or respect in the community. Also, they roughly *correspond* to what Weber seems to have meant by social stratification: income *approximates* wealth as education and occupational prestige approximate social honor. Occupational position results from educational attainment and provides income (Bogue, 1969:429), but occupation represents a person's place in social strata because of the various conditions associated with work. Finally, gender and ethnicity are often included as additional indicators because they reflect differential access to wealth, power, and social honor.

Social class standing is strongly associated with health, and for good reasons. Middle- and upper-class persons more likely work in occupations whose physical conditions are relatively safe and whose psychical conditions are less stressful compared with lower-class occupations. In addition, such work usually offers benefits such as health insurance and incentives to maintain personal health. Income provides the means to pay for health care not covered by insurance, and education is associated with greater knowledge of preventative health care practices and the utility of medical services. Thus, upper- and middle-class persons are less likely to engage in risky lifestyles such as smoking, drinking excessively, or not wearing seat belts (Blaxter, 1990; Leigh, 1983; National Center for Health Statistics, 1992). Social class differences thus result in differentials in morbidity and mortality even after accounting for lifestyle differences (Dutton, 1989; Marmot & Theorell, 1994).

In the United States, rates of chronic illnesses such as ischemic heart disease, hypertension, gastric ulcers, and diverticuli of the intestines were substantially higher for those with an annual family income of less than $20,000 or more (National Center for Health Statistics, 1985). Prevalence rates of acute illnesses among those making less money exceeded those for individuals making more money. In addition, persons in the United States making less than $10,000 per year visited the hospital 1.7 times per year compared with 0.7 times for those making more than $10,000 (National Center for Health Statistics, 1985). Similarly, 14 percent of those with incomes under $10,000 suffered some degree of physical limitation due to chronic illness whereas only 8 percent of those making $25,000 or more had such an experience.

A much smaller proportion of women sought annual breast exams among those who made under $10,000 compared to those making more than this amount. In England, women in professional occupations were far less likely to smoke (24.6 percent) than women in semiskilled or unskilled occupations (56.2 percent) (Mascie-Taylor, 1990). Nearly 60 percent of the former breast fed their infants, but only 24 percent of the latter did so. In the United States 18 percent of persons with more than 12 years of education smoked compared to 32 percent of those with less than 12 years of education (U. S. Bureau of the Census, 1994:144).

Food consumption and nutritional status are substantially affected by social class background. In general, those of higher standing in the class order more likely enjoy food in sufficient amounts and of sufficient quality to possess not only a desirable lifestyle but also good health. In fact, even those of middle- or upper-class background are less likely to experience so-called overnutrition.

Social Class and Stature

Height is considered to be a measure of long-term nutritional status during childhood. Once adulthood arrives, the individual carries with him or her a permanent record of nutritional status and thus socioeconomic experiences in childhood. Height is highly correlated with socioeconomic status and some economic historians have used data on height as a surrogate measure of income (Komlos, 1994). In addition, average height increased in periods of prosperity and decreased during periods of economic decline (Floud et al., 1990; Komlos, 1994). Some have found, however, that economic development sometimes exacerbated income inequalities, which, in turn, were associated with downturns in height (Streckel, 1994). Floud et al. (1990) have found that urbanization may have intervened so as to have seriously weakened the income–height relationship.

Social Class and Obesity

Sobal and Stunkard (1989) reviewed the results of 144 studies conducted during the past 40 years regarding the relationship between obesity and socioeconomic status (SES) in developed nations. They reported an inverse relationship between SES and obesity in women (in 93 percent of these studies), whereas only half (52 percent) of the studies of men observed an inverse relationship. Nearly one third (30 percent) of the male studies found a *positive* relationship between SES and obesity. As smoking exhibited a high negative relationship with SES and smoking is positively associated with lower weight, this and other lifestyle factors not taken into account may explain the differing findings for men versus women (Sobol & Stunkard, 1989).

Turning to developing countries, Sobal and Stunkard (1989) discovered that 91 percent of the studies found a direct relationship between SES and obesity. Eighty-six percent of the studies report the same relationship for men.

In developing nations, lower-class groups may suffer lower body weight because of lack of food "coupled with higher energy expenditure" (Sobal & Stunkard, 1989:266). Obesity has been considered a lifestyle choice in these countries; obesity reflects the status associated with not having to work hard to survive.

In developed countries, SES may also promote lifestyles that bear on obesity. As Sobal and Stunkard (1989) noted, upper-SES women were more likely to diet and engage in exercise programs than were lower-SES women.

In the United States class differences appear in food purchase, food intake, and nutritional status. Engel first suggested that as incomes increase, the proportion of that income devoted to food purchase grows smaller (Engel's Law) (Ferguson, 1972:46–49). There is little advantage to purchase more food, once a household achieves a sufficient level of consumption. A related observation is also true. Those with less money tend to spend a greater proportion of it on food. Few exceptions have ever been found to these claims. The relationship between income and proportion spent on food continues to hold true in the United States. According to the U.S. 1988 Continuing Consumer Expenditure Survey, those persons with annual incomes of less than $5,000 devoted about 82 percent of their budget to food; those making between $10,000 and $15,000, 22 percent of their budgets; and those making more than $50,000, only 8 percent (Senauer et al., 1991).

Significant percentages of both blacks and whites living in poverty consumed less than 70 percent of the Recommended Daily Allowances (RDAs) for calories, calcium, iron, and magnesium. However, these percentages exceeded by 6 percentage points or less those for blacks and whites not living in poverty (see Senauer et al., 1991). Regarding nutritional status, among three- to five-year-olds living below the poverty level 14 percent had impaired iron status compared to only 4 percent of the nonpoverished from the same age group (Senauer et al., 1991:225). Twenty-nine percent of poor men aged 55–74 had low serum vitamin C levels compared with only 6 percent of the nonpoor from this age group (Senauer et al., 1991:227).

Results from several recent HANES (Health and Nutrition Examination Survey) studies indicated a low prevalence of malnutrition in the United States. Data from trends in hospital diagnosis, for example, indicate that nutritional deficiencies have remained at between 5 and 6 per 100,000 persons during the period 1980–1987. Furthermore, anemia has declined significantly from 61 to 59 per 100,000 (Elixhauser, Harris, & Coffey, 1995). This situation reflects a dramatic improvement over the conditions found by the 1968 Ten State Study, which indicated high levels of several types of deficiency disease such as anemia (McLaren, 1976a). These improvements resulted from WIC (Supplemental Feeding Program for Women, Infants, and Children) and other federal government interventions, rather than a significant increase in upward mobility.

Hunger and Poverty

The Food Research and Action Center (FRAC, 1991) sponsored and coordinated hunger studies in seven of the nine Census Bureau divisions and all four Census Bureau regions. Based on these surveys, FRAC estimated that among families with children under 12 years of age, 12 percent experienced hunger in 1989. An additional 28 percent of the surveyed families were considered at risk of hunger. Hunger was measured by asking one head of household eight questions regarding such things as whether and how long a period of time the family "ran out of money for food," "adults eating less because of insufficient money for food," and "the child goes to bed because there was not enough money for food" (Samets, 1991). When compared with families with nonhungry children, families with hungry children reported these children suffered more health problems, lowered school attendance, and symptoms of low energy (e.g., fatigue, irritability, dizziness).

Education and Nutrition

Education has become an important class indicator because it reflects (1) prestige, (2) access to economic opportunities, and (3) exposure to modern, scientific ideas. Persons with education tend not only to be more highly respected, but to have a greater chance of obtaining employment that will increase life chances (and change lifestyles, thus enhancing social honor). Such persons will more likely seek out and utilize sources of information that lead to self-improvements in preventative health care measures (e.g., getting more exercise, lowering dietary fat).

Education has provided strong competition for income in Third World country studies aimed at distinguishing families with malnourished children from families without such children. Among poor families, mothers with more education or who are more literate tend to have fewer malnourished children. Some have argued that the importance of maternal education lies in its status-enhancing qualities, giving her more power and control in the household (Bateman & McIntosh, 1994; Blumberg, 1988).

Others note, however, that the effectiveness of nutrition intervention programs had not always shown itself among the better educated of poor women. In a number of intervention studies, nutritional knowledge and improved infant health occurred most frequently among the least well educated women (Zeitlin, Ghassemi, & Mansour, 1990). This suggested that specific health care education may possibly play a more pivotal role than overall education in intervention. Perhaps possession of such specialized knowledge enhanced poor women's status and thus her power, but earlier research on so-called Mothercraft Centers indicated that new knowledge about how traditional sex roles ought to be changed has no impact on the distribution of decision-making power (McIntosh, 1975). Increasing specialized knowledge may only have its intended effects in societies in which status boundaries and sex roles are less rigid.

Occupation and Food

Since occupation is a chief source of prestige, it may well be an important determinant of lifestyle, beyond the dictates of income or education. Some research and discussion confirmed this assertion (see Gerstl, 1961; Zablocki & Kanter, 1976). Bourdieu (1984) used occupation as a key marker of class position but argued that the construction and maintenance of occupational status depended on both economic and cultural capital. These writings suggest not only that certain groups consume more goods but that they consume particular mixes of goods. "A higher status group will consume more theater and ballet, but less bowling, more wine and liquor, but less beer" (Zablocki & Kanter, 1976:271). Bourdieu (1984:176) pushed these differences to the extreme with his rubric of the "taste of necessity" versus the "taste of luxury."

Occupations are an important determinant of lifestyle because of occupational cultures that may be said to involve similarities in tasks, work schedules, perceived demands on energy, training, career patterns, worldview, and absorptiveness in terms of intrusion into the private time of individuals. These have a major impact on the way persons lead their lives outside of their occupations.

Occupational cultures lead to differences in the type of leisure activities pursued, in the way children are raised, and in the types of relationships that are maintained with nonimmediate kin. Research and theoretical development in the area of occupations and occupational cultures remain underdeveloped, but this aspect of social stratification has potential value for studying food behavior.

A number of studies have demonstrated the potential in examining occupational variables. These studies often contained rather primitive measures of occupation and do not tap elements of occupational culture. They have remained, however, an indicator of intriguing possibilities. One study, utilizing data from the U.S. Department of Agriculture's Nationwide Food Consumption Survey 1977–78, found significant differences in nutrient intake by occupation. Managers, clerical workers, and salespersons tended to have lower intakes than farmers, craftsmen, and blue-collar workers (Keplinger, 1981). Farmers had the highest intake levels of all. Turning to women, Keplinger (1981:71) found that housewives had the highest intake of all occupation groups, followed by female professionals, craftsmen, salespersons, and service workers in declining order. Similar patterns were reported by McIntosh and Shifflett (1981). These differences may result from actual differentials in the energy demands of the work involved in the various occupations. Alternatively, higher levels of food intake among those with lower status occupations may reflect differences among occupational cultures.

Cox, Huppert, and Whichelow (1993) found that while a significant percentage of adults in England had reduced white bread and increased whole grain bread consumption from 1984 to 1991, significant differences by class remained. In 1991, while 55 percent of men employed in nonmanual occupations consumed "whole meal" bread, 67 percent of those involved in manual labor consumed white bread. While a number of these intake differences may be due to differences in income and activity levels associated with the occupation, occupational cultures may play an important part as well.

As discussed earlier, Bourdieu (1984) argued that the objective conditions of class position generate systems of social practices and perceptions of these practices as well as products used in such practices. He referred to the capacity to make such judgments as taste (Bourdieu, 1984:170). Furthermore, "taste is thus the source of the system of distinctive features which cannot fail to be perceived as a systematic expression of a particular class of conditions of existence, i.e., as distinctive life style by anyone who possesses practical knowledge of the relationships between distinctive signs and positions..." (Bourdieu, 1984:175).

Practices and tastes are internalized through a lifetime of socialization. Of particular interest is Bourdieu's (1984) differentiation between the taste of necessity versus the taste of luxury. Taste of necessity consists of those practices and perceptions that result from one's limited class circumstances. However, such taste is not defined by its possessors as that of necessity, because socialization has left the individual with the perception that such necessities are in fact virtues.

Those in dominant positions view dominant practices associated with the taste of necessity as "vulgar because they are both easy and common" while portraying their own tastes and lifestyle in more ascetic terms (Bourdieu, 1984:176).

Bourdieu (1984) provided data on the spending habits of various occupational groups to illustrate his framework of tastes. His analysis rung true when contrasting the rather aggregate differences in the spending practices of skilled manual workers, foremen, clerical workers, teachers, senior executives, professionals, engineers, and industrial and commercial employers. He found expected differences in the proportion of household budgets that these occupational groups spent on food and in the frequency of eating meals at restaurants. Attention to expenditures for specific food items, however, weakened his argument considerably. Despite his claims that one group spent either more or "distinctly less" than another on particular food items, these differences were rarely more than several percentage points. For example, Bourdieu (1984) claimed that class fractions vary significantly in terms of the amount and types of meats they purchase. However, even for expensive meats such as mutton and lamb, while foremen spent the least amount (1.3 percent of their incomes), those in the professions, whose relative expenditures for these meats exceeded all other groups, devoted only 3.2 percent of their incomes to mutton and lamb.

As discussed in the chapter on culture, no one has attempted to replicate Bourdieu's (1984) research in the United States, although Lamont (1992) provided a partial replication. Sobel (1981), however, supplied some supporting evidence for general effects of occupation on lifestyle choices. He treated consumption (purchase) as an indicator of lifestyle in the United States. While he examined a variety of expenditures, two food-related purchases—food purchased for household use and food purchased away from home—were pertinent. Using factor analysis, Sobel (1981) placed goods purchased away from home into a "visible success" factor and food purchased for home use into a "maintenance" factor. He also looked at other factors, including one described as "higher living." He then attempted to predict these factors, using education, occupation, and income. His results tended to confirm the notion that differing lifestyles are associated with differing socioeconomic and occupational groupings. Sobel's (1981) use of occupation, however, was somewhat primitive in that he utilized broad categories of occupation. Further research is needed to more clearly identify specific lifestyles with specific occupational cultures in the United States.

Finally, several qualitative studies have examined class differences in food behavior, using both occupation and income as indicators of class background. Charles and Kerr (1988) studied women's household food responsibilities in a sample of 200 families in England. They found that women from households in which the husband held either skilled or unskilled manual labor positions paid greater attention to the price of food and perceived that they often had to purchase poorer quality foods than women whose husbands held higher-status occupations.

DeVault (1991) reported similar findings for a smaller sample of families living in Chicago. Both studies found that middle- and upper-class families used meals at home as a means of feeding guests and experienced concern over costs related to these kinds of meals. Women in lower class homes were concerned with having enough money to feed their own families.

Charles and Kerr (1988) also detected class differences in the importance of family meals and in the structure of meals. Middle-class families saw that meals were not only an opportunity for all members of the family to be present at a single event, but also a chance for parents and children to interact and for parents to socialize their offspring. Lower-class families were more likely to practice the dictum "children should be seen but not heard." These families ate meals more frequently while watching television and were less likely to reside in a dwelling with sufficient space so that all family members could eat together (Charles & Kerr, 1988). The middle-class households studied by DeVault (1991) placed much more emphasis on meals and new foods as sources of family entertainment and adventure and actively sought new information sources as a means to these ends. This orientation was conspicuously absent in the lower-class households, although some effort was made to obtain new recipes from friends or coworkers.

Gender and Social Class

Social stratification has to do with unequal distribution of resources. Gender is an important element of social stratification. Gender differences evidence themselves in divisions of labor inside the home and in the economy at large. Such gender differences tend to disadvantage women in terms of the access it gives them to wealth, power, and prestige. Placement in the division of labor itself, however, depends on prior levels of these resources. So the issue is not simply one of differences in achievement. We saw in an earlier chapter that women are also disadvantaged relative to men in terms of occupation and earnings.

Gender and Nutritional Consequences

Women in the Third World experience lower enrollment rates in both primary and secondary schools when compared with men and, not surprisingly, illiteracy rates from 10 to 15 percentage points higher than men (World Bank, 1993:300–301). Their labor force participation was also less than that of men; these inequalities tended to reduce women's decision-making power at home. Women with less control over household resources had less control not only over their own health but that of their children as well (Bateman & McIntosh, 1994; Blumberg, 1988). In industrialized societies such as the United States, households in which both heads participated in the labor force were at low risk of poverty in contrast to female-headed households, which were at high risk (Senauer et al., 1991). Worldwide, women fare more poorly than men in terms of prevalence and severity of three out of four of the major nutritional deficiencies, which include protein energy malnutrition (PEM), iron deficiency, and goiter (iodine deficiency) (Leslie, 1995). While some debate occurs over whether families systematically regulate and lessen the amount of food that women receive, little doubt exists as to specific effects of insufficient nutrition in women. In a comprehensive review of the existing literature, Hamilton, Popkin, and Spicer (1984) show that women's fecundity and fertility and lactation during pregnancy are affected. Low birth weight, which is associated with infant mortality, is also more likely, and the combination of frequent births and poor nutrition greatly increase the chances of complications and maternal death as a result of childbirth.

Ethnicity and Nutrition

Drawing on a variety of data regarding health conditions in the United States (National Center for Health Statistics, 1992), significant ethnic differences in nutrition-related illnesses and health practices were evident. For example, the infant mortality rates for blacks and American Indians exceeded those for Anglos and Mexican Americans; those for Japanese Americans were less than the Anglo/Mexican American rates. Death rates for blacks by specific causes such as heart disease and cancer surpassed those for whites. A greater percentage of blacks than whites smoked, and blacks were somewhat less likely to seek medical attention than whites. Hispanic and black women were less likely to have a Pap test than Anglo women. Many of these differences resulted from differential resources. Blacks earned less money than whites, and many lived in areas without health care facilities in close proximity (Woolhandler et al., 1989). Anglos were more likely than blacks and Hispanics to have either full or partial insurance coverage (Paulin & Weber, 1995). Furthermore, after controlling for income only some of the ethnic differential in health disappeared.

Differences in food intake and nutrition status, as reported by Senauer et al. (1991), tended to vary more by race than by poverty. Nayga and Capps (1994a, 1994b) analyzed data on food consumption and nutrient intake from the most recent Nationwide Food Consumption Survey (1987–88). Their weighted least squares regression and logit models showed that ethnicity matters when considering food consumption, even after controlling for income, employment status, residence, gender, age, and a number of other factors. Their results indicated that whites ate more beef, but less pork, poultry, and fish than blacks; Hispanics consumed more beef than non-Hispanics. Blacks had lower intakes of nutrients such as food energy, saturated fats, dietary fiber, vitamin A, thiamin, riboflavin, calcium, and iron but higher intakes of protein, cholesterol, and vitamin C than whites.

Asians and Pacific Islanders consumed greater amounts of riboflavin, carotene, protein, iron, and vitamin C, but lower amounts of fat, saturated fat, and calcium than whites. Hispanics took in less fat, saturated fat, riboflavin, calcium, and copper, but had higher cholesterol, dietary fiber, and folate than non-Hispanics.

DEVELOPMENT VERSUS EXPLOITATION IN SOLVING WORLD FOOD PROBLEMS

The association of starvation and malnutrition with poverty has led to efforts to alleviate food and nutrition problems through reducing poverty. Economic development schemes represent the standard long-term solution proposed, but some have argued that development simply elevates the entire class system without altering its fundamental inequalities. As these critics of the class system contend that inequalities cause the human misery associated with lack of adequate food, their solutions emphasize either redistribution or development plus redistribution. In this section of the chapter, we move away from static comparisons of class differences to discuss how theories of economic and political change provide an understanding of both nutritional improvement and decline. Two major approaches apply: economic development theory and world systems theory. The former is applied by various aid agencies such as the U.S. Agency for International Development, the World Bank, and the UN Economic and Social Development Office as well as many academics. World systems theory and related dependency theories have emerged from academic extensions of Marxism, although the Economic Commission for Latin America made a major contribution during the early, developmental stages of these approaches. The literature on economic development is both voluminous and well developed; less well known is world systems theory and its application to world food problems. I will thus spend more time elaborating the latter.

Economic Development Theory

Classical versions of economic development theory focused on labor productivity and capital accumulation. As the theory developed further, capital formation became the key element in growth and development. Capital accumulation was said to serve as the means for increasing investments in expanding economy. The new willingness to invest was explained by cultural changes such as the Protestant ethic (Weber, 1968) or by a "social climate" that, first, favored risk-taking and, second, rewarded amply successful risk-taking (Schumpeter, 1950).

Economic development was initially linked with laissez-faire or capitalist economics, but the Keynesian revolution of the 1930s argued for a central role for governments as the source of capital investments and labor improvement.

Much of the writing on economic development utilized English history to shape its models. Several key events thought to signal such development have been identified. In addition to new orientations regarding capital investment, development moved forward through industrialization. The development and spread of industry was thought to be the engine of wealth creation, its benefits spread throughout the entire economy. Rising wages improved the standard of living through increased purchases of food and better housing. The expenditure of wages fueled further economic expansion.

More recently, observers have noted the importance of capitalist expansion in agriculture as a necessary precursor of industrial growth (Mellor, 1966). Expanding trade, along with profit-seeking orientations, led landowners to innovate through crop rotation and improved plows in order to expand output.

Labor's importance in these theories largely had to do with its supply. Sufficient numbers were necessary for both agricultural and industrial production. In cities a large pool of potential workers kept wages down, a necessary condition in the early days of industrial development. In the countryside, an oversupply of labor in agriculture meant labor inefficiencies (underemployment), so the development process required that underemployed agricultural labor be shifted to urban areas. In England, labor left rural areas involuntarily, largely through the same Enclosure Act that gave capitalist agriculturists access to even greater amounts of land on which to expand production. The English model has largely inspired development theory although recent versions have added Keynesian variables and concerns for import-substitution strategies.

Economic development has been defined as permanent economic growth accompanied by structural change. Proponents argue that without it, living standards cannot improve. A great deal of evidence generated by economists over the past century suggests that as incomes grew, absolute expenditures for food increased. Furthermore, Engel's Law describes the tendency for the proportion of income spent on food to fall as income rose. However, as wages rose those with lowest incomes decreased the proportion of income devoted to food at a much slower rate than middle- and upper-income families. Perhaps more importantly, with increasing income the composition of the diet changed. Meat, fruits, vegetables, and fats played a more prominent role, while complex carbohydrates from grains or fibers declined dramatically (Caliendo, 1979). For instance, the shift from a low-income diet to a high-income diet may have involved a decline by as much as 50 percent of the proportion of calories in the diet obtained from carbohydrates. Dewey (1979, 1980, 1981) provided examples of such findings.

However, a number of studies point to nutritional decline in the face of economic development. The introduction of cash cropping where subsistence farming was once practiced is one such instance (Gross & Underwood, 1971). Others have argued that very high economic growth rates over a long period of time are necessary to make significant improvement in the diet of the poor in underdeveloped countries (Milikan, 1971). More recent findings, however, have challenged these pessimistic views. A series of longitudinal studies have found that participating in commercial agriculture improved incomes, which, in turn, led to greater food expenditures (Bouis, 1994; von Braun, 1994). The increased money spent on food led to increased children's food intake and to improvements in those children's physical growth (i.e., height and weight for age) (Kennedy, 1994; Mebrahtu, Pelletier, & Pinstrup-Anderson, 1995).

It is difficult to reconcile these contradictory findings. Several explanations, however, should serve further study. First, the industrial revolution did not improve diets overnight. In fact, some have argued that diets worsened (Scholliers, 1992). Perhaps wages and diets improved later, or perhaps these changes were precipitated by labor unrest. Second, world systems theorists and dependency theorists argue that the kind of economic changes experienced by England and other Western countries occurred in places that were free from domination by more powerful countries. Countries attempting to mimic the English experience today not only have to compete with more advanced industrial societies but are held in check by those societies in order to preserve the wealth differentials between them. This will be explored in more detail in a later section. Before addressing these ideas, the role of nutrition in development theories needs brief discussion.

Nutrition and Economic Development

Most of the economic development literature that takes nutrition into account at all generally has treated it as a *consequence* of changes in supply and demand. Berg (1973, 1987) and others, however, viewed nutritional status as a *cause* of development as well. For example, researchers found that malnutrition and hunger affected concentration and ultimately, the intelligence of school children (Barrett & Frank, 1987; Popkin & Lim-Ybanez, 1982). The implication of these findings was that such children were less well prepared as adults to function competently in jobs that call on mental abilities. Others demonstrated links between work output and malnutrition, finding that poorly nourished laborers produced less and had lower endurance (Basta & Churchill, 1974; Viteri, 1982).

A number of economists argued that significant levels of malnutrition can retard economic development (Berg, 1969; Berg & Muscat, 1971; Call & Longhurst, 1971; Cook, 1971; Oshima, 1967; Schultz, 1967). They based their arguments on the implications drawn from aggregating the impacts of lessened work productivity, lessened learning capacities, and premature deaths. Correa (1969) and Correa and Cummins (1970) developed aggregate estimates of working capacity from caloric intake data and suggested that slight increases in energy intake could raise economic growth rates by 5 percent. Cook's (1971) analysis provided no aggregate estimates but instead argued that the monetary cost to Jamaican society of each child dying in infancy was $110 and each child dying during the first to fifth year of age was $190. He concluded that a significant number of premature deaths represented a significant waste of resources and thus retarded development. Given the lack of certain kinds of data and the questionable reliability of the data used in these studies, such estimates were more suggestive than precise.

Dependency and World Systems Theories

Market solutions remained the orthodox position in discussions of the "world food problem." Economists and others observed that industrial capitalism improved the European diet in both quantitative and qualitative terms. Thus, industrialization and urbanization were promoted in the 1950s as solutions to Third World food problems. By the 1960s, urbanization had achieved a high rate, but industrialization performed more feebly. Greater emphasis was given to agricultural development and improving the lives of the "poorest of the poor."

At the same time, some observed that development in the Third World would have to embark on a course different from that taken in Western nations; the global environment in which the West developed was different: it was less competitive. The European conquest of the New World involved rather stiff competition for trade routes and calories, but this involved a contest among a small number of equals in a world where countries more powerful than European nations did not yet exist (see Meneig, 1986).

Others such as Frank (1978) and Wolf (1982) observed that Western development occurred through the de-development and impoverishment of the nations that now make up the Third World. This perspective, referred to as dependency theory, argued that underdevelopment is created and sustained through dependent economic and political ties between powerful, Western nations and weak, non-Western nations.

Building on Marx and dependency theory, scholars such as Immanuel Wallerstein (1974, 1980) and Chase-Dunn (1989) have described the world in terms of a capitalist world system. This view essentially takes Marx's ideas regarding the mode of production and class exploitation and applies them to relationships both between and within nation states. The class system is recapitulated at the nation-state level by observing that certain *core* states control the means of production worldwide, resulting in among other things the exploitation of *semiperipheral* and *peripheral* states. Core states include those who are the most technologically advanced, most politically and militarily powerful, and richest. Semiperipheral states have a function similar to that of the middle class: core states exploit them, while, in turn, they exploit the peripheral states.

Furthermore, a nation's position in the hierarchy is not fixed. The competitive dynamics of the world system creates new winners and losers; over the long haul nations that exercised great economic and political power exhaust their potential and begin a decline that leads them to semiperipheral, if not peripheral, status. Spain and Portugal were core nations in the fifteenth and sixteenth centuries but lost this position and eventually fell to the peripheral level by the middle of the twentieth century. Other nations are able to move up; Japan, a peripheral power 150 years ago, recently entered the core. In the past 20 years, Korea, Taiwan, Thailand, and Brazil have escaped the periphery to join the upper reaches of the semiperiphery (or what some have described as the semicore).

A World History Lesson

The world system developed from the European need for greater food supplies than it could generate itself (Hugill, 1993; Wallerstein, 1974). Food shortages resulting from wars and epidemics led European states to finance the search for shorter routes to the Far East and the exploration of Africa. The motivation for these investments was staples, not luxury goods. Others hold to the older argument that the desire for more spices drove the efforts to reach the Far East more efficiently. Spices represented both practical as well as symbolic needs. Sugar, salt, and other spices facilitated the preservation of meat and other perishable foods. Some spices had medicinal value (Mintz, 1985). Great demand for spices as gifts and symbols of a luxurious life was also evident (Schivelbusch, 1992:6). Great displays of wealth were expressed through confectioner objects made from sugar at a time in which sugar was relatively expensive (Mintz, 1985). Others gave away great quantities of imported pepper (more than an individual could possibly consume in a year's time) as an indicator of extreme wealth and generosity (Schivelbusch, 1992).

Wallerstein (1974) argued that the development of the world system facilitated and was later abetted by capitalism. Mintz's (1985) study of sugar production in the Carribean supported this view. The nature of sugar refining required a tightly controlled workplace and highly disciplined labor force. Entrepreneurs were able to achieve these conditions by means of slavery. The principles of industrial capitalism developed from the refinery experience and were exported to England, where entrepreneurs applied them to textile production (Mintz, 1985).

The emerging world system transformed farming in other ways. The demise of feudalism was completed in Western Europe, leaving behind yeoman farmers (Wallerstein, 1974). These later became the capitalists of agriculture. Eastern Europe's feudalism was revived, with peasants forced once again into serfdom. Wheat and timber were the major products of this part of the system (the semiperiphery). The remainder of the world (the periphery), when colonized, provided raw materials often by means of slave labor.

An unintended result of the new world system was the "Colombian Exchange," the interchange of food items between Western Europe, Africa, and the Americas. The written history of these exchanges has generally described them as mutually benefitting. The Old World (core) and Africa (periphery) obtained the potato, maize, tomato, chili pepper, and sweet potato from the New World (periphery); the New World and Africa received wheat, red meat from domesticated animals, dairy products, lettuce, cauliflower, citrus fruits, figs, and bananas from one another and Europe (Davidson, 1992; Sokolov, 1991). At the same time, the core states probably garnered most of the rewards. In exchange for wheat seed, they acquired two of the most efficient grains and tubers available on the planet: maize and potatoes.

The success of the emerging core states in incorporating New World societies into the world system occurred in part because of superior technology: the core's representatives brought with them gun powder, armor, and horses. Invasions of core states by armies of the periphery was far less likely; the periphery lacked sailing vessels and navigation knowledge needed for such an undertaking. Europeans had, in addition, a major advantage lacked by Amerindians and others in the periphery, namely biological weapons in the form of European weeds and animals, which, in effect, generally aided their carriers while harming their new hosts (Crosby, 1986; McNeil, 1976). The purposeful introduction of animals (pigs, goats, cattle) and accidental introduction of weeds slowly transformed the physical environment, rendering it more useful to the Europeans and less so for the "aboriginals."

Diseases such as smallpox, measles, typhus, diphtheria, and mumps from Europe, and malaria and yellow fever from Africa, decimated local populations. Such catastrophes rendered the more numerous Amerindians helpless when they faced the smaller numbers of invaders. In addition, whole groups were obliterated by these diseases.

Europeans practiced extensive rather than intensive agriculture, and the relatively "empty" continents of Africa and the Americas permitted this type of agriculture on a wide scale. Relatedly, much of the large-scale migration of Europeans to the Americas was motivated by the vision of a place that permitted the production of food sufficient to stave off famine. European crops and animals flourished in much of the periphery where land was available in quantities to insure enough production for survival (Crosby, 1986). In addition, settlers adopted crops such as maize and Amerindian farming techniques to broaden their survival repertoire.

The core states were strengthened by the incorporation of the periphery into the world system. The periphery began to provide cheap raw materials, food stuffs such as sugar and coffee, and fuel. Furthermore, Europeans imported the best of crops native to the periphery to improve the health of their populations. Maize and potatoes, second only to rice in terms of energy production, and tomatoes, chili peppers, peanuts, and manioc, which provided important sources of vitamins, were all introduced into European agriculture (McNeil, 1976). Cheap sugar became an important energy source of the working class diet (Mintz, 1985).

Health and the World System

A number of writers argued not only that health declined after colonization, but that health in pre-colonial Asia and Africa outstripped that experienced by Europeans (Cohen & Purchal, 1989; Rau, 1991). Regarding Africa, the combination of slavery for some and forced entry into the world market for others created local population shortages and thus a reduced labor supply to produce food. In addition, the death rate rose with the introduction of new diseases such as smallpox, measles, and syphilis. Undernutrition occurred for the first time. Unfortunately, much of the data on which these assertions are based derive from anecdotal observations made by travelers and missionaries. Little documentation regarding changes in the amount of food eaten or in the number of deaths actually exists.

However, countries in the periphery or semiperiphery that once were colonies experienced conflicting inputs into their population's health. On the one hand, the colonial government wished to impart the superiority of Western civilization to "uncivilized natives," and on the other, to improve the labor productivity of the native labor force (Manderson, 1989). These efforts came too late to prevent the deaths of millions in Central and South America and Africa. In fact, the greatest impact of colonial public health efforts occurred late in the colonial experience; after the Second World War, efforts to eliminate malaria, smallpox, yellow fever, and other diseases led to substantial declines in mortality rates (Phillips, 1990).

Ironically, the Europeans may have also introduced deficiency diseases to some societies that heretofore had no such experiences. The imposition of taxes and cash crops drove living standards well below subsistence levels, according to this view. While the evidence supports the notion of "impoverishment," less sufficient support for the view that aboriginal populations had little experiences with dearth and deficiencies prior to European contact is available. Despite the relatively low intake of animal protein, Southeast Asians had attained average heights congruent with those of Europeans by the seventeenth century; only after improvements in the European diet in the eighteenth century did its citizens' stature increase relative to that of Southeast Asians (Reid, 1988:48). In contrast, Chastanet's (1992) study of the Sahel found evidence that famine conditions existed prior to the arrival of the French. At best, colonialism can be said to have greatly exacerbated already difficult circumstances for large numbers of non-Europeans. In addition, the core rid itself of epidemic famine and endemic deficiency diseases partly through the greater variety of cheap foods made available through exploitation of the periphery.

The World System and World Food Production

Harriet Friedmann (1978b, 1990, 1991) has described the consequences for both food production and nutrition during a specific period in the world system. A new international food regime took hold after the Second World War. It was based on two interconnected interests of the leading core state, the United States. First, the problem of food surpluses had arisen out of the prosperity of the postwar period: excess food needed a market. Second, food and aid were necessary in a world in need of rebuilding so as to lessen the chances of fascism through the unguided regrowth of Germany and Japan and to deal with the rise of socialism in a devastated Europe and in the nations emerging from colonialism. Food aid was formalized through Public Law 480 of the Agricultural Trade Development and Assistance Act of 1954. While the European community invested in agriculture, most Third World countries chose cheap food policies by accepting the low-cost grain made inexpensive by U.S. subsidies.

One result of the international food regime was to further change the international division of labor. Cheap food from the United States, coupled with efforts by Third World governments to develop their industrial sectors, while ignoring their agriculture sectors, reduced the demand for local products. These various events drove many indigenous producers out of business entirely or into work for wages. Wheat became the means of proletarianization (Friedmann, 1991).

The world system also introduced capitalistic production and relations to peasants. Many were forced into cash crop production initially through the imposition of taxes (Rau, 1991; Wells, Miller, & Deville, 1983; E. Wolf, 1969). In order to pay taxes as well as increases in taxes, which were demanded in cash, former subsistence farmers shifted their production practices (and crops) toward cash crops. In other cases, "entrepreneurs," with the help of the state, displaced peasants to establish plantations (Stonich, 1991). Both taxation and displacement strategies remained at work in the world (Enge & Martinez-Enge, 1991; Whiteford, 1991; Williams, 1991).

Other organizational changes that have occurred in the postwar period involve the development of agri-food industries—companies that not only produce production inputs such as fertilizers and insecticides/herbicides, but also treat food as a raw material for food products (Winson, 1993). These corporate giants link periphery production of raw foods (sugars, oils, meats) to core production of finished goods (supermarket food items; McDonald's hamburgers). The agri-food industry has also pursued research that has permitted the creation of chemical substitutes (e.g., sweeteners) to replace food items with high price volatility (Friedmann, 1980).

The consequences of industrial food products include food items excessively high in fats and simple carbohydrates. The diet of U.S. citizens and some Western Europeans, which is based on these industrial foods, has been linked to heart disease and certain cancers.

Predicting Food Production and Nutritional Health from a Position in the World System

Thus far I have discussed the implications of the world system for food production and health. Based on the logical conclusions of the theory and descriptive, as well as more rigorous empirical, accounts of specific world system impacts on various countries, we can predict the consequences of position (core, semiperiphery, periphery) in the world system. Adequacy of food production, percentage of the household budget spent on food, ability to build a productive agricultural sector that at the same time requires employment of only a fraction of the population, general health, and nutritional health all reflect the impact of world system membership. Using existing data, I will endeavor to make a preliminary determination of the validity of these predictions.

The core relies primarily on industrial and service production to generate gross domestic product. These goods are produced for both domestic and foreign consumption. According to the theory, the industrial goods are exported primarily to the semiperiphery. Consumer goods go to both the semiperiphery and periphery. The semiperiphery exports raw materials to the core and industrial and consumer products to the periphery. The periphery largely produces primary goods for self-sufficiency and export. The export crops are frequently of less nutritional importance, coffee, sugar, and sisal.

While agriculture no longer represents the dominant sector of core economies, its industrialization has made it so productive that the core outproduces the periphery and semiperiphery in primary goods production. Abetted by price supports, the core undersells the rest of the world system's membership. As we have seen, as agriculture further industrializes, it increasingly exports "finished" food products and develops biotechnological substitutes for food ingredients. Thus, agriculture in the semiperiphery and periphery may remain relatively "backward," employing relatively higher proportions of their populations in a relatively unproductive, noncompetitive sector of their economies.

The core and older members of the semiperiphery have undergone both the demographic and epidemiological transitions. The demographic transition occurs when a society moves from a state of high mortality and high fertility to one of low mortality and low fertility (Bogue, 1969). Industrialization receives most of the credit for these changes, but public health measures have also been given mention. Income improvement from industrialization leads to better diets; capital intensive rather than labor-intensive agriculture requires fewer workers. As family members' health improves, fewer of them are needed as labor.

The second transition, dubbed the epidemiological, occurs when a society moves from a state in which deaths result primarily from acute, infectious diseases to one in which they result mainly from chronic illnesses (Omran, 1971). Acute diseases occur across the life cycle but cause especially high mortalities among younger age groups. Modern medicine and public health programs have together eliminated many of these diseases from advanced countries. These countries now experience most of their mortalities from chronic illnesses that more likely strike during middle and old age (Mosley & Cowley, 1991). Such illnesses, while less treatable by modern medicine, are believed preventable through lifestyle changes (Omran, 1971; Popkin, 1993; Rogers & Hackenberg, 1987). The advantages of the transition lie in longer life expectancy and much lower infant and child mortality. The disadvantages lie with the disabling, debilitating conditions experienced by those who develop chronic illness. In the West, the longer a person lives, the greater his or her probability of experiencing a chronic illness and the apparent greater probability of having disabilities (Crimmins, Saito, & Inegneri, 1989).

Modernization leads to the adoption of both Western medical practices and Western lifestyles, resulting in the epidemiological transition. Countries moving from the underdeveloped to developed state should thus exhibit a tendency of lessened acute diseases and increased chronic illnesses. The timing and stages of the process might vary from one society to the next. Acute illness might disappear more rapidly than chronic illnesses replace them, but the general pattern should be observed.

World systems theorists as well as critics of the Western impact on the non-Western world observed that (1) the impact of the West, during colonial times, was to add to the list of acute illnesses experienced by the colonized as well as to introduce food shortages; (2) the West created a chronic state of underdevelopment in non-Western societies thus locking them into a high mortality, high acute illness state; and (3) by introduction of its lifestyles, the West increased in the incidence of chronic diseases in the Third World (Sklar, 1991). The affected underdeveloped societies experienced the worst of both worlds' high mortalities. The poor suffered from acute disease and the well-to-do, Westernizing segments suffered from chronic disease (see Campbell et al., 1992). Perhaps the middle class experienced high death rates from both types of illnesses, although this was not the pattern undergone by the West.

A unique feature of world systems theory revolves around the ideas produced by the concept "semiperiphery." The semiperiphery consists of a middle category, or "middle class" of countries that are among neither the richest nor the most powerful but, at the same time, have higher levels of wealth and more power than the least wealthy, least powerful countries. This category increases the credibility of world systems theory, for a significant number of countries fit this classification, including India, Indonesia, Egypt, and Mexico (Arrighi & Drangel, 1986; Kick, 1987; Smith & White, 1992). The theoretical importance of the semiperiphery lies in its use in explaining the stability of the world system: the few core states are not placed in the position of the sole exploiters of all other countries. While not benefitting to the same degree as the core from the system of exploitation, semiperipheral countries benefit sufficiently so as to resist collusion with peripheral states in overthrowing the entire world system.

Having identified the empirical and theoretical benefits of the concept of "semiperiphery" for world systems theory, one may legitimately inquire as to "application" benefits. In what ways does the hypothesized existence of a semiperiphery enhance understanding of health and nutrition conditions in the less developed world? One hypothesis to consider is that semiperipheral societies are more likely to exhibit increasing chronic illnesses and declining acute illnesses of either the core or the periphery. This, however, is both theoretically and empirically simplistic. Some of the semiperipheral societies are former core states; others are upwardly mobile with potential for future core status (Brazil, China [PRC]); others are static; still others are declining. Ghana, at one time a member of the semiperiphery, has fallen into peripheral status (Kick, 1987); Mozambique, it could be argued, has experienced a similar fate in more recent times.

Predicting the disease patterns of this state of affairs thus becomes more difficult. Do rates of chronic illness decline and rates of acute illness increase with declining status in the world system? Does the rate of status change (either upward or downward) affect the rates of change in disease patterns? These are not only interesting theoretical questions but ones whose answers have practical importance for intervention strategies as well. Exploration of these questions, however, is limited by the availability of cause-specific death rates. Perusal of the World Health Organization's yearly publication of available mortality statistics provides data for only a handful of less developed countries. Lack of such data is a concomitant of a low-income country (Ruzicka and Lopez, 1990). Data do exist for countries that make up the semiperiphery as well as the core, permitting partial tests of such hypotheses. Tables 5.1–5.6 provide data on deaths caused by common acute and chronic illnesses, along with indicators of development such as gross national product (GNP) per capita, percent employed in agriculture, percentage gross domestic product (GDP) from industry, and so on.

Countries were selected from the World Bank data set for these tables on the basis of the completeness of overall data availability. The classification of countries in world systems categories was based on the results of empirical work by Kick (1987), Arrighi and Drangel (1986), and Smith and White (1992). It should be noted that these efforts resulted in a more complex conceptual scheme than the standard core, semiperiphery, and periphery categories employed by others and that the schemes classify several countries differently. As the Arrighi and Drangel (1986) categorization was based largely on GNP and Kick's (1987) was based on interrelations between countries involving trade; military, cultural, and diplomatic treaties; conflict; and others, the Kick classification was adhered to except where it contradicted Smith and White's (1992) scheme, which was based on more recent data. World systems theory places more emphasis on exploitation (interrelationships) than on income differences.

World systems theory seeks to show not only that countries of both the periphery and semiperiphery have worse standards of living than core countries, but also that these living standards were worsened because of their unequal relations with the core. The literature suggests deteriorating diets and health in the Third

World countries that make up the periphery. To follow the logic of the world systems approach, weak members of the semiperiphery should also experience decline relative to the core, but not to the same degree as with the periphery. Upwardly mobile members of the semiperiphery should demonstrate improving conditions.

Position in the World System and Development

Countries of the periphery have the lowest national incomes of any nations and often experience negative economic growth (see Table 5.1). Sectoral productivity growth is generally low, and, except for El Salvador, more than half to two-thirds of their populations are employed in agriculture. This sector is sufficiently weak such that these countries must not only import food but receive it in additional amounts as foreign aid. Needless to say, most countries of the periphery export little or no food (see Table 5.2). Yet agriculture accounts for more than one-third of GDP in many countries. The data in Table 5.2 suggest that in the low-income economies of the periphery, food purchases consume between 24 and 61 percent of household income; cereal purchases alone absorb anywhere from 8 to 38 percent of income.

Low-income countries of the semiperiphery vary a great deal in terms of both the percentage of the economically active portion of the population employed in agriculture (40 to 65 percent) and percentage GDP from agriculture (18 to 31 percent). While Thailand, India, and Ecuador export more cereals than they import, most of the countries in the semiperiphery rely on both food imports and food aid to supplement domestic supplies. The proportion of the household budget devoted to food ranges from 19 to 51 percent; the amount devoted to cereals, 7 to 21 percent.

Upper-income countries in the semiperiphery have fewer persons working in agriculture (the range is between 12 and 62 percent), less of their GDP derives from agriculture (9 to 21 percent), and they require somewhat less food aid (with several exceptions).

In the semicore, percentage GDP from agriculture ranges from 9 to 27 percent and the proportion of the population working in agriculture, with the exception of China, ranges from 11 to 23 percent. Per capita incomes are higher than most found in the semiperiphery (save for China) but are below those in the core (with the exception of New Zealand). Again excepting New Zealand, semicore citizens devote a similar proportion of income to food as those living in countries of the semiperiphery. The economies of core states involve fewer persons employed in agriculture (2 to 6 percent), depend less on income from agriculture (percentage GDP from agriculture ranges from 2 to 9 percent), yet generally export far more food than they import. For several core countries such as the United

Table 5.1. Basic Economic Indicators of Selected Countries from Segments of the World Capitalist System

	GNP		Percent GDP from:		Percent economically active population in agriculture	
	Per capita (in dollars) (1990)	Average annual growth rate (%) (1965–1990)	Agriculture (1991)	Industry (1991)	(1980)	(1993)
Periphery						
Tanzania	100	−0.8	61	5	91.5	85.6
Ethiopia	120	−1.6	47	13	99.8	72.8
Nepal	180	2.1	59	14	93.0	91.3
Burundi	210	1.3	55	16	92.8	90.8
Bangladesh	220	1.9	36	16	74.8	66.5
Lao PDR	220	—	—	—	75.7	70.3
Mali	280	−0.1	44	12	85.5	79.2
Kenya	340	0.3	27	22	81.0	75.5
Sri Lanka	500	2.5	27	25	53.4	51.2
Senegal	720	0.1	20	19	80.5	77.7
Cameroon	850	−1.0	27	22	69.8	58.4
El Salvador	1,080	−0.3	10	24	42.5	35.0
Semiperiphery						
India	330	3.2	31	27	69.7	65.4
Indonesia	610	3.9	19	41	57.2	45.8
Egypt	610	1.9	18	30	45.7	39.0
Bolivia	650	−2.0	—	—	46.4	40.0
Philippines	730	−1.2	21	34	51.9	45.4
Ecuador	1,000	−0.6	15	35	38.6	28.1
Thailand	1,570	5.9	12	39	70.9	62.3
Chile	2,160	1.6	—	—	16.4	11.6
Mexico	3,030	−0.5	9	30	36.6	21.7
Semicore						
China	370	7.8	27	42	74.2	65.2
Brazil	2,940	0.5	10	39	31.2	22.6
Korea, Rep.	6,330	8.7	8	45	36.4	21.7
Israel	11,950	1.7	—	—	6.2	3.8
Greece	6,340	1.1	17	27	30.9	22.5
New Zealand	12,350	0.7	9	27	15.9	10.7
Core						
United Kingdom	16,550	2.6	—	—	2.6	1.8
Italy	18,520	2.2	3	33	12.0	6.0
France	20,380	1.8	3	29	8.6	4.5
Canada	20,440	2.0	—	—	5.3	2.8
United States	22,240	1.7	—	—	3.5	2.1
Germany	23,650	2.2	2	39	6.9	4.1
Japan	26,930	3.6	3	42	11.2	5.5

Source: World Bank (1993); Food and Agriculture Organization (1994).

Table 5.2. Cereal Imports, Exports, Aid, and Proportion Household Budgets Devoted to Food Cereal Expenditure of Selected Countries for Segments of the World Capitalist System

	Cereal imports (thousand metric tons)	Food aid in cereals (thousand metric tons) (1990/1991)	Cereal exports (thousand metric tons)	Percent household income spent on all food cereals	
				1980	1985
Periphery					
Tanzania	130	24	7	64	32
Ethiopia	802	894	0.2	50	21
Nepal	5	1	5	57	38
Burundi	31	3	0	—	—
Bangladesh	1,631	1,356	0	59	36
Lao PDR	44	0	0	—	—
Mali	226	37	20	57	38
Kenya	330	63	50	39	16
Sri Lanka	918	200	0.4	43	18
Senegal	784	39	0.1	50	15
Cameroon	532	9	32	24	8
El Salvador	324	84	0.3	33	12
Semiperiphery					
India	13	217	1,354	52	18
Indonesia	2,795	45	34	48	21
Egypt	7,807	1,525	151	50	10
Bolivia	380	229	6	33	—
Philippines	1,848	81	30	51	20
Ecuador	481	98	1,410	30	—
Thailand	521	104	5,700	30	7
Chile	605	11	582	29	7
Mexico	5,433	239	57	35	—
Semicore					
China	13,431	134	9,077	61	—
Brazil	6,332	16	4	35	9
Korea, Rep.	10,411	—	5	—	—
Israel	1,635	2	1	22	—
Greece	753	—	1,535	30	—
New Zealand	223	—	32	12	2
Core					
United Kingdom	2,799	—	6,144	12	2
Italy	8,466	—	3,126	19	2
France	1,206	—	29,456	16	2
Canada	477	—	28,962	11	2
United States	2,833	—	86,863	13	2
Germany	3,544	—	6,554	12	2
Japan	27,918	—	420	16	4

Source: World Bank (1993); Grant (1991); Food and Agriculture Organization (1993).

States, food exports constitute a major source of export income, while percentage household income devoted to food purchases ranges from 12 to 19 percent.

Position in the World System and General Health

Low birth weight, low life expectancy, high under-the-age-of-five mortality, and high population growth characterize the periphery, with the populations of the semiperiphery enjoying longer life expectancy (aside from notable exceptions such as India and Indonesia) (see Table 5.3). Advancing semiperipheral countries such as Chile, Thailand, and Mexico experience relatively low under-five mortalities, while more stagnant members such as Ghana, Indonesia, and Bolivia have much larger under-five mortality rates. These latter countries remain better off than those in the periphery. Countries of the semicore perform even better than those of semiperiphery in these matters. The core, of course, provides its average citizen with the very highest of life expectancies, lowest under-age-five mortalities, and low population growth.

The percentages of children born underweight vary a great deal but are somewhat higher in both the periphery and the semiperiphery compared with the semicore and core rates. These percentages range from 9 to 39 percent in the periphery, 7 to 30 percent in the semiperiphery, 5 to 9 percent in the semicore, and 5 to 7 percent in the core. The under-age-five mortality rates generally exceed 100 per 100,000 in the periphery, while in the semiperiphery most fall in the range 20 to 96 per 100,000, with three countries with rates above 100. In the semicore, the range is 11 to 69; in the core, it is 6 to 11 per 100,000.

Data on the incidence of tuberculosis have recently become available for a very large number of countries. These data lend some weight to the epidemiological transition hypothesis, as Table 5.4 and weighted regional averages discussed by the World Bank (1993) demonstrate. The annual incidence of tuberculosis is 220 per 100,000 persons in sub-Saharan countries, most of which are members of the periphery. Excluding India and China, the rate for Asia and the Pacific is 202; for Latin America and the Caribbean, the rate is 92. The average for the core is closer to 20 per 100,000. Finally, the data in Table 5.3 suggest a monotonic relationship between health care expenditures and health: the more expended per capita by both the public and private sectors, the lower the low birth weight and under-age-five mortality rates.

Turning to causes of death, again application of world systems theory suggests that the epidemiological transition has already occurred in the core, begun (but perhaps arrested before completion) in the semiperiphery, and barely underway, if at all, in the periphery. Given the lack of data for cause of death for almost all countries of the periphery, and incomplete data for members of the semiperiphery, claims about causes of death across the world system must be made with care.

Table 5.3. General Health and Demographic Indicators of Selected Countries from Segments of the World Capitalist System

Position/country	Percent infants with low birth weight (1980– 1988)	Under 5 mortality rate per 1,000 live births (1990)	Life expectancy at birth (1990)	Average annual population growth rate percent (1980– 1991)	Annual incidence tuberculosis per 100,000 population	Health expenditures per capita (official exchange rate dollars) (1990)
Periphery						
Tanzania	13	165	49	3.0	140	4
Ethiopia	—	197	48	3.1	155	4
Nepal	—	135	56	2.6	167	7
Burundi	9	180	47	2.9	367	7
Bangladesh	28	137	56	2.2	220	7
Lao PDR	39	171	50	2.7	235	5
Mali	17	200	48	2.6	289	15
Kenya	15	83	59	3.8	140	16
Sri Lanka	28	22	73	1.4	167	18
Senegal	11	156	48	3.0	166	29
Cameroon	13	125	55	2.8	194	24
El Salvador	15	52	69	2.0	110	61
Semiperiphery						
India	30	127	58	2.1	220	21
Indonesia	14	111	59	1.8	220	12
Egypt	5	96	64	2.5	78	18
Bolivia	12	125	60	2.5	335	25
Philippines	18	62	64	2.4	280	14
Ecuador	11	42	70	2.1	166	43
Thailand	12	36	68	2.5	173	73
Chile	7	20	73	2.7	67	100
Mexico	15	38	70	3.2	110	89
Semicore						
China	9	43	69	1.5	166	11
Brazil	8	69	66	2.0	56	132
Korea, Rep.	9	10	72	1.1	162	377
Israel	7	10	76	2.2	12	494
Greece	6	13	76	0.5	12	358
New Zealand	5	11	75	0.7	10	925
Core						
United Kingdom	7	9	75	0.2	10	1,039
Italy	7	11	77	0.2	25	1,426
France	5	9	77	0.5	16	1,869
Canada	6	9	77	1.2	8	1,945
United States	7	11	76	0.9	10	2,763
Germany	6	9	76	0.1	18	1,511
Japan	5	6	79	0.5	42	1,538

Source: World Bank (1993).

Table 5.4 contains death rates by cause (note that in regard to the periphery, only for Zimbabwe, several Central American countries, and Sri Lanka are recent data available). The death rates, whether due to diseases of affluence or poverty, are all relatively low in Zimbabwe, although the rates of death from infectious diseases, TB, malaria, and acute upper respiratory diseases all exceed those reported for core countries. It should be remembered that Zimbabwe is a relatively affluent country compared with other countries in the periphery as well as in the semiperiphery. Sri Lanka is also unusual in that it suffers relatively low rates of mortality from both the diseases of poverty and of affluence. Nicaragua's highest death rates result from the diseases of poverty, although the rates for diseases of affluence suggest problems as well. Lacking sufficient data for the periphery, the semiperiphery must bear the brunt of this analysis.

Older members of the semiperiphery, such as Colombia and Argentina, exhibit much lower death rates from the diseases of poverty than from those of affluence; newer members, such as Thailand and the Philippines, experience lower deaths from most diseases of affluence and high to very high death rates from various infections.

Countries in the semiperiphery exhibit additional patterns that suggest developmental distortions whose causes may lie within world systems' dynamics. In some such countries, remarkable gains in health have occurred, often without similar improvements in GNP (Caldwell, 1986). In others, where GNP is relatively high by periphery standards, such as Saudi Arabia, Iraq, Iran, Libya, Ivory Coast, and Morocco, infant mortality is high and life expectancy low. Caldwell (1986) found that several conditions seem to differentiate the "high" versus "low" health achievers: commitments to both female education and public health and activist governments willing to put high priorities on universal education and health care (see Table 5.4). Such actions may only be possible by those countries not tightly integrated into exploitive relationships with core states. Semicore countries generally have higher rates of death from the diseases of affluence than countries of both the semiperiphery and periphery, but lower death rates from the diseases of poverty. Core countries have very high death rates from the diseases of affluence and very low death rates from diseases considered the product of poverty.

Position in the World System and Nutritional Health

Beginning with widespread patterns in deficiency diseases, we find a pattern that roughly coincides with the world system framework. For instance, Africa and Southeast Asia have greater numbers of persons at risk of malnutrition than the countries of the Eastern Mediterranean. Two-thirds of the 40 million cases of xeropthalmia (vitamin A deficiency) occur in Southeast Asia; most of the rest occur in Africa. A similar pattern is observed for the anemias, of which there are 1.5 billion cases worldwide. Over 40 percent of the population of areas of the world that

Table 5.4. Death Rates (per 100,000) by Cause for Selected Countries from Segments of the World Capitalist System

Columns 2–11 (Heart through Liver disease) fall under **Diseases of Affluence**; columns 12–23 (TB through All malnutrition) fall under **Diseases of Poverty**.

System/country	Heart M	Heart F	Cancer M	Cancer F	Cerebro-vascular M	Cerebro-vascular F	Athero-sclerosis M	Athero-sclerosis F	Liver disease M	Liver disease F	TB M	TB F	All infectious diseases M	All infectious diseases F	Malaria M	Malaria F	Cancer of stomach M	Cancer of stomach F	Acute upper respiratory M	Acute upper respiratory F	All malnutrition M	All malnutrition F
Periphery																						
Zimbabwe	11.7		22.7		9.6		0.7		4.1		8.7		19.6		3.7		3.7		4.9		11.5	
Nicaragua	19.0		27.3		21.9		0.8		6.4		6.6		73.8		1.2		2.9		23.3		5.8	
El Salvador	20.5		35.4		23.7		0.2		6.5		2.5		61.0		0.0		6.1		19.6		7.4	
Jamaica	34.5		90.2		95.9		4.3		4.1		1.2		49.7		0.0		13.7		17.7		17.7	
Panama	41.8		56.3		23.0		0		4.5		5.4		34.2		0.1		5.8		13.1		6.1	
Costa Rica	53.9		77.0		26.0		1.6		8.5		2.7		23.4		0.1		3.1		10.8		3.1	
Sri Lanka	31.6	10.8	28.2	27.6	18.2	11.9	0	0	8.4	1.2	1.7		42.2	27.0	—	—	2.7	3.7	0.1	0.1	5.2	6.0
Guyana	59.3	33.1	28.8	31.0	31.8	55.8	2.1	1.9	19.2	6.2		0.4	19.9	11.3	—	0.2	5.3	3.6	0.9	1.1	4.8	6.5
Semiperiphery																						
Egypt	37.2	28.0	25.6	18.2	20.7	17.1	9.9	10.0	10.5	5.6	3.1	1.9	96.4	101.4	0.0	—	0.6	0.8	1.0	0.7	1.7	1.8
Ecuador	25.3	21.6	45.0	51.8	26.2	24.9	1.3	2.1	12.2	4.3	12.1	9.5	65.0	57.3	0.7	0.6	13.8	11.3	1.0	0.7	16.2	16.5
Colombia	66.2	56.5	57.3	63.3	34.9	41.8	3.2	4.1	4.1	1.9	6.7	3.7	34.9	28.5	1.3	0.9	13.9	10.4	0.4	0.3	10.5	9.4
Thailand	18.9	15.2	3.9	2.5	8.3	5.1	—		5.5	1.9	18.5	11.1	68.0	49.6	—	—	0.8	0.5	47.1	39.6	2.9	3.2
Chile	67.7	63.4	102.7	105.9	49.3	54.8	6.3	10.1	27.2	10.8	6.7	2.5	21.5	16.9	—	—	24.2	13.0	0.1	0.1	2.6	2.2
Mauritius	148.6	98.5	51.1	57.1	94.2	75.2	0.4	0.2	22.5	3.6	2.0	0.4	18.0	11.3	—	—	8.0	7.4	0.2	0.4	14.6	9.6
Semicore																						
Argentina	110.5	74.1	160.3	120.9	81.1	79.2	20.4	30.8	16.6	5.2	4.9	2.1	29.5	23.9	0.0	—	13.6	7.8	0.1	0.1	5.5	4.9
Korea	46.1	36.3	99.3	55.9	63.3	57.2	1.7	1.7	39.1	8.7	17.7	6.8	22.1	10.6	0.0	—	34.0	19.8	0.3	0.3	1.0	1.1
Ireland	289.1	209.3	219.8	197.8	75.5	99.7	11.6	15.6	3.5	2.7	1.4	1.4	6.0	5.5	0.1	—	14.5	10.3	—	—	1.7	1.7
Core																						
United Kingdom	337.8	267.0	300.4	262.2	101.8	163.0	5.3	10.3	7.1	5.5	0.9	0.4	5.1	4.6	0.0	0.0	20.9	13.4	0.1	0.2	1.6	3.4
United States	232.1	206.9	215.5	180.0	49.9	72.0	7.0	10.9	14.4	7.3	0.8	0.4	12.6	13.0	0.0	0.0	6.8	4.4	0.1	0.1	2.2	3.2
Denmark	387.8	342.8	315.2	284.8	93.6	122.6	37.8	45.6	19.2	8.7	0.9	0.3	10.5	5.6	—	—	13.4	9.2	0.6	0.3	5.1	4.9
Japan	51.0	48.0	216.4	139.3	95.6	103.0	1.5	2.0	19.1	8.5	4.4	1.3	11.9	7.7	0.0	—	49.6	28.1	0.7	0.9	1.7	1.9

Source: United Nations Statistical Office (1980, 1990); Pan American Health Organization (1992). M, male; F, female. For most periphery countries, data were available only for both sexes combined.

principally constitute the periphery (Southeast Asia and Africa) experience anemias; only 13 percent of the persons in Latin America suffer from this disease (see World Health Organization, 1990, for these and other data.)

On the other hand, countries in Latin America have reached a point where both obesity and wasting (the condition of being seriously underweight for age and sex) afflict equal numbers of persons. This would seem to confirm the idea that as countries in the semiperiphery move toward corelike conditions, their health problems become more corelike. Popkin (1993) provides evidence that countries such as Japan and Korea Westernized their diets with increasing income.

Country-by-country comparisons can be made from Tables 5.4 and 5.5. Death rates from malnutrition are moderate in Zimbabwe, high in Guyana, and lower in Thailand, Chile, and Argentina (three upwardly mobile members of the semiperiphery). The percentage of children suffering from either underweight, wasting, or stunting (being underheight for age and sex) are all higher in countries of the periphery, somewhat to considerably lower in the semiperiphery, and low to nonexistent in the core. Half or more of the children in many countries of the periphery experience stunting. With the exception of India, Indonesia, and the Philippines, most semiperipheral countries exhibit stunting rates of less than 40 percent. A somewhat similar pattern for wasting and underweight appears.

Prevalence of iron deficiency is generally high in some countries of the periphery with rates of 24 percent in countries like Nepal to 66 percent in Bangladesh. Others, like Ethiopia and Sri Lanka, experience rates under 10 percent. A somewhat similar pattern is observed for countries that constitute the semiperiphery. With the exception of India, which has a deficiency rate that exceeds two-thirds of its population, less than half of the populations of countries in the semiperiphery experience iron deficiency. The pattern of the prevalence of iodine deficiency is less clearly demarcated by position in the world system. Percentages of affliction vary from 10 to 72 percent among countries that make up the periphery, with the preponderance of proportions at 30 percent or greater. Rates in the semiperiphery, excluding Egypt, Bolivia, and Ecuador, generally fall below 20 percent. Again, if several prominent exceptions such as Ethiopia, Cameroon, and El Salvador are ignored, the prevalence of anemia in pregnant women ranges from 30 to 80 percent in countries of the periphery (averaging about 49 percent). The range in the semiperiphery is 20 to 88 percent with an average of 35 percent. In the core, anemia in pregnant women is less than 20 percent and averages close to 15 percent.

World systems theory, as we have argued, suggests that the core markets its lifestyle patterns to both the semiperiphery and the periphery to increase its shares of various commodity and finished goods markets. Van Esterik (1989) has suggested that core countries export their habits to other countries when a profit is to be made. Thus, bottle feeding, a creature of core technology, has rapidly diffused into the periphery, often via the concerted efforts of transnational corporations.

Table 5.5. Indicators of Malnutrition in Children and Women for Selected Countries from Segments of the World Capitalist System

Position/country	Under-weight children (percent)	Wasting 12–13 months (percent)	Stunting 24–59 Months (percent)	Iron deficiency (percent)	Iodine deficiency (percent)	Prevalence of anemia, pregnant women (percent)
Periphery						
Tanzania	57	5	46	25	40	80
Ethiopia	38	19	43	6	34	6
Nepal	—	14	69	24.1	46.1	33
Burundi	38	6	48	7.2	56.0	68
Bangladesh	71	16	65	66.0	10.5	51
Lao PDR	37	20	40	37.0	—	62
Mali	31	11	24	4.6	20	65
Kenya	—	10	42	6.0	15–72	57
Sri Lanka	38	13	27	3.8	19.3	62
Senegal	22	8	28	—	33	55
Cameroon	17	2	43	—	59	8
El Salvador	36	15	6	8.6	48	14
Semiperiphery						
India	41	27	65	69.0	7.3	88
Indonesia	51	9	67	—	20	74
Egypt	13	1	31	22.4	70	47
Bolivia	13	2	38	18.6	61	36
Philippines	33	14	48	37.5	14.9	48
Ecuador	17	4	39	46.0	36.5	46
Thailand	26	6	22	11.0	14.7	52
Chile	3	1	10	20.0	18.8	20
Mexico	—	6	22	—	17.0	41
Semicore						
Brazil	5	2	31	—	14.7	34
Korea	—	2	18	—	—	—
Israel	—	—	—	—	—	25
Greece	—	—	—	—	—	24
New Zealand	—	1	3	—	—	22
Core						
United Kingdom	—	1	2	—	—	19
Italy	—	1	2	—	—	10
France	—	0	6	—	—	18
Canada	—	1	5	—	—	—
United States	—	2	2	—	—	17
Germany	—	—	—	—	—	12
Japan	—	—	4	—	—	—

Source: World Bank (1993); Grant (1991); Levin, Pollitt, Galloway, & McGuire (1993).

There is some evidence, however, that only better educated women are affected by infant formula marketing efforts (Guilkey & Stewart, 1995). The core itself, however, has shifted (at least its middle- and upper-class members have) back to breast feeding. A cultural lag thus results.

The data in Table 5.6 indicate that while breast feeding has declined in some countries of the periphery such as Tanzania, Kenya, and Sri Lanka, in others over 80 percent of all mothers breast-feed until the twelfth month. However, "modern" infant feeding has taken hold in some parts of the semiperiphery, most notably among its Latin American members. Asian members maintain more traditional patterns of infant feeding. Again, this may reflect length of time that a country has belonged to the semiperiphery.

The comparison of differences across the world system fails to provide definitive evidence for the theory's predictions. This will require multivariate analyses of the larger data sets from which the tables in this chapter were drawn. Without better data than what currently exist, the most sophisticated of analyses will fail to resolve the issues raised here. Before discussing the impact of the world system on lifestyle, especially food choices, existing multivariate studies of how the world system impacts life chances should be briefly reviewed.

Multivariate Studies of the Effects of the World System

A perusal of Table 5.7 indicates the range of dependency measures created by dependency and world systems theorists. The table by no means reflects the entirety of available studies or fully represents the range of their results. Note that the effects of dependency include not only economic growth but also income inequality and the meeting of basic human needs (as represented by child mortality, life expectancy, and food availability). Only the study by Burns et al. (1994) includes measures of nutritional status as outcomes. Still, dependence on exports, disarticulation, and transnational corporate penetration not only negatively affects economic growth and income equality but also increases mortality and decreases both life expectancy and food availability. A very recent study has found that available calories per capita and childhood health interventions have *declined* over time as debt and investment dependency have grown (Bradshaw, Noonan, Gash, & Sershen, 1993). While data that provide estimates of changes in nutritional status are not available for most countries, Burns et al. (1994) found that increases in external debt as a percentage of exports increased the percentage of household income spent on cereal, which in turn increased the percentage of children under five years of age who suffered from stunting or wasting.

Note that despite reference to the world system, the focus is on the periphery. Variables such as transnational corporation penetration probably reflect core influences on the periphery, but various measures of trade dependency may reflect both dependence on the core and semiperiphery. Neither the effects of the semi-

Table 5.6. Prevalence of Breast-feeding in Selected Countries
from Segments of the World Capitalist System

Position/country	Percent of mothers breastfeeding 1980–1988		
	3 months	6 months	12 months
Periphery			
Tanzania	100	90	70
Ethiopia	—	97	95
Nepal	92	92	82
Burundi	—	95	90
Bangladesh	91	86	82
Lao PDR	—	99	93
Mali	91	—	82
Kenya	96	82	67
Sri Lanka	95	81	68
Senegal	94	94	82
Cameroon	92	90	77
El Salvador	—	—	—
Semiperiphery			
India	—	—	—
Indonesia	98	97	76
Egypt	90	87	81
Bolivia	—	—	—
Philippines	—	74	—
Ecuador	86	74	48
Thailand	83	79	68
Chile	81	57	20
Mexico	62	52	36
Semicore			
China	—	65	55
Brazil	66	58	34
Korea, Rep.	58	40	27
Israel	—	—	—
Greece	—	—	—
New Zealand	—	—	—
Core			
United Kingdom	26	22	—
Italy	—	—	—
France	—	—	—
Canada	53	30	—
United States	33	24	—
Germany	—	—	—
Japan	72	52	—

Source: Grant (1991).

Table 5.7. Multivariate Analysis Testing World–Dependency Effects on Basic Human
Needs (Life Chances)

Dependency measure	Outcome

A. Disarticulation
  1. Differentiated sectoral development (high percentage) of labor force concentrated in traditional (nonmodern) sector
Example: Stokes & Anderson (1990)
	A. Basic human needs
	  1. Increased child mortality
	  2. Increased crude death rate

B. Investment dependence
  1. Multinational corporation penetration (investment stock per capita and per total domestic capital and per total domestic capital stock)
  2. Investment flows (change in amount of investment as a ratio of changing GDP)
Example: Wimberly (1991a, 1991b)
	B. Basic human needs
	  1. Increased infant mortality
	  2. Decreased life expectancy
	  3. Decreased food availability (available protein and calories per capita).

C. Export dependency
  1. Proportion of GDP of exports
Example: Gacitua & Bello (1991)
	C. Economic growth and basic human needs
	  1. Increased food availability (protein and calories per capita)

D. Debt dependency
  1. Change in the ratio of external debt to the value of exports
  2. IMF pressure (index of numbers of debt renegotiations, restructurings, use of extended fund, etc.)
Examples: Bradshaw et al. (1993); Burns et al. (1994)
	D. Economic growth and basic human needs
	  1. Decreased food availability (calories per capita)
	  2. Immunization
	  3. Under-5 mortality
	  4. Underweight, wasting, stunting

periphery on the periphery nor the impact of the core on the semiperiphery has been considered in these studies. Yet world systems theory clearly suggests such effects.

A review of these studies indicated that dependency lowers the rate of economic growth, illustrating the difficulty low-income countries have in escaping the periphery. At the same time, life chances (basic human needs), measured as life expectancy, infant mortality, and per capita food availability, varied in the manner predicted by the dependency hypotheses. However, Firebaugh (1992) and Firebaugh and Beck (1994) found that direct foreign investment increases both growth and well-being.

The World System and World Culture

World culture, to the extent that it permeates and influences states, emanates from the core. Sklar (1991), among others, has argued that global culture is spread through the ever increasing globalization of the mass media via satellite linkups, the spread of VCRs, and the development of transnational news and advertising by transnational corporations. The most widely viewed television programs in the Third World originate in the United States. Less than 15 years ago, citizens of peripheral countries had to "settle" for taped copies of older American television programs. Thanks to satellites, Third World viewers can watch the *same* shows at nearly the *same* time that U.S. viewers do. Sklar's (1991) critique involved the cultural dependency that world culture creates. The industry that has led the penetration of Second and Third World societies is processed fast foods (Sklar, 1991:151). Such franchising is perceived as nonthreatening to local interests as well as, perhaps, local culture.

Sklar (1991) presented several case studies of global consumerism. The first was the Nestle corporation's marketing of infant formula and the second, the cola wars in the Third World. Both involved transnational corporations' attempts to change perceptions and behavior in order to sell particular products. The infant formula controversy is discussed in Chapter 10. The apparent association between GNP per capita and lower rates of breast-feeding discussed earlier should alert us to the possibility that Westernization has caused this change in health behavior.

The cola war illustrates what Sklar (1991) and others referred to as "induced wants or needs." The idea is that to sell a product to individuals who do not desire to consume it, their perceptions have to be changed. The potential consumers must not only be made aware of the product but also come to see its consumption as highly desirable. The Coca Cola and Pepsi companies, perpetual competitors for the American market, have extended their struggle for soft drink hegemony to the Third World. As Sklar (1991) noted, these two companies have spent more on advertising in any given country of the periphery than many of the same countries spend on education.

CONCLUSION

Lack of food represents the very essence of poverty; it is, among other things, the lack of wherewithal to obtain food. In the United States, for example, the poverty line that connotes eligibility for a number of assistance programs is based in part on ability to afford a sufficient amount of food. At the same time, food offers an avenue for the expression of status: families in many societies have this opportunity through mechanisms such as having guests for dinner and eating in expensive restaurants. These observations appear universal in applicability. Because of the universal importance of food, it also provides a means by which some states can bring others into conditions of dependency, as reflected in trade arrangements and the provision of food aid.

The application of theories of social stratification to the distribution of food and nutrition has already reaped many benefits, but this application has frequently resulted in simplistic, superficial results. This, in part, occurs because non–social science researchers have plucked social stratification concepts from theory. In addition, the full range of a theory's implications is often ignored in the push to draw dichotomous contrasts between well-to-do and nere-do-well classes on the one hand, and rich and poor countries, on the other. In both instances, the experience of the middle becomes blurred and potentially mistaken for that of the top. Middle class income, education, occupations, and lifestyles differ from both those above and below them (Bourdieu, 1984). It is evident that countries of the middle (the semiperiphery) also differ from countries above and below them. Further studies of the "middle" will surely uncover differences heretofore ignored.

Social stratification studies also tend to take on a static character, ignoring the element of mobility. Some have found that "downward drift" of social status leads to poorer physical and mental health among individuals. A similar outcome may result when an entire class or country experiences socioeconomic decline.

Differences in access and use of food, on the one hand, and resulting well-being, on the other, arise from both the possession of differential amounts of resources and lifestyle-based choices. The latter may result from what Bourdieu (1984) described as "tastes of necessity." At the same time, within similar class fractions, lifestyle differentiation may provide members with the "distinction" they seek. These, too, tend to restrict choices of foods. Restrictions caused by lifestyle choices and resource constraints interact to affect life chances in ways that we have only recently begun to explore (see Blaxter, 1990).

Resource domination and lifestyle promotion by the core in its relationships with the periphery and semiperiphery have had demonstrable effects on food availability, food choices, and lifestyles. However, the exact nature of these changes and what effect they may have on countries' experience of the epidemiological transition have only begun to be explored.

6

THE BODY AND SOCIOLOGY

INTRODUCTION

Bodies produce and consume food and, through this consumption, experience consequences. From one point of view, this statement describes an apparent series of physical and physiological processes. However, as sociologists well know, food production and consumption involves culture, social organization, and technology. Furthermore, distinct social consequences result from various nutritional as well as bodily states. Therefore, sociologies of food and nutrition that do not account for the social aspects of the body are likely to be profoundly lacking.

With rare exception, however, sociologists tended to take the body for granted. Goffman (1959, 1963) and other interactionists argued that the body serves as a significant vehicle for interpersonal communication. Foucault's repeated insistence that bodies were the site of social control and Elias's location of the civilizing process in human bodies have spawned greater attention, and Giddens (1985, 1991) has explicitly worked toward incorporating bodies into his sociology. Perhaps the most direct and compelling arguments for a sociology of the body came from Bryan S. Turner (1984, 1987, 1992). He and others have maintained a steady flow of papers and books that attempt to develop such a sociology along various theoretical lines.

Recent work includes *The Body and Social Theory* (Shilling, 1993) and *The Body Social* (Synnott, 1993). This chapter reviews first the traditional approaches to the "physiological body" found in both functionalism and medical sociology. The remainder of the chapter deals with a series of alternative theoretical perspectives on the body in terms of their varying relevance to sociologies of food and nutrition.

THE PHYSIOLOGICAL BODY

When social scientists have examined the body, they generally have assumed a physiological entity with modes of health and ill-health and with physiological needs.

Early Theoretical Approaches

Many sociologists have viewed an interest in biology and/or psychology as reductionist and have argued that necessary and sufficient explanations of social behavior require social variables. An example of such thinking can be found in discussions of human needs by Collins (1975) and Turner (1988).

Beyond these writings, however, is the legacy of psychologism that treats biological needs as a source of human motivation. The Freudian legacy and its combination with Marxism by Adorno, Marcuse, and Habermas come to mind. Instinctual drives involving hunger, thirst, and sexual appetite are generally suggested as illustrations. However, when specific drives are further examined in terms of their effect on behavior or social structure, the sex drive has received the most attention.

Needs and Motivation

Early "motivation theories" contained a clear recognition of the importance of physiology/biology in human motivation. Turner's (1988) review of early motivation theories found that behaviorism (Watson), the exchange theory of Simmel, Mead's interactionist version of behaviorism, and Freud's theory all contained explicit reference to physiological needs. However, it was clear that beyond some effort to acknowledge these needs, their nature was not clearly spelled out. The degree of explanation given varied from theorist to theorist. For example, Freud devoted considerable attention to sex and other drives, in contrast to Mead, who noted that needs propel people to act. The act and its social nature clearly interested Mead more. Thus needs were recognized as *the* base or *one* of the bases for action and interaction, but most theorists, like Mead, were interested in resulting social behavior. In addition, or perhaps because human needs were viewed as constants, they were universal in number, impact, relative importance, and so on.

Parsons and Shils's (1951) accounts of action systems occasionally delved into the personality system where biological needs were channeled into socially acceptable drives, relying on a Freudian conception of the process. Giddens (1984) has drawn from Freud's notions of the unconscious but has largely "sociologized" human needs into "unconscious needs for ontological security" and "unconscious needs for a sense of trust." Collins (1975) posited the "need for group membership" and Turner (1988) has combined Giddens and Collins so that ontological security, trust, and group membership constituted the three basic needs underlying the motivation for social interaction.

As important as all the work on developing models of social action is, the denial of physiology and its role in motivating interaction removes from sociology important subject matter. People do not live by interaction alone and they do not become part of a group simply because they need group membership. There are other perhaps even more fundamental reasons, some of which are biological, others of which are unique to the human animal, and others which are socially derived. Functionalism, despite its many shortcomings, has, as one of its utilities, recognition of needs and how these needs have something to do with social structure and social interaction. One of the most explicit accounts of needs and their relations to the social world is contained in Malinowski's (1944) *Towards A Scientific Theory of Culture.*

Marx and the Body

Use and Exchange Value of Bodies

Bodies (labor) have use value and exchange value. The use value of something has to do with its ability to satisfy a want (Cohen, 1978). The use value of a body thus is its ability to satisfy its wants as well as the wants of others.

A commodity has use value and can be offered in exchange for other things, but the body itself may also become a commodity for exchange. The slave's body or portions of the prostitute's body seem straight-forward applications of this logic. Similarly, the dancer's or model's labor is valued and so is the visual display of the dancer's or model's body. Here labor and the body itself are not so easily separated.

Developing the Body's Use Value

Blane (1987) noted that Marx examined the value of labor power from three approaches. Labor power involved the value of those goods and services necessary to sustain the worker at some subsistence level, to raise the next generation of workers, and to provide for laborers while they are in training. As Blane (1987) and others pointed out, Marx argued that subsistence was not a universal standard that transcended time and place but rather varied with "historical" and "moral" circumstances. Blane's (1987) analysis suggested, at least in a particular period in the late nineteenth- to early twentieth-century in England, that these circumstances included falling commodity prices in conjunction with stable wages (which were due to the successful pressures of organized labor to maintain current wage levels). These particular circumstances led to greater purchasing power and thus improved diets.

Alienation and the Body

When Marx spoke of alienation, he referred to a separation from, "productive activity (nature, products, other people)....[The worker] cannot develop mentally or physically...he mortifies his body and ruins his mind" (Ritzer, 1991). While Marx recognized needs and conditions in which needs were not met, he argued that those were relative to the mode of production. This in turn suggested that needs were relative to the mode's standard of living and that deprivation was relative as well.

Discussions of alienation in Marx and Marxist writings, in general, have focused on the separation of the products of work from a conscious identification with those products. Alienation thus separated self from the fruits of one's efforts. Yet in one sense, it is the body that becomes alienated in that the body and its operation become separated. As O'Neill (1985) noted, alienation further occurred to the extent that the body becomes a part of a mindless machine, stamping out products.

As the body itself becomes a commodity, then is it not possible for individuals to become alienated from their bodies? This occurs in the form of self-denial, in the "mortification of mind and body." Unable to "express species powers and needs, alienated workers are forced to concentrate on natural powers and needs" (Ritzer, 1991:181). This leaves humans "freely active" in the pursuit of "animal functions; eating, drinking, and procreating" (Ritzer, 1991:181) Bodily alienation, on the one hand, implies the willing participation in an economy that debases the body, exposing it to noxious conditions, subjecting it to physical and mental stresses and strains. On the other hand, *forced* pursuit of animal functions leads potentially to gluttonous excess in eating and drinking. Are the social origins of overweight and excessive drinking to be found in the modern conditions of alienation?

Perhaps the origins of excessive eating and drinking lie in the increasingly alienating production process. Current studies of obesity focus on differences in the self-appraisal of "overweight" versus "normal weight" individuals, under the assumption that the weight causes the low self-appraisal rather than the obverse. Similarly, excessive drinking is thought by some to result from poorly developed self-images. If our extension of Marx is correct, then weight or drinking problems that stem from excessive intake may occur because of the alienating conditions of the work these individuals do.

Medical Sociology

Social epidemiological studies characterize a great deal of early and current work in medical sociology (Wolinsky, 1980). These studies have made major contributions to the understanding of the origins of chronic illness (see Mechanic, 1962; Suchman, 1965). More recently medical sociologists have examined the relationship between body awareness, or the individual's self-monitoring of internal bodily states, and seeking health care (Hansell, Sherman, & Mechanic, 1991). Social scientists concerned with nutrition have sought the determinants of adequacy of diets, where bodily needs determine adequacy. A similar approach is taken by those wishing to determine the interrelationships between body size and shape and social relationships. Specifically, studies of the impact of social class and marital status on obesity and obesity on status and marital attainment come to mind (Sobal, 1984a, 1991a; Sobal & Stunkard, 1989). Still others have examined social support and stress effects on immuno-competence (Kaplan, 1991; McIntosh, Kaplan, & Kubena, 1993a). Some of these ideas from medical sociology have made their way into research in the sociology *in* nutrition effort.

Body Biochemistry

Medical sociologists have found that certain social factors, such as social support, stressful life events, social class background, and cultural heritage affect physiological states such as the sympathetic adrenal-medullary, pituitary adrenal-cortical, and immune systems (Kaplan, 1991; McIntosh et al., 1993b, 1994a; Vogt, 1988; see also McIntosh, Kaplan, Kubena, Bateman, & Landmann, 1996). Furthermore, similar variables affect nutrient levels in the body. For example, thiamine, pyridoxine, folate, total iron-binding capacity, serum transferrin, hemoglobin, and hematocrit were all affected positively by various indicators of objective and subjective forms of social support (McIntosh et al., 1989a). Subsequent analyses of these same data indicate that particular stressful life events negatively affected these measures of nutritional status. The physiological mechanism by which social experiences impact body biochemistry have yet to be identified.

Body Size and Composition

Sociologists and psychologists tend to study perceptions of body weight and their social psychological outcomes. Jeff Sobal and his colleagues (1992) have continued to pursue the links between fatness/obesity and social relations, attempting to determine whether weight problems develop only after the individual marries or is a factor in determining whether the person gets married. The marital causation model received some support in their analysis of data from the National Survey of Personal Health Practices and Consequences but only in the case of men; that is, men gained weight after marriage.

McIntosh et al. (1989a) have examined the effects of the various forms of social support on body mass index, percent ideal body weight, midarm muscle mass, triceps skinfold, suprailiac skinfold, and abdominal girth. The findings, after controlling for physical disabilities and sex, indicated that support in the form of companionship and confiding relationships was associated with less excess body weight, less body fat, and more muscle mass. Again, the mechanisms are unclear, but social relationships may affect long-term food intake and amount of activities/exercise, resulting in body weight outcomes.

Follow-up analyses indicated the presence of simultaneous effects between body size and body composition and social support. Thus, social relations may affect and, at the same time, be affected by these aspects of the body. Such work and the work of Sobal, while still in its infancy, remain intriguing. As interesting as this work might seem, sociological theories applied to the body and its accompanying features and needs offer the opportunity for medical sociology to make reciprocal contributions to sociological theory (Turner, 1992) and perhaps for similar contributions from food and nutritional sociology.

Current approaches to the sociology of the body, while cognizant of the physiological aspects of the body, are more inclined either to supplement this view or ignore it altogether and settle on political-economic, phenomenological, symbolic, and socially constructed aspects of bodies.

The Political Economy of the Body

A "political economy of the body" contained O'Neill's (1985) wisdom regarding production and consumption. O'Neill extended Marx's discussions of the body and its needs, adding insights from additional perspectives such as phenomenology. O'Neill thus began with the recognition that bodies have real needs. "We are chained, then, to the alternating pleasures and pains of the body's satisfaction" (O'Neil, 1985:92). In a modern economy, however, the difference between authentic, or primary, needs and secondary (inauthentic) needs has become blurred.

The productive body is more than a factor of production. It is fetishized, with its "stress, relaxation, health, illness, beauty, and spontaneity" reified (O'Neill, 1985:100). The body is an extension of machines in production and an extension of products in consumption. Both as producers and consumers, people are taught to "disvalue their biological bodies...tolerating not only poor working conditions, but impossible expectations...disvalue it only to revalue once it has been sold grace, spontaneity, vivaciousness, bounce, confidence, smoothness, and freshness" (O'Neill, 1985:101).

Finally, production is work; consumption is work. Both are the results of the commitment of time and energy, and both are perplexing, disappointing. O'Neill is particularly cognizant of the particular strain on women's bodies as both producers and primary consumers in this regard.

The Body as Commodity

Many of the critical writings on culture, social class, and social change have included discussion of the "commodification of everything." Such a perspective argues that, in market economies, all objects of value to human beings have a price, and they have been incorporated into the economy.

Baudrillard has argued that while the body and its experiences represent rights and pleasure, they also serve as a "mode of subjugation" (Kellner, 1989). In societies where design and consumption are paramount, the body and its sexuality have been subjected to design.

Ewen (1988), basing his analysis on Lukacs, argued that objects that serve to gratify human needs were refined and turned into commodities. A modern world consisted of two economies: a real world of goods and services and a world that specialized in the manufacture of "thin air" in which "less is more" was the creed. In women's fashions, less is more prevailed in that those articles of clothing thought most fashionable were those that exposed more of the body while using less material. Commodities were developed for their value as display, for communicating status and self-worth. Thus, bodybuilding equipment was advertised in terms of "self-absorbed careerism, conspicuous consumption, and a conception of self as an object of competitive display" (Ewen, 1988:194).

Bodies are sites for the display of fashion in that they serve as a mechanism for exhibiting clothing, jewelry, perfume, and so on. Further, bodies themselves may be the fashionable objects and the clothing and other accoutrements may then serve to highlight or mask some aspect of the body. The face, breasts, and legs come to mind.

Contemporary views of the female breast provide illustrations of both commodification and alienation. Surgeons and women themselves engage in activities designed to enhance the exchange value of breasts through surgery, exercise, and careful choice of attire. It is easy to argue that the results of such efforts are confined to the pages of men's magazines such as *Playboy*, but a review of the covers of *Cosmopolitan* during the time period 1990–1993 reveals that women themselves place high value on breast appearance. The size, shape, and complexion of breasts have become one of the primary mechanisms for assigning female beauty. Every cover of *Cosmopolitan* during this time period centered on the head and body of an attractive, well-dressed, made-up, and coiffured woman. The dress always exposes a portion of the woman's breasts; generally more than less.

Furthermore, breasts are commercialized by a surgical industry willing to enlarge or reduce their size for cosmetic rather than medical reasons. The fashion industry commercializes breasts by means of the cut of the neckline of dresses and blouses and the construction of the brassiere. The bra has made its latest fashion statement through a configuration that pushes the breasts together and upward. One company sells such a bra for $23. Not so long ago, the construction of the bra reflected an interest in lifting and separating breasts.

Breasts have use value as well as exchange value in terms of their ability to provide both human sustenance and pleasure. Their multivalent character creates situations of conflict regarding their appropriate use. Their conflicting values have led some to decide that drawing on their use value for infant feeding may permanently lessen their exchange value (Schmitt, 1986).

Women may find their breasts alienating because they may perceive that the value of their breasts derives largely from the size and shape. Those not already estranged from this aspect of their bodies may develop this condition as the process of aging renders their breasts less attractive. Women may experience further alienation through the discovery that breast-feeding is unpleasant and painful for some and impossible for others (Van Esterick, 1989). Finally, many women find that this source of both use and exchange value potentially contains hidden dangers in the form of cancerous lumps.

The potential conflict between the breast as a source of nutrients and as a symbol of sexuality and a device of sexual pleasure is illustrated by a recent court case. A New York woman was charged with child abuse for breast-feeding her two-year-old. The alleged abuse was defined by the view that breast-feeding a two-year-old was inappropriate and "physically impossible" and thus must have been motivated by twisted sexual desires ("Officials," 1992).

The discussion of the phenomenological approach to the body also develops the idea of alienation in the context of the body but at the interpersonal level. This approach permits a more credible explanation of various "body disorders" such as obesity, anorexia nervosa, and bulimia.

THE BODY AND THE SELF

Sociologists, instead of developing theories of personality, have focused on the idea of "self," which is thought largely to be the product of social interaction. The self is thus not body nor personality, but rather the person's view of herself or himself. As the self has social origins, this viewpoint is based on what others think (Collins, 1988).

The self, however, is thought to be multiple: people hold multiple views of themselves rather than a unitary one. The self's "me" arises from the roles each person plays in society and, at the same time, represents the potentially restraining expectations of others. These include gender, occupation, age, life cycle, and a myriad of other roles that each person in society plays. Interaction is possible because a person can "take the role of the other," that is, empathize with other persons by mentally taking on *their* roles, and because of the "generalized other" or the ability to empathize with people in general.

The Body Self

One of the selves identified by William James is the "body self," one's image of one's body. This image largely derives from the individual's perceptions of how those with whom he or she interacts view his or her body as well as expectations associated with a more generalized view of human bodies. Thus, an individual's perception of whether she is slim and attractive depends, in part, on the views of others. Some argue that an individual's interpretation of others' views is less harsh than those actual views. Thus, a person may consider himself slimmer than others see him (Collins, 1988). However, this is not the case when it comes to body assessment: women tend to view themselves as larger than they actually are (Gordon, 1990).

In a study conducted at the University of Pennsylvania, Fallon and Rozin (1985) found that female students tended to overestimate how much they actually weighed. Furthermore, when asked to select the picture of a human form from a set of drawings that looked most like their own and the picture of a figure that approximated one that they aspired to, they consistently chose a larger figure than their current size to represent how they saw themselves and a smaller figure for their desired body size. Finally, women selected a figure they perceived most attractive to men that was, in fact, smaller than the ideal figure chosen by the male students in the study.

Rosenberg (1981) argued that almost all psychological pathologies involve low self-esteem. This suggested that a healthy self is one that holds itself (or its selves) in high esteem. Further, it suggested a set of significant others that provide the individual with positive images. The generalized other in Western societies placed an emphasis on fitness and slimness. Without the supportive views of others, living in such a milleau may create distorted body images and thus low self-esteem. Allon's (1979) research on women in weight-loss groups supported this view. As Bordo (1993) observed, distorted body images are extremely widespread, leading us to conclude that many women have low self-esteem. As we shall see, this may not necessarily be the case.

Body image distortion and accompanying low self-esteem in women may also occur as women compete for roles traditionally held by men. Parents, while expecting their daughters to remain feminine, emphasize the necessity of becoming independent, self-reliant, and self-supporting. This may create pressure on women to value a more "male" type of body—less curvaceous and more tubular (Garner, Garfinkel, & Thompson, 1980; Gordon, 1990). This perspective assumes that women believe that in order to compete with men, they have to look like them. These pressures and the difficulty of easily achieving a male body may lead to eating disorders. The self thus becomes divided between a "male" and a "female" self and by "male" and "female" expectations of others, particularly family members.

Indeed, Brumberg (1988) observed that in certain historical periods in the United States, young women have received encouragement to become competitive and aggressive in the pursuit of independent careers. In such times it became fashionable for young women to adopt the "tubular" look, but it is misleading to conclude that only when women strive for equality with men do eating disorders occur. Brumberg (1988) found that anorexia among young women during the nineteenth century resulted not from pressure to compete *with* men but, in a sense, *for* men. That is, the women were pushed in the direction of the upwardly mobile marriage, achievable only through a thorough-going femininity.

Others have embraced the divided-selves diagnosis of disorders. In his book *The Alcoholic Self,* Norman Denzin (1987) argued that alcoholics have divided selves: an alcoholic self (the self when intoxicated) and a sober self. Deep contradictions thus developed in the mind of the alcoholic, which led to emotional problems and a disembodied self. If the self relied on others for definition, a divided self produced contradictory expectations and evaluations. In addition, the alcoholic increased her or his dependency on others while maintaining the belief that he or she was an independent, functioning person (Denzin, 1987:135). This, in turn, led to resentments over the unsatisfactory relationships that resulted from a divided self.

Finally, some have approached bodies and selves through stereotyping. Certain characteriological aspects of others' identities are associated by types of bodies and particular features of those bodies. The desirability of a female self may hinge on the size and shape of breasts. Certain stereotypes about character develop with regard to the kind of body one has. A desirable body is a desirable self; thus a slim but not skinny body is honest, self-reliant, hard working, sociable, and intelligent (Jackson, 1992). At the same time, individuals with such bodies experience higher self-esteem and fewer affective disorders.

Jackson (1992) has reviewed the "appearance" literature, noting that the research in this area distinguishes "facial" from "body" appearance. To summarize, males placed more stock in facial attractiveness than females, a finding for which there was some cross-cultural support. Similarly, both males and females in many cultures preferred certain body, as well as body part, shapes and sizes to others. Such preferences also changed as the prevailing economic and cultural circumstances undergo change. Cultural preferences in bodies exhibit social class influences as well, which are discussed more fully in Chapter 5.

Research on the divided self has not, however, incorporated ideas about body stereotypes into research on anorexia and bulimia. The literature on obesity, however, is replete with references to negative stereotypes held by the victim and others. These result in the incorporations of stereotypical attributes into the self. At the same time, however, investigators have not dealt with the means by which the overweight attempt to overcome negative stereotypes in their associations with others. It is possible that persons who experience "overweight" without problems of low self-esteem may have successfully elevated other selves to the forefront, lessening the importance of their body self. Allon's (1979) work indicates that the most important service that the weight loss groups or significant other might provide individuals of "nonnormal" weight status is an appreciation of the individuals' other selves. Work on eating and body disorders has attempted to capture the sufferer's body image but has not focused on either the other components of the self or the image that others, particularly family members, have of this body. Researchers of body disorders have neglected the whole area of body stereotypes.

The Lived Body

While symbolic interaction theory points to the importance of a body self as part of self-image, the Merleau-Ponty (1962) approach to phenomenology brings together mind and body in a unity such that speaking of a "self" as composed of the mind and its parts is no longer sufficient. Life experiences become the lived body, emphasizing the idea that humans experience the world not directly through the mind alone but directly through the senses. Life is lived; it is experienced through the body. The body acts on the world; the world in turn acts on the body.

More specifically, the phenomenological approach to the body makes the following assumptions. First, while the body is a physical entity, containing physiological structure and processes (Korper), it is also a "lived body" (Leib) in that the world is experienced through the body rather than apprehended by the mind. Second, people experience the world through their senses; they thus experience only what their senses permit and sensual perception is not always fully accurate. Experience contains a certain amount of ambiguity and indeterminacy. The body is simply not an accurate measuring device that records perceptually reliable data. Third, perception is conditioned by social interaction and culture. However, much of what is learned and shared occurs through the observation of the bodies of others. Fourth, thoughts are conditioned by bodily experiences in the world. Fifth, the self is integrated with the experiential body and is said to be "embodied." And sixth, the body is both subject and object to its owner and object to other bodies (Ostrow, 1990; Turner, 1992).

One useful aspect of the phenomenological approach lies in its ideas concerning bodily learning. Phenomenologists argue that infants begin to learn about their world, not through their own bodily experiences, but by observing the bodily experiences of others and comparing those with their own. Learning to like foods the body might ordinarily reject involves watching another ingest them. By watching the ingestion and observing the facial expression of the ingestee, the observer learns whether the food in question is sour or sweet. Spurling (1977:52) describes this sort of an experience as "a crude kind of role taking in perception." These shared perceptions may involve neither speech nor conscious awareness.

The taste system evolved to protect individual members of a species from ingesting poisons. The "hedonic" value of food is monitored by the hindbrain with "acceptance/rejection reflexes" available to deal with a potential item of food (T. R. Scott, 1990:46). Unconscious facial expressions communicate to the ingestor as well as to others the food's hedonic value. Taste aversions that develop in infancy carry over into adulthood. Behavioral manipulations by researchers demonstrate that the aversions and preferences can be altered; at the same time, an organism can overcome an aversion in order to meet a psychological need (T. R. Scott, 1990).

Learning food preferences from experiences and interpreting those experiences likely begins in infancy as the child learns about its bodily experiences and their interpretation. This occurs through observing the reactions of others to specific foods and nonfoods. Mothers and fathers may unconsciously transmit cues about foods via their facial and other body expressions. They may also purposely attempt to teach their child about a desirable food by means of both verbal encouragement and facial expression. Similarly, they may attempt to drive home the undesirability of an item as food by means of the look on their faces.

Psychologists have found that children develop an early sense of satiety in light of sufficient intake of food. Internal cues regulate ingestion and cessation, based on the experience of either hunger or satiety. Environmental influences of sufficient strength, however, may override these internal regulators. Research shows that overcontrolling parents can impede both the development and functioning of internal signals (Birch, 1990:129).

As individuals age other social beings become important. For example, in the presence of someone of highly desirable body weight, individuals may curtail their intake. Recent research showed if such an individual announces they are on a diet this may to lead to further reductions in intake by those around them (Logue, 1991). However, in some cases the opposite effect can occur. Two groups of research subjects each shared a lunch table with a model who announced that she was on a diet. In the first group, the model proceeded to eat a quantity of food greater than expected for someone dieting. In the second case, the model consumed an amount thought more appropriate for the circumstances. Subjects exposed to the "overeating" model ate significantly more than subjects exposed to the "just-right eating" model (Logue, 1991).

Body Habits

The body takes up space and moves through it. Body schema involves an implicit "picture" the body has of itself in time and space (Moss, 1978). The experience of space becomes an important part of the world of a particular human being (body). For example, the space close to the refrigerator is more important than the space further away from it. Routes toward resources that meet perceived bodily needs (e.g., hunger) thus take on familiar pathways. An individual probably gets to the refrigerator in much the same way each day; the same route to the grocery store is driven. However, the individual who travels these routes daily does not consciously select them but rather gets from one point to the next through habituated body movements. The body has captured the essential relationship between it and the environmental conditions in question. Only when the route becomes blocked or some other impediment arises does conscious action take over. Here too a certain amount of the body's movements are "sedimented." Individuals need not remind themselves that in order to walk, one foot must proceed the other. The body knows how to walk without conscious prompting.

Along similar lines, Leder (1990) described what he calls an "absent body." Absence occurs in two ways. First, at any given time people are unaware of their bodies in the manner described above. Similarly, they are generally unaware of the thousands of bodily processes that go on underneath the skin. Thus, they do not notice when their last meal begins to be digested or when nutrients enter the bloodstream. They do become aware of "corporeal states" such as hunger or thirst. These, in turn, draw attention to food and drink, sources of gratification heretofore "absent." Digestion may also appear to us perceptually through means of an "upset stomach." This first type of absence is called "disappearance"(Leder, 1990).

The second distinction has greater interest to sociologists. The term "disappearance" refers to alienation of self from body. This can happen in several ways. When the body experiences illness or injury, the individual feels a sense of separation. The body is no longer familiar; it has become an alien presence. The experience of hunger, starvation, or deficiency disease appears to have an alienating effect through the discomfort the body feels, as well as the loss of ordinary skills, aptitudes, and the ability to concentrate. In such cases the individual not only experiences bodily estrangement but also estrangement from others as the effects of the condition transform the individual's ability to successfully interact (see Cravioto & DeLicardie, 1972; McIntosh, 1975).

Other bodily changes lead to alienation, to a loss of the "taken-for-grantedness" of one's body. Adolescence and aging involve changes in the body that frighten and appall (Leder, 1990). Weight gain at almost any age for females alienates them from their bodies. But unlike puberty and aging, which are defined as "normal," weight gain may create a sense of bodily alienation that remains a part of the sufferer's life for as long as that person lives. However, even the loss of weight alienates those who have come to take for granted a particular body size. Thus, after losing a substantial amount of weight, individuals continue to behave as though the weight were still there. For instance, they give obstacles a wider berth than necessary under their new, slimmer circumstances. Young adults, who until recently were considered obese, find themselves at a loss when it comes to engaging in social activities they experience, perhaps, for the first time. While some of this has to do with what to say, much has to do with body comportment. How should a person sit on the first date? How much should one eat? Even mild forms of alienation occur when one spills, say, coffee in one's lap, particularly in the presence of another, or when a person discovers that a portion of breakfast has attached itself to his shirt or her blouse.

Under the examination of a physician, the individual may suddenly feel the body as alien (Leder, 1990). Perhaps the most significant form of bodily alienation occurs via the gaze of others (Bordo, 1993; Leder, 1990). Women report a long-term alienation from their breasts because of the fixation and perpetual stares of men. This may lead to an alienation from the act of breast-feeding (Schmitt, 1986). Women, in fact, may learn a perpetual sense of "disappearance," which then leads to biological dysfunction. Self-consciousness about one's breasts may contribute to the problem of "lactation failure" experienced by many women. Continued self-awareness of body and its size may lead to anorexia nervosa. The gaze of others may be so powerful as to lead to a misperception of one's own body size and shape. In fact, Bruch (1988) argued that a diagnosis of anorexia nervosa requires the presence of distorted body image. Other research indicates, however, that a distorted body image is widespread among the female population of the United States (Bordo, 1993; Jackson, 1992). This more general misperception may result from habituated perceptual reactions to an unrelenting and pervasive male gaze.

Body Image

Body image, as opposed to body schema, involves an explicit picture of the body in the mind (Moss, 1978). Body image represents an image not based soley on experience, but on objective observation. In fact, the "objective" picture of the body we believe ourselves to have occurs much later in the development process (Moss, 1978). The body image, instead, is based on "lived experiences" in which the body acts on the world and is acted upon. Part of this lived experience involves the physical experience of, for example, the hands as they manipulate the environment. These "prereflective" experiences become the basis of the explicit, reflected body image individuals later develop. This "reflective appropriation" of "prereflective experiences," however, also involves interaction with others. Through intimate/elaborate relations, body parts of others are incorporated into the person's body image.

A number of pathologies involve body image distortion. Severe obesity often involves alienation from the body. The individual literally divides the head from the body; the head becomes useful, desirable, "me"; the body becomes useless, undesirable, "it." Body ownership is thus disrupted and depersonalized. As already mentioned, some claim that body image distortion characterizes anorexia nervosa. Gordon (1990) and Bordo (1993) argued that the distorted body images experienced by anorexics occur because of cognitive rather than perceptual failure. Gordon (1990) also suggested that more accurate body images are produced only through confrontation.

Finally, Turner (1992) derived a different perspective on anorexia nervosa. Instead of focusing on body distortion or alienation, he combined the notion that the mouth served as the main bodily mechanism for communication with ideas concerning communication while in the sick role. He, like Brumberg (1988) and Bordo (1993), acknowledged conflicting pressures on young women who seek escape by means of the sick role. He extended the notion of sick role by arguing that it sometimes involved miscommunication between the sick and the well. In instances in which women lose the ability to speak when confronted with contradictory expectations, in the realm of the body, women lost their ability to communicate through eating, breaking a communicative link with their mothers.

WHEN BODIES COLLIDE

The symbolic interaction approach has attempted to capture the effects of interaction with others in self development. The dramaturgical offshoot has viewed the body as a potential tool in manipulating the impressions of others, on the one hand, and as a source of embarrassment, shame, and stigma, on the other. Interactionists such as Denzin (1984) and Schmitt (1986) have treated the body as an embodied self, formed through interactions with others. Schmitt (1986) built an approach to "embodied identities" from work by Stone (1962) on the importance of appearance in interaction and on the work of Denzin (1984), which identified four "body structures" (physical, lived, enacted for self, enacted for others) and their connections with emotions. Applying this framework to the narrative data presented in *Breasts: Women Speak about Their Breasts and Their Lives* (Ayalah & Weinstock, 1979), Schmitt (1986) identified eight types of "breast identities" in women's breast talk. These include age-related, deviant, health-related, physical appearance, sexual, and womanhood (Schmitt, 1986). More than half of the women in this study chose either the physical appearance or the sexual as their primary breast identity; some selected multiple identities.

A key theme in Schmitt's (1986) work is the notion that women develop breast identities, which are in part an outcome of interacting with other persons who include breasts in the formation of their image of women. Women have resources that enable them to control, with varying degrees of success, the image that others develop of them, including their breasts. Others can subvert these efforts, and regardless of the woman's efforts, some kind of breast image develops as others evaluate them. Even "breastless" women have a breast identity.

Breast-feeding received only infrequent attention in the examples provided by Schmitt (1986); however, the breast identity of motherhood ranked third in importance (behind physical attraction and sexual) and was generally accompanied with feelings of pride. Other women who associated with motherhood identity could experience embarrassment when discovering negative evaluations of them for their breast-feeding in public. Van Esterick (1989) provided additional examples of such embarrassment, as well as of reactions by males who upon viewing such behavior reacted with disgust perhaps because it detracted from their belief that breasts exist principally for men's pleasure. Many women reported what Schmitt (1986) referred to as "ambivalent breast-me's." These women considered their breasts attractive but resented the apparent assumption by many males that their breasts were the only important aspect of their selves.

The contemporary link between the cultural importance of motherhood and breast feeding developed in the late nineteenth century in Europe with the emphasis of the home as a haven from a heartless world (McIntosh & Zey, 1989). Homes would provide a place in which, unlike the marketplace, people could live and interchange by higher standards than those of the jungle. Women were said to possess and encourage this higher behavior. It was in this context, as well as the maternal duty to lower the infant mortality rate to help meet the person-power needs of the state, that breast-feeding became a concern (Perry, 1992). The importance of breast-feeding was supported by means of social control. The medical community turned its attention to such matters, arguing that motherhood represented women's natural heritage and efforts by women to escape their nature would only lead to disastrous consequences such as the disease of hysteria. In addition, the contract wet nurse industry in England and France was outlawed (Perry, 1992; Sussman, 1982).

While much distinguishes the symbolic interactionism from existential phenomenology, their separation becomes more difficult when applied to empirical cases. In dealing with anorexia nervosa, both perspectives begin with the idea of body image. The phenomenologist deals with the experiences of eating and not eating. Symbolic interactionists look at the perceptions of one's own body in relation to the perceived body experiences of others. The latter would include the experience of height, weight, and shape as well as of various body parts. The interactionist approaches body image as more of a cognitive artifact determined through the exchange of symbolic representations. The interactant develops a body image as a result. From the perspective of the phenomenologist, anorexics experience an unacceptable body. Their bodies appear to them larger than they do to others. In fact, however, distorted body images characterize many nonanorexic women as well. This literature, however, provides little phenomenological insight into how these distortions come to take such a powerful hold on women. Perhaps the idealized body images have become "sedimented" through early observation of maternal self-dissatisfaction. If this is the case, why do only women develop such perceptual distortions? Perhaps these misperceptions arise from the frequent observation that other women critically assess their own bodies as well as those of other women, often displaying displeasure through their bodies. Perhaps Schmitt's (1986) discussions of embodied selves lend support to the view that bodies move from states of "absence" to "disappearance" under the critical gaze of others.

The interactionists focus more attention on the exchange of symbolic representations regarding expectations of body dimensions and their links to natural versus deviant behavior. These perspectives also overlap considerably. Becker's (1963) classic account regarding learning to become a marijuana smoker contains both perspectives. Becker examined the verbal exchanges that transpire as experienced users attempt to instruct novices. Novices are told, for instance, that the smoke must be inhaled in order to get high and are instructed regarding the symptoms associated with being high as well as how those symptoms should be interpreted. However, the account implies that this instruction involves experts who engage in smoking themselves in order to consciously demonstrate techniques and experiences. Unconscious body instruction undoubtedly accompanies these conscious efforts as well as the novice noticing facial expressions and body demeanors of their guides. The learning of drinking behavior probably involves even less conscious instruction and more conscious mimicking than does the learning of the ingestion of illicit drugs.

SYMBOLIC APPROACHES TO THE BODY

Structuralists and semiologists, for the most part, have shown an interest in the body's symbolic rather than its material characteristics. Once again we find Mary Douglas as well as Piero Camporesi in the forefront.

Douglas's work on the body is found in her *Purity and Danger* (1991) [1966] and *Natural Symbols* (1973). In the latter work, Douglas contrasted the physical body with the social body (society) and argued that the physical characterizations a people give the body are cultural constructs rather than physical reality. She followed Mauss's lead in declaring that in regard to the body, "there can be no such thing as natural behavior" (Douglas, 1973:65). Thus, eating, sleeping, having sex, and bodily elimination are all learned behaviors. While breathing may constitute innate behavior, social circumstances define and limit "proper" breathing—not breathing too loudly, especially while one is asleep (snoring); breathing into the ear of only "appropriate" persons.

Furthermore, according to Douglas (1973, 1991 [1966]) the social categories that pertain to the body reflect how society itself is viewed. Societies consist of structure and boundaries. The perceived structure and boundaries of the body will thus reflect societal structure and boundaries. Each society experiences particular problems, some of which threaten boundaries and some of which threaten structure. The body symbolizes these threats symbolically through distinctions of what Douglas (1991) [1966] calls "social pollution." One kind of social pollution has to do with group survival or fear of contamination by outsiders. Groups ritually distance themselves from nonmembers by speaking of the defilement that awaits its members who come into contact with the bodily excrement of members of other groups. "Unclean" foods pollute the body and thus the group as well. In India castes are separated, in part, by occupation. The preparation of food, however, threatens this separation in that it involves the effects of several castes: blacksmiths, carpenters, rope makers, and peasants. Responsibility for cooking must thus be assigned to those whose hands are ritually pure (Douglas, 1991 [1966]:127). This strict division helps to maintain the separation of social groups into a rigid hierarchy.

Taking an entirely different perspective was Jean Baudrillard (1981), who argued that Marx's political economy has been superseded by the "political economy of the sign." In Baudrillard's idealism, the sign was more real than the object it represented; in fact, signs represented a kind of hyperrealism. Signs, instead of reflecting authentic needs, imposed inauthentic desires.

Fashion has become a major commodity in postmodern society; driven by the frantic forces of capitalism, it personifies "planned obsolescence—not just the necessity for market survival but the cycle of desire itself, the endless process through which the body is coded and recoded" (Faurschou, 1987:10). Thus fashion, as a system, is coded, fettished beauty. Beauty is no longer subjective, but is homogenized into a code, "a system of endlessly but equally differentiated signs...its ultimate goal closure and perfection, a logical mirage suturing all social contradictions and divisions of the level of the abstract. This is the glamour of fashion, the glamorized body of disembodied perfection" (Faurschou, 1987:11).

SOCIALLY CONSTRUCTED BODIES

Many social scientists take the body seriously only to the extent that groups define bodies by means of a set of fundamental social categories. Perhaps the most critical of these classificatory distinctions is that of gender. The bodies of women and men have clearly distinct external and internal features, although not all societies find these of particular importance. In one sense, at least, the biological basis for these apparent differences is slight: only 1 out of 46 chromosomes distinguish females from males (Synnott, 1993). These perceived differences, however, take on monumental importance. Thus, men are said to be strong; women, weak; women are passive; men, aggressive. Bodies are said to represent desire and irrationality, while minds represent reason and rationality. Here the whole body is said to be feminine while the mind is masculine. The interpretation of bodies has a long history. Bodies have thus been described as alien, as confining tombs, as the enemy, as machines, and as self.

The senses themselves bear a heavy cultural load. Most cultures greatly restrict touching because of what it symbolizes. However, most cultures appear to place the least restrictions on married couples. Even here strongly sanctioned rules may apply regarding, for example, what body parts may come into contact during sexual intercourse, as well as how much force may be applied in touching. Touching in public is highly restricted as is the touching of members of the same as well as opposite sexes. Detection of inappropriate touching leads to application of deviant labels and other forms of punishment.

One version of the social constructionist approach involved the application of Foucault's (1977, 1978) ideas regarding bodies and power. Bordo (1993:24–25) argued that "mass cultural representations" were imposed upon bodies, based on race, ethnicity, gender, and these images homogenized by "smooth[ing] out all racial, ethnic, and sexual 'differences' that disturb Anglo-Saxon, heterosexual expectations and identifications." These images also normalized; that is, they served as a standard by which bodies were measured, judged, "disciplined," and "corrected." Drawing on Foucault, Bordo (1993) argued that homogenization and normalization were not simply imposed by the powerful on the powerless; rather, those "below" engaged in self-monitoring, judging, and correcting.

This approach has clear application to the cult of slimness that holds most Western women in its grip. Men idealize slimness and expect it in "their women." "Over and over, extremely slender women students complain of hating their thighs and stomachs (the anorexic's most dreaded spot); often they express concern and anger over frequent teasing by their boyfriends" (Bordo, 1993:154). The discourse on anorexia reflects both the constructed dualist tendencies in representing the body as well as the extreme of self-monitoring, disciplining, and correcting. Anorexics report they desire to "kill off appetite," the constant dread of being overwhelmed by appetite, and of "feeling caught" in their bodies (Bordo, 1993:147).

Postmodern Bodies and Selves

Both postmodernists and some of those who support the notion of advanced or high modernism have given the body and its connection to the self a prominent position in their perspectives. Giddens (1991), for instance, argued that lives were now oriented around the building of lifestyles and that the body represented a major tool in the arsenal of those building a lifestyle and a set of selves to go with it. Exercise and weight reduction represented two of many strategies that may be employed. Fitness and eating disorders occurred because of the contradictory messages of a postindustrial environment: be fit in order to be a productive worker while at the same time be a self-indulgent consumer (Scheper-Hughes & Lock, 1987). Producer selves were taught to delay gratification and subliminate desires, while consumer selves were encouraged to give in to desire, to indulge on impulse (Bordo, 1993:96). Thus, women were under pressures to be slim, to forego the same rich foods that others proclaim as a part of a respectable middle class diet.

Glassner (1990) has pointedly argued that the current fitness craze is a postmodern phenomenon. Fitness is postmodern for it involves a pastiche—a borrowing from diverse imagery of healthfulness, vitality, confidence, vigor, and relaxation. It provides a sense of control over something in a world in which the forces that affect our health seem less under control than ever before. Fitness retains a modern theme in its optimism that through exercise, life can get better; it is postmodern in its escapist notion that the ills of modern society can be avoided through separation of one's body from it all (Glassner, 1990). At the same time, exercise helps fashion by creating postmodern selves—selves that "undo" principal dualities of human identity such as gender (postmodern exercise routines contain the same prescriptions for male and female participants; health products no longer differentiate male vs. female treatments/substances); both the inner and outer bodies are joined—the appearance of one affects the appearance of the other; acts that are undertaken for vanity's sake and acts undertaken for health's sake become interchangeable; exercise is meant to be work—it's hard work to achieve the body you desire—accomplished during leisure time (Glassner, 1990; see also, Willis, 1991). Today's gyms are postmodern for they combine the sweat and hard work with a relaxed, clean-smelling atmospheres. Old gyms smell like old gyms!

Obsessions with body and self were viewed by observers such as Mestrovic (1992) as an example of narcissism. Giddens described anorexia as a "pathology of reflexive self-control, operating around an axis of self-identity and bodily appearance, in which shame anxiety plays a preponderant role" (1991:105). Anorexia is an option late modernity provides in the context of continued exclusion of women from the same opportunities as men. This form of mastery, as Giddens correctly observed, is not the same as authentic self-mastery. At some point, the anorexia itself takes over, the woman no longer makes the decisions about eating. Furthermore, authenticity involves positive self-image, not shame, self-destruction, and body alienation. Nonanorexic females who strive for fitness do so as a recognized means of achieving equality with their male counterparts; furthermore, anorexia shuts others out, while those merely "obsessed" are so for social reasons: they want to affect how others view them and they often engage in fitness pursuits surrounded by others (Glassner, 1988).

While Mestrovic (1990, 1992) has not commented directly on problems of obesity and anorexia, his discussions of modernity, postmodernity, stress, and illness suggest that both of these problems result from the malintegration of the dualistic tendencies of individuals and society. Individuals and the societies of which they are a part contain a mind and will through relationships with others and the consciousness. At the same time, desires largely unconscious and infinite reside within the individual and have a collective counterpart at the societal level. Societies, as well as individuals, reflect tension between representations and endless desires. A healthy society maintains a balance between the two poles. A society that might manage to eliminate desires removes the source of altruism as well. It is clear from Mestrovic's (1992) discussions that complete elimination of desires is neither desirable nor practical. The heart or body is more powerful than the mind or rationality; thus, at most the mind holds the heart in check to some degree.

In Mestrovic's view (1990, 1992) the postmodern world is characterized by anomie and egoism. Rapid alteration in social arrangements such as a rising unemployment rate detach individuals from a significant source of connections to society through the loss of colleagues and workmates (Mestrovic & Glassner, 1983). Egoistic suicide occurs when individuals maintain loose ties to social structure, such as membership in Protestantism as opposed to Catholicism, or when significant ties are lost, such as through divorce or widowhood. Modern societies are characterized by weaker controls over individuals. Egoism or unchecked, infinite desires thus become more prominent. Under such conditions, overconsumption and the search for new experiences to ward off boredom become paramount. On the one hand, obesity may be a result of underchecked egoism. Anorexia, on the other hand, may reflect the anomie that occurs when institutions fail to control behavior. Economic anomie appears to be the chief cause of many current problems: when material desires get the better of economic realities, other forms of anomie result. The greed that this represents is found in the selling of junk bonds and the other economic scandals of the era. Indices of such anomie include individual and corporate bankruptcies, surges in prices for goods such as food, and jail terms for corporate wheeler-dealers (Mestrovic, 1990).

Anorexia may also result from the general lessening of controls. Some have suggested that anorexia results from excessive controls by families. However, another interpretation suggests that the anorexic is someone troubled by weakening conventional controls of kin and friends. In a world that seemingly lacks control over desires, the individual turns inward in an attempt at self-control. The desires at work reflect the desire for bodily perfection, a goal that is unachievable.

The Body Fights Back: Body Skirmishes and Body Wars

If addictions are diseases produced by demands of bourgeois society, then their renouncement represents a means for the body to reassert control. If alcoholism includes the inability to "drink one drink" or to keep one's hands off a glass of liquor, then developing the ability to stay away from alcohol and not take that first drink represents personal victory. Alcohol treatment such as the principles of Alcoholics Anonymous (which have been incorporated into many treatment center programs) provides such a means. AA is no revolutionary organization designed to emancipate the individual from the repressive society that led to the alcoholism but adjusts the fit of the individual to society. Like traditional psychoanalytic theory, the AA program assumes an alcoholic's id needs firmer control by an ego that is backed up by significant others (a sponsor; home group members).

Some feminists have argued that anorexia nervosa is a successful tool in a woman's bid for independence from patriarchy (Bordo, 1993). There is little evidence that anorexics strive to escape male control and that at some point in the development of anorexia, the individual loses control of symptoms (Brumberg, 1988). Some have insisted, however, that anorexia is a political position, a protest against contradictory expectations regarding women's roles and against male control. Orbach (1979) argued that the refusal to eat constitutes the bodily expression of sentiments women feel unable to express in words. Thus, in J. C. Scott's (1990) terms, anorexia is a "weapon of the weak." Not all such weapons effectively halt repression, but they do afford the expresser some sense of dignity (J. C. Scott, 1990).

Others have taken an approach that calls on women to overthrow societal obsessions with slimness through self-acceptance, size and weight regardless. Bodybuilders find that one of the attractions of their sport lies in the sense of empowerment that developing a powerful body provides (Bordo, 1993).

Naomi Wolf (1991:290) declared that a "woman wins by giving herself and other women permission to eat; to be sexual, to age, to wear overalls, a paste tiara, a Balenciagen gown, a second-hand opera cloak, or combat boots, to cover up or to go practically naked, to do whatever we choose in following or ignoring our own aesthetic." Baudrillard's (1989) recent work dwelled on nihilism and the futility of expecting the explicitness and alienation of bourgeois society to disappear. Instead, he called for an anarchistic attack on the system by overheating it: by consuming more and more without regard to need or purpose. Stuff until the system bursts!

CONCLUSION

The sociology of the body has advanced on many fronts, some of which have been reviewed here. A number of these demonstrate great potential for varying approaches to food and nutrition. Thus far these applications have not ventured beyond the links between body image and eating disorders. However, this chapter has attempted to extend the phenomenological approach to the body to food socialization and breast experiences. Much more, however, can obviously be accomplished through study of the connection between lifestyles and food in a manner similar to Bourdieu (1984). As will be discussed in Chapter 9, the state's increasing interest in the nutritional health of bodies has led to increased surveillance of its citizen's diet and physical condition.

Bodies are essential for sociologies of food and nutrition. Human action occurs in a physical context, which both facilitates as well as limits the nature and extent of that action. Bodies provide individuals with the means of mobility, communication, and survival. All existing modes of production ultimately require human bodies situated at key points in production processes. It is the body that requires food, necessitating modes of production to begin with.

Bodies are also projects for the development of the self. The body represents a major avenue of study and understanding for those interested in the relationship between the worlds of food and nutrition and the social world. Changing cultural explanations of food's impact on both the exterior and interior of the body affect the food choices that individuals make as well as the nutritional consequences of those choices. In the advanced modernity of Western cultures, people pursue particular body shapes in order to shape their identities, regardless of their often unintended health effects.

The projects occur, however, within a network of relationships with others that may direct or attempt to divert the individual's body work. Social network studies indicate that connections to others may have unanticipated, positive benefits for body health. At the same time estrangement from one's body may lead to estrangement from others. Finally, estrangement from significant others may result in alienation from oneself, particularly one's body self among females.

The experience of body alienation deserves far more attention than it has thus far received (Shilling, 1993). All of the perspectives developed by social scientists regarding the body contain some reference to this phenomenon. Women are particularly prone to this because of the great importance placed on the body self for women. Thus, the social definitions and increasing exchange value of breasts have led many women to view their breasts as alien appendages. Others find their body size and shape deeply troubling; still others experience alienation from their body selves because of the difficulty they find in controlling their appetites (Bordo, 1993).

7

THE SOCIOLOGY OF FAMINE

INTRODUCTION

Famines have both historical and contemporary relevance. Their occurrence often has far-reaching consequences for segments of populations; major cataclysms cause their occurrence. Only recently has their sociological significance received attention. The argument exists that despite the appearance of famine as having largely medical consequences and ecological causes, significant social causes and consequences play a part as well. The world system and the state are major actors in the development and unfolding of famines. Indigenous class structure, community, family and individual roles suffer temporary and, possibly, long-term alteration as a result.

DEFINITIONAL MATTERS

Most would agree that famines are due to a lack of *access* to sufficient food, either because there is a true lack of that food or because it is maldistributed. To help distinguish a famine from a mere shortage that results in hunger, excess deaths have to appear (Alamgir, 1981). In other words, there has to be above the more "normal" pattern of malnutrition-related deaths. How many deaths constitute an excess? Part of this may be related to temporality—how long there are "excess deaths"—for there normally are fluctuations in death rates that reflect seasonal and other cycles. DeWaal (1989) countered the view of excess death, arguing that (1) not all famines are alike, (2) excess deaths is a Western-imposed standard, and (3) local peoples have their own definitions of famine, which center on the degree to which their lives are permanently disrupted.

Both DeWaal (1989) and Arnold's (1988) views are attractive, for they emphasize social consequences. The disagreement over excess deaths may require empirical tests to ascertain at what point a food shortage becomes a famine. Deaths may increase in some linear fashion with worsening food shortages, making it difficult to ascertain at what point the shortage becomes a famine. Perhaps

159

in light of such a continuum, there are no famines, only shortages that differ by degree. Alternatively, medical criteria might be invoked such that once the hunger, malnutrition, or death rate (or some combination) affect a given proportion of the population, a food shortage epidemic (famine) might be declared. Given DeWaal's (1989) perspective, cultural definitions might serve as a means of determining when a situation has reached "famine" proportions. "People know a famine when they see it" would reflect this position. A weakness, of course, lies with the relativism this approach *might* introduce. This too is an empirical question.

The issue of the relativism of famine arises in another context as well. The possibility exists that what counts as famine in a given culture may vary; so too may causes vary. In some instances, climatic change may have brought the disaster, where in others, human actions, either conscious or unconscious, precipitate the famine. Multiple causes are both possible and likely.

Having made the conventional distinction between "human-caused" and "natural" disasters, it is of some interest to note that several disaster researchers consider all disasters human caused in the following sense: Humans make choices regarding where and how they live. Thus, they could choose, for example, to live in areas less prone to droughts or floods. Famine thus results from bad choices. I find this argument somewhat disingenuous in that the choices available regarding where human beings can live and secure a livelihood are usually extremely limited. The issues of definition and relativism are taken up again in Chapter 10, which discusses the differences between objectivist and social constructionist approaches to social problems like hunger and famine.

Before dealing with the issue of what causes famine, a methodological note is in order. Most of the work done on famines involves case studies of a single famine. Sen (1981) is unique in this regard as he relied on case materials from six famines that occurred in this century. A more recent study, however, departed from this single-famine tendency. Dirks (1993) compiled data on famines from the Standard Cross-Cultural Sample to test a series of hypotheses regarding famine. His sample consisted of nearly 200 societies (as opposed to nation-states), and his data were drawn from both ethnographic and historical materials. He carefully separated starvation (endemic and epidemic forms) from famine. He also distinguished occurrence, severity (the degree of community breakdown), persistence (the frequency of famine occurrence during the past 50 years), and recurrence of famine (the appearance of at least one famine in each of the two preceding centuries) (Dirks, 1993:31).

Dirks's (1993) research is useful for two reasons. First, he tests hypotheses relevant to our assessment of causes of famine. Second, his definition of famine (insufficient food + sharp increase in mortality + social disruption) squares with Arnold's (1988) and will serve as the definition of famine that will drive this chapter's discussion. Having committed to a definition that, in essence, differentiates famine from chronic malnutrition, we will also consider the possibility that famines are merely more acute versions of malnutrition and are the result of similar circumstances. Data from the World Bank data set will be used to examine this possibility.

THE CAUSES OF FAMINE

A variety of causes of famine have long been identified and debated. A brief review is worthwhile, and it should be noted that many of these same arguments appear in current discussions of the "world food crisis" (which usually is described as a world food shortage). This similarity should heighten our concern for the definitional problems associated with the concept of famine.

Climate

Climate change is associated with many famines of the past. The Little Ice Age of the fourteenth century caused crop failure and production shortages sufficient to bring famine to Europe (see I. Wallerstein, 1974:34–36).

During the 1970s, academics tended to place great emphasis on the "vagaries of the earth's climate in assigning causes of famine" (Devereux, 1993:35). While this may overstate the case, climatic changes frequently precipitate a famine. Several years of drought or flooding can greatly reduce available food supplies. Furthermore, monsoon rain failure preceded every major famine in India during the nineteenth century (Arnold, 1988). The recent famines striking countries of the Sahel have been blamed on the cooling of temperatures in Northern Europe (Cox, 1981). DeWaal's (1989) argument, based on the perceptions of locals, was that the 1984–85 famine in Sudan was caused by drought, not politics or the economy. Furthermore, Dirks (1993) examined the ethnographic/historical record for reported causes of the famines in his sample and found that factors such as drought, warfare, and crop failure were among 19 identified causes. Many of these causes were mentioned less than 10 times; drought, however, received 41 out of the 114 mentions (Dirks, 1993). Clearly, those who experienced these famines believed that insufficient rainfall was to blame.

Immanuel Wallerstein (1974) argued that the numerous changes of the fourteenth through sixteenth centuries were not only caused by cooler temperatures but by economic crisis as well. Arnold (1988) argued that Europe still suffers from drought and flooding yet has not experienced a famine in over a century. So climatic change may be a necessary condition for some *types* of famines but insufficient alone as an explanation (Devereux, 1993). This suggests that poor weather may devastate those communities already in disarray because of either political or economic circumstances. Drought apparently triggered the great Russian famine of the late nineteenth century, but it came at a time of extreme economic vulnerability; peasants were already stretched to the limit as a result of recently enacted land reform and taxation policies (Robbins, 1975). The combination of drought and economic stress proved insurmountable.

Finally, the issue of the relationship between long-term climatic change and dearth has yet to be fully explored (Matthews, Anderson, Chen, & Webb, 1990), but the consequences of these forces may tell us more about the social response to scarcity (in terms of migration and innovation) than about famine itself.

Ecology

A related argument to climate suggests that external forces such as insects, plant disease, and a deteriorating environment cause famines. Soil degradation due to overcropping, overgrazing, and deforestation led to reductions in food output (Stewart, 1988:143–148). The historical record indicates, however, that ecological constraints, while present in many cases, generally are not a sufficient condition for famine. For example, Franke and Chasin (1980) argued that the ecological destruction of the Sahel, often claimed as the cause of famines in that part of the world, was itself the product of international socioeconomic forces.

Population

Population pressure leads among the most widely held explanations of famine. Malthus rendered this view so effectively that famine is frequently referred to as a "Malthusian check" to indicate that while overpopulation causes famine, reductions in population are achieved through increases in the death rate, partially achieved by famine.

Malthus argued that human passions inextricably lead to geometric rates of population growth while food supplies lag behind, growing only arithmetically. The history of famines does indicate that in some cases differences between the numbers of persons and the amount of food necessary to feed them have resulted in famine. In many cases it was the shortage of agricultural *producers* relative to the remainder of the population that produced famine. According to Wallerstein (1974), the crisis in Europe in the fourteenth to sixteenth centuries was largely due to insufficient agricultural labor.

Critics of the Malthusian approach to famine have suggested that population pressures on food supply lead to innovations in agriculture that increase food supply. Known as the Boserup (1965) hypothesis, production intensifies by increasing the amount of labor per unit of land and the amount of land under irrigation. Julian Simon (1977) argued that not only does population pressure result in increased food stocks, but that without such pressure the overall rate of societal invention tapers off. This is "necessity is the mother of invention" with a vengeance.

He and others have argued more recently that, in fact, the prospects for the planet in the next century are bright: "If present trends continue, the world in 2000 will be *less crowded* (though more populated), *less polluted, more stable ecologically, and less vulnerable to resource-supply disruption* than the world we live in now" (Simon & Kahn, 1984:1).

A recent study by Kellman (1987) found little evidence for the classical Malthusian model of gloom; the "induced model" (Kellman's version of Boserup) also received little support outside the European experience. In other words, during the past 100 years, population pressures have *not* increased rice, wheat, or other grain production in Asia, Central America, South America, or the underdeveloped nations.

A variant of the Malthusian argument, developed by Seavoy (1986), asserts that peasant societies remain at risk of famine because of their preference for large families. Reflecting the moralism of Malthus, Seavoy (1986) characterized peasants as work averse, arguing that children are viewed as a means of lessening parental burdens. Dirks (1993) provided no direct test of Malthus but evaluated Seavoy's (1986) claims instead. He finds that societies that place a higher value on children are no more likely to suffer from famine than those who place a lower value on children. Dirks (1993) did, however, support Seavoy's (1986) contention that population density is related to famine severity.

The World Bank data set provides some support for the hypothesis that population pressure results in malnutrition. We find that a few of the host of various indicators of malnutrition are significantly related to population growth or population density. Countries whose populations grew during the decade 1980–90 experienced higher percentages of pregnant women with anemia ($r=0.472$; $n=72$) and greater percentages of children suffering from moderate to severe stunting ($r=0.234$; $n=55$). However, if we consider the indirect effects of population growth on factors that directly affect malnutrition, a stronger case can be made. Population growth decreases the percentage of GDP devoted to both public and private health care efforts.

Despite these findings, we are left without compelling evidence for a causal factor for famine. Population pressure is not the whole story. As Devereux (1993) concluded, in an argument consistent with the Boserup (1965) hypothesis and with Cohen's (1989) assertions, famine may cause population growth.

The Entitlements Arguments

Advanced by Sen (1981), famines are seen as caused, in part, by entitlement failure. This view holds that starvation occurs because people have lost their "right" to food. Rights to valued resources are granted by entitlements, which in turn derive from economic, political, or religious institutions. Most of Sen's analysis focused on economic rights. Such rights derive from property ownership (land) or labor. Land can be used to grow food or rented out to obtain income and thus purchase food. Labor can be exchanged for food or salary. Entitlement failures occur during economic crises in which jobs are lost, food prices rise, and property is converted into cash to purchase food. Famines thus occur as people lose resources that give them the right to eat.

Sen's (1981) findings support his hypotheses. Support by other research, however, is somewhat mixed. O'Grada (1989) argued that while it is unclear whether Ireland experienced a crop shortage during the 1840s, Ireland was a net exporter of grain during this period. He argued that low wages kept Irish peasants from obtaining sufficient food and fuel. Dirks (1993) took up Sen's entitlement theory through a series of indirect tests. His data did not measure entitlement failure but do measure attributes of entitlement, the loss of which would increase the probability of famine. He began with ownership and argued that societies with communal ownership of land and tools are at lower risk of famine than those with private ownership of such resources. He also argued that societies in which reciprocal exchanges supersede exchanges through trade are less famine prone. Finally, he agreed with Sen's hypothesis that the dependence of food entitlement on social rank constitutes a "famine hazard." Dirks (1993) found support for the first hypothesis: Societies that place property rights with individuals instead of communities are more likely to experience famines. Regarding the second hypothesis, he found that while societies that rely on trade rather than reciprocity experience famines of greater severity, they were no more likely to experience either more frequent or more persistent famines.

To test the entitlement failure hypothesis, we would need, at a minimum, data on the worsening of economic circumstances for vulnerable segments of the population. The World Bank data contain no such indicators. However, the data do indicate that countries with lower rates of economic growth experience higher rates of poverty, which are associated with higher rates of malnutrition.

The Failure of Entitlement Failure

Some critics have argued that Sen underestimates the importance of absolute food shortages during a famine (Nicholson & Esseks, 1978). Arnold (1988) suggested that Sen is overly "legalistic" in his interpretation of entitlements. Sen recognizes that governments do intervene either to prevent famine or to alleviate its consequences after onset but offers no suggestion as to what "entitles" recipients to such welfare (see Dreze & Sen, 1989).

Famines occurred in peasant societies, which have been described as having "moral economies" in which the "right to survive" was frequently a fundamental norm resulting from the impact of famine (Scott, 1976; Thompson, 1971). Thus noneconomic entitlements ought to be investigated. However, a point often overlooked in Sen's work suggests that the primary victims of famine in this century are precisely those outside of subsistence relationships: landless laborers or small-scale farmers who depend on the market. Others supported this view by suggesting that famines result from major structural changes in society (Millman & Kates, 1990). While the United States has experienced no famines, hunger occurs when the economy is weak. This relationship may hold without the presence of major structural changes.

Furthermore, Sen and many other observers of famine have taken a static view. Walter (1989) argued that in England, as wheat prices escalated (his measure of scarcity), marriage and fertility rates lessened, thus absorbing the brunt of scarcity. He employed these findings to explain the lack of substantial impact of scarcity on mortality rates. Livi-Bacci (1991) used these adjustments made by individuals and families to argue that population growth need not result in famine. The severity of recent famines suggests, however, that lowering the nuptiality and fertility rates would have been insufficient responses to scarcity.

Finally, Sen and others convey an image of passive acceptance: Victims accept their fate because of their lack of entitlement. L. Tilly (1983) outlined the consequences of "entitlement failure" as the result of structural change and notes that food rioters express their outrage in terms of such failure. J. C. Scott (1976) traced revolutionary activity in northern Vietnam to famine conditions, which largely resulted from the imposition of the market on the peasantry.

Sen's analysis also pays little attention to other normative relationships such as those that bind members of communities together and citizens to a state, although again he recognized that states have intervened (Dreze & Sen, 1989:6–7). Such relationships may provide "entitlements" beyond those guaranteed by economic institutions.

Political Famines

"The Almighty created the blight, but the English created the famine."

In a recent monograph, Varnis (1990) claimed that famines in the postcolonial world are politically induced. Governments respond to crises in different manners, some of which may lead to famine out of "benign neglect or callous disregard." Varnis (1990) noted that famine-proneness results during economic transitions, particularly those involving the introduction of the market. Such transitions, as well as national politics, benefit some regions, urban areas, and certain ethnic groups while harming others. He stresses that it is the food policies pursued by the government, not the changing structure of the economy, that induces famine in the modern world.

Varnis (1990) chose post-Selassie Ethiopia as a case study of famine. The study begins with the takeover of that country's government by the communists. While Varnis attributed part of the problem to Soviet foreign policy, demonstrating that dependency theory's ideological blinders have led it to ignore socialist forms of dependency, the main culprit was the Ethiopian government itself. This government combined militarism with socialism to produce a command economy. To support the larger, more active government, taxes and procurement quotas were increased at a time during which population growth increased food demand. At the same time, food security for rural dwellers was considered a low priority. Furthermore, the famine actually worked to consolidate governmental efforts at centralizing the food procurement system and later became a tool in the political–military struggle with dissident groups. Government policies were also partially responsible for the ineffectiveness of Western aid.

According to Robert Conquest (1986), the Ukrainian famine in the 1930s occurred not simply from benign neglect or callous disregard but rather represented a means used by the Soviet government to further collectivization, as well as eliminate a class of peasant known as the kulaks. The kulaks were middle peasants who prospered by money lending. Ideologically, the group was designated not only as the peasant equivalent of the bourgeoisie but also as an enemy of socialism.

The U.S. government has stood accused of using starvation as one of many tools in dealing with Native Americans (unsafe food was another). While the intentions were no more benign than those pursued by socialist governments, U.S. policies were less effective in terms of numbers killed than were either the Soviet or Ethiopian governments.

A final example is Kampuchea (formerly Cambodia). The Kampuchean government surmised that to achieve socialism, all Western (and thus capitalist) influence first had to be eliminated. This was accomplished by the forcible displacement of urban dwellers to rural areas and the extermination of those individuals, as well as others identified as having the stamp of Western influence (such as knowledge of a foreign language or wearing glasses). Methods of dispatch ranged from outright execution to starvation.

Warfare

Historically, surrounding the enemies' position in order to cut off the food supply was considered effective strategy. Alternatively, shutting down the supply lines of invading armies can insure their defeat. The U.S. government's inability to inhibit the flow of material down the Ho Chi Minh Trail led to an eventual North Vietnamese victory. Famine has accompanied many of the major conflicts, for example, the purposeful starvation of the Dutch by occupying German forces during the Second World War. More recently, armed conflict in Africa has involved both purposeful and inadvertent famine. As Devereux (1993) described, war can set off a famine through three mechanisms. First, food production may be disrupted by drafting a significant portion of the agricultural labor force into military service or by destroying infrastructure such as irrigation systems. Second, interdiction of highways and other transportation modes can disrupt the distribution of food. These efforts can render ineffective attempts by third parties to provide food aid to those in most need. Third, military expenditures during peacetime have absorbed significant portions of government budgets, leaving little in the way of funds for agricultural development or food purchases during emergencies.

World Systems Theory and Dependency Theory

According to one view, food scarcity and famine resulted from "a great overriding cultural phenomenon, the world-wide spread and diffusion of a particular cultural system, that of North Atlantic capitalism" (E. R. Wolf, 1969:276). Colonizing states compelled the populations (or portions of those populations) into the market: they were forced to sell a specified amount of what they produced and were expected to purchase and/or produce what they needed to subsist. Wolf (1969) observed that the deprivation fostered by this system may be sufficient for riots or revolts, but full-scale revolutions aimed at transforming the system occured only when middle peasants were sufficiently squeezed or when rural revolutionaries linked up with urban rebels.

World systems theorists have made a similar argument regarding the effects of core relations with the periphery. While colonies have largely disappeared, left behind are weak nation-states unable to deflect or soften the impact of capitalism. The argument continues, noting that core countries export their "contradictions," which in Marxian terms means that the most egregious forms of labor exploitation no longer permitted within core countries now occur in the Third World. Furthermore, the "threat of capital flight to the periphery" serves to dampen the demands of labor unions and other labor representatives (Chase-Dunn, 1989:221).

The penetration of capitalism into the Third World results in dependency, destruction of indigenous industry, and placement in trade relations whose terms are sufficiently unfair to cripple agricultural development. Frank (1978) and others have described this process as "de-development."

Harriet Friedmann (1991) has focused on food as it becomes a commodity in the world system. She has developed a concept called the "international food order," which describes food relations between the core and periphery after the Second World War. This order is driven by food surpluses produced by core countries (which occur to placate domestic farmers who would otherwise become restive over low prices). These surpluses are placed on the international market at relatively cheap prices, broadening the market for American grain exports, opening new markets in the Third World, and creating a dependence on cheap foods by peoples heretofore self-sufficient in food production. Local producers in the periphery obtain competitive prices for their foods in the domestic markets of core countries. Countries with hungry and malnourished persons frequently export the very nutrients that would alleviate these problems (Christenson, 1978).

Critics of capitalism frequently point to China, Cuba, and Nicaragua as examples of hunger reduction and elimination of malnutrition. Certainly these cases should not be ignored. They suggest that when core country influence is excluded and resources are more equitably distributed, improvement in food production and distribution are possible. At the same time, the glowing accounts of socialized food production overlook evidence that in some socialist countries chronic shortages occur. Furthermore, the former Soviet Union for years has permitted a private market to exist alongside the socialized one in order to alleviate shortage problems. The Chinese have permitted a similar arrangement in more recent times.

Bradley et al. (1990) and Dirks (1993) both attempted to test hypotheses consistent with world systems–dependency theories, using indirect measures of external influence such as the introduction of new crops, intensification of land use, and increase in the use of labor and trade. The general argument suggests that prior to incorporation into the world system, peasants establish an equilibrium with their environments that entails using sustainable agricultural practices and seeking subsistence rather than market goals. These orientations are disrupted by the imposition of new crops, the loss of a subsistence crop, expansion of resource exploitation, and market relations. Dirks (1993) found, however, that such changes, while frequent during the past 100 years, are not significant predictors of famine occurrence. However, expanded land use was significantly related to famine severity in the predicted direction.

Returning to the findings from the World Bank data set discussed in Chapter 5, we find that higher levels of malnutrition occur largely in countries in which poverty is high. Those countries have not only low rates of economic growth but also increasing levels of debt dependency (foreign debt/value of exports). Thus, the world systems–dependency theory arguments receive some support.

CONSEQUENCES OF FAMINE

One clear consequence of a famine is the loosening, if not destruction, of traditional social patterns. Less evident, however, is the permanence of such change.

Among those social relationships altered by famine include those between patron and client. Patrons either refuse to maintain obligations to help clients or lack the resources to do so. The normal safety net for many peasants thus disappears, as does the patron's ability to achieve certain goals. How such disruptions affect trust and the reestablishment of a long-term patron–client relationship has never received study.

Certain occupational classes likely suffer more than others. Whole occupations may disappear as the goods and services they provide become luxuries. Among the hardest hit include barbers, clothing makers, and other artisans and tradespersons.

Gender Roles

One group highly affected by famine is women. Many of women's most important roles cannot be successfully accomplished, particularly those having to do with agricultural production and storage. Enactment of food preparation roles also becomes difficult. As women are primarily responsible for food production and consumption activities, they would appear to be rendered irrelevant by famines.

However, famines also opened up jobs to women that they normally do not fill, such as road construction. These "opportunities," however, did not signify upward mobility, were temporary until the famine ended, and were not necessarily desirable from a subsistence point of view (Arnold, 1988).

In some circumstances, husbands abandoned their wives or sold them into slavery. Those abandoned frequently resorted to prostitution in order to survive (Arnold, 1988). Such events represent personal calamities but not permanent alterations of social structure per se.

Finally, while researchers such as Ogburn and Thomas (1922) documented long-term consequences for family formation and family dissolution caused by economic change, studies of disaster have detected few such impacts on either families or the economic well-being of the communities involved (Friesema, Caporaso, Goldstein, Lineberry, & McCleary, 1979; Wright & Rossi, 1981). Famines may thus cause less social change than might be expected.

Social Mobility

Other changes reflecting downward mobility taken alongside those mentioned above may as a whole represent a deepening of inequality. In addition to the increase of persons in servitude, others descend the status ladder through the loss of land ownership. Repeated crop failures frequently lead to indebtedness; in addition, the need for resources for simple survival drive many to sell the little land in their possession.

Downward mobility is a likely prospect for many during a prolonged period of dearth. To survive, savings and assets will be progressively drawn down, starting with household goods such as cooking utensils and extra livestock. As the period of hardship lengthens, productive assets are sold. This may include the sale of land and productive animals (Webb, von Braun, & Yohannes, 1992). The wealthy may in fact increase their resources during such periods, as they take advantage of those desperate to convert assets into food (Colson, 1980). These strategies parallel those undertaken by households in ancient Greece during times of famine. Households began by drawing down nonessential resources but, as the crisis continued, were increasingly forced to convert capital assets into emergency food supplies. Gallant (1991) noted that the strategy, pursued to its extreme, left families unable to recover financially after the crisis had ended.

In some cases, these changes result in the proletarianism of agricultural labor as landless peasants exchange work for resources. In many instances, however, instead of rendering relationships more capitalistic, semifeudalism is the likely outcome.

Social Deviance

Case studies of famine often allude to increases in social deviance. Sorokin (1975) [1922] provided data for periods during food shortages indicating increases in property crimes. Ethnographers describe reports of increased theft in peasant societies in times of famine. Others note that prostitution and the sale of children increased during such calamities. Sorokin (1975) [1922] characterized these increases in terms of a moral breakdown caused by the physiological changes that result from hunger. The physical and psychological changes described by Keys, Brozek, Henschel, Micklesen, and Taylor (1950) lent some credence to this argument. However, it is equally likely that long before such changes occur, individuals and groups come to perceive theft as a reasonable response to their predicament. Such individuals may have lost or never possessed the informal safety net enjoyed by others.

Survival Responses

Dirks (1980) argued that response to famine varies with the level of deprivation experienced. Initially, victims drew heavily on existing social relations for aid. Investments in relationships, established for the very purpose of coping with dearth, were drawn upon. Locally, food sharing, once a symbolic necessity in some communities, was restricted to immediate kin. Similarly, in situations of deprivation involving nonkin groups such as military units, individuals limited sharing reciprocity to dyadic groups (Dirks, 1980). Part of these cooperative efforts were devoted to guarding against theft. As the participants exhausted their supplies and energy, the family itself no longer functions as a source of protection and redistribution: individuals began to fend for themselves (Dirks, 1980). Children and elderly members were sent away in hopes that relatives living outside the famine zone will take them in.

Social Protest

The histories of many countries include riots, strikes, and demonstrations over the lack of food or its price. Tilly, Tilly, and Tilly (1975) and Bouton (1993) documented numerous food riots in France during the nineteenth century resulting from food exports from areas experiencing food shortages.

There may also be organized attempts to influence governmental policy, although this is rare in peasant societies, given the normal relationship between "citizen" and government. In this century, as governments are increasingly held accountable for what happens to their people, such organized efforts might have a bearing on elections or where these elections are held, or cause a shake-up in government from the top.

Food riots occur not during famines but during times in which dearth and famine are anticipated. The so-called Flour War in France took place nearly 60 years after the last famine in that country (Bouton, 1993). These and other riots appeared as a response to changes in state policy regarding state guarantees or state entitlements: A policy of laissez-faire replaced governmental regulations over the flow of food in and out of communities. Food riots during the latter part of the twentieth century have resulted from similar economic environments: reduction in governmental price controls and other safety-net programs in response to pressure from the International Monetary Fund (Walton & Seddon, 1994). In exchange for a rescheduling of external debt repayments, countries were persuaded to reduce or eliminate social programs as a means of reducing the governmental budget. As a result, 39 countries experienced 146 food riots during the period from January 1976, to October 1992; more than 10 riots per country took place in Peru, Argentina, Bolivia, and Brazil (Walton & Seddon, 1994).

Is there any evidence that food riots and social protests become revolutionary forces of change? The answer is unclear. Certainly famines are associated with revolutions in a temporal sense in that they frequently occur at the same time, but they seem to lack sufficient causal force on their own. Only when coupled with general economic crises, loss of legitimacy by a government, failure of governmental policies, and dissolution of elite alliances, did states break down and revolutions occur (Goldstone, 1991). Revolts in China occurred after repeated famines led to the "loss of the Mandate of Heaven," causing dynastic but not structural change (Yates, 1990).

Shepard (1975) argued that the Ethiopian monarchy fell because of its inadequate response to famine. However, the participants in the overthrow were not those most affected by the dearth. Famine victims may engage in civil disorder and theft but generally lack the physical strength and endurance to involve themselves in long-term, well-organized actions aimed at political change (Dirks, 1980).

Many countries have experienced famine without undergoing a revolution, and a number have undergone a revolution without having had famine. Thus, famine is neither a necessary nor sufficient cause of revolutions.

Famines as Stress

The impact of stress on the health of ordinary individuals is a much studied topic. Stress is found to adversely affect mental health and physical health. Some researchers have suggested, however, that individuals react differently to stress. Some may "rise to the occasion" and grow personally as a result of a famine experience.

Antonovosky (1987) noted that those concentration camp inmates who survived did so by a willingness to take risks and engage in innovative behavior. Research on the long-term effects of the Great Depression revealed that women who entered the labor force at that time experienced not only an elevation of status but also better physical and mental health 50 years later (Elder & Liker, 1982).

Do famines ruin the lives of the survivors? Do they carry away permanent damage and scars? Or do many of the survivors benefit in a fashion similar to those who underwent the Great Depression? The answers await further research.

WHERE IS SOCIOLOGY?

Sociologists appear among the last to take an interest in famine (if Sorokin's work is taken as an outlier), whereas medical scientists, geographers, economists, and anthropologists have written about famine for decades. This is somewhat surprising, given the involvement by sociologists in disaster research since the 1950s. Organizational sociologists and social psychologists have studied the impacts of natural disasters such as floods, hurricanes, and tornadoes (Dynes & Tierney, 1994; Haas & Drabek, 1973). Sociologists ought to take particular interest in organizational responses to disasters in terms of the effectiveness of such efforts, as well as the formation of new organizational structures during such crises. Extant literature on famine makes little mention of local- or state-level efforts to stave off famine or to lessen its effects. Recent work discussed efforts made by households and the social networks that represent a resource upon which locals draw (DeWaal, 1989). Yet we know from histories of China that both the Chinese state and local governments developed contingencies. In fact, social disruption occurred more frequently during times the Chinese state responded ineffectively to crises (Stavis, 1981).

While we should not wish for more famine, sociologists ought to consider the sociological significance of such human tragedies. They may then utilize their appearance as an opportunity to understand the impact of such events on social structure, as well as the response of social structure to such events. This would not only provide the discipline with insights regarding social organization but would also contribute to a more effective organizational response to disasters in general.

Sociologists should also take part in the search for the causes of famine; the World Bank data lend some credence to population pressure and world systems arguments. As more data become available, the entitlement hypotheses can receive a more direct test. In addition, sociologists can study the impact of inequality and changes in inequality not only on malnutrition but also on the development of famine.

8

FOOD AND SOCIAL CHANGE

INTRODUCTION

A major preoccupation of social scientists and historians is the explanation of the large scale, lasting changes that societies undergo over time. This interest has led to debates over explanans (what it is to be explained), causes, directional trends, and the role of human agency in change. Ideational and materialist camps point to values, technology, scarcity, economic forces, or exploitation as "engines" of change and identify changes in levels of living, culture, technology, resource redistribution, or social and other forms of complexity as outcomes.

Those who have taken a close look at history have noted the importance of fundamental resources in models of social change that utilize technology and population variables; some have gone as far as to implicate specific resources, such as energy, as key variables. Despite these examinations, most analyses have failed to observe that food (and its consequences for survival and well-being) lies at the heart of many social change theories. Concepts such as technology, surplus, and price and income frequently serve as surrogates for food production, food availability, and nutritional health.

For example, population size is principally determined by fertility and mortality processes, both of which depend on the food supply in quantitative and qualitative terms. Furthermore, much of the technology said to propel societies through history consists of agricultural innovations that permit populations to grow, economies to develop, and modes of production to alter. Recent theories of social change have begun to incorporate concerns for "human capital," that is, human beings in whose capacities and aptitudes can be invested in order to achieve greater productivity. Once again, food and nutrition serve as important factors and in this case as inputs to increase productivity. Finally, theories of revolution either explicitly or implicitly include deprivation as a necessary (but insufficient) condition. Much of such deprivation concerns insufficient food. While recognizing this is so, few revolutions actually occur during famines. Even *severe* deprivation apparently is insufficient; furthermore, the very severity of such deprivation may actually decrease the likelihood of revolution.

The goal of this chapter is to identify those theories that contain food implicitly or explicitly, determine continuities and discontinuities in the role that food is said to play in the theories and research on food and social change, and suggest ways through which such theories might be extended.

WHAT IS SOCIAL CHANGE?

Social change is defined here as relatively permanent changes in social structure, function, and process over time in a persisting identity (Nisbet, 1969; see also, Moore, 1974). Nisbet (1969, 1972) is from the functionalist camp, and his definition reflects this approach. The definition can be defunctionalized by removing the word "function" from it; the definition remains useful. Nisbet and Moore note that such definitions separate social change from personality change and individual changes that occur during the life cycle. The concern shown for defining social change and distinguishing it from structure and process is no mere semantic exercise, but rather is an attempt by observers to have the capacity to sift through the prehistorical, historical, and contemporary record to isolate social change and its causes.

In addition to identifying social change, a major theoretical concern lies in identifying forces of change. The candidates are few, but debate continues unabated over whether demographic pressures, technology, exploitation, or some combination of these forces represent the "engine of change." Of nearly equal interest is the issue of whether social change, particularly at the societal level, has a direction. Issues of whether direction equals progress, regress, or no moral movement also continue to interest these scholars. Finally, some have attempted to determine the degree, if any, that human beings can alter the nature and direction of that change.

This chapter attempts to show the critical role that food and nutrition continue to play either directly or implicitly in these debates. As with most theories of social change, the links between food and societal change serve as the focus. Richard Applebaum (1972) developed a taxonomy of theories of social change which I find as a useful jumping-off point. He argues that four main kinds of theories of social change exist: evolutionary, equilibrium, conflict, and cyclical. I will ignore the cyclical models as have most contemporary theorists.

EVOLUTIONARY THEORIES

Among the oldest and most hotly disputed approaches to societal change is the collection of perspectives designated evolutionary. Evolutionary theorists generally posit general trends in societal change over long periods of time. For example, societies are said to grow larger in size (population) and more complex (greater division of labor). Frequently, these trends are categorized into stages (Sanderson, 1990; Wright, 1983). Societies are thought by some to "move" along these trend lines or through these stages at varying rates, while others take a more multilineal view arguing that the trends or stages represent movement in a general direction, like the upward-spreading branches of a tree, representing the prehistorical/historical experience of societies as a whole. In addition, these trends are said to be unidirectional; most evolutionary theorists either argue against or ignore regressive tendencies.

Two main types of evolutionary theories stand out. These are the materialistic and the ideological. The majority of the theories, especially the contemporary ones, take the materialist view and so will this chapter. However, as the chapter on food and culture indicates, consumerism as a form of ideational change implicates food. In addition, the material approaches have split into two major camps: population-push and technological-pull (Matras, 1979).

Both population-push and technological-pull theories posit stages through which societies and/or civilization have passed. Technological rather than demographic factors differentiate these stages, and the majority of the stages are distinguishable by their food-producing technology. Table 8.1 provides some prominent illustrations of conceptual schemes of stages.

Population-Push Models

Population theories are similar to ecological theories in that they assume, under normal circumstances, an equilibrium between a given population size and the environment in which it operates. Much of the interchange between population and environment is physical and biological (Miller, 1978), but in human populations cultural and social factors play important parts in balancing human demands and environmental output. The culture component of technology provides the means by which the population meets its needs; culture, at the same time, works to minimize the impact of resource extraction on the environment's ability to regenerate. A variety of forces occasionally disturbs this equilibrium. Overuse of the environment, for example, results in its degradation (Geertz, 1963; Wilkinson, 1973) and may also lead to declining population size (Meadows, Meadows, Randers, & Behrens, 1974). Animals are as capable of overpopulation as people, resulting in their starvation, inability to produce offspring, and so forth (Wynne-Edwards, 1962).

Malthusian models propose that populations suffer the consequences of lack of control in the face of relatively inflexible conditions. Evolutionists argue, however, that human populations learn how to intensify the exploitation of resources through the application of new technology. Thus, most of those who hold

Table 8.1. Evolutionary Stages and Their Principal Technology

Name	Stages and their technology					
Lewis Henry Morgan	*Savagery* Lower-Middle-Upper Fishing, bow, pots, fire, and Arrow	*Barbarianism* Lower-Middle-Upper Domestication of animals and plants	*Civilization* Alphabet and writing			
Leslie White	*Agricultural revolution* Domestication of plants	*Fuel revolution* Harnessing of inanimate sources of power				
Colin Clark	*Hunting and gathering*	*Horticulture*	*Agriculture*	*Industrial*		
Gerhard and Ann Lenski	*Hunting and gathering* Spear	*Horticultural* Spear thrower Plant domestication	*Advanced horticulture* Bronze	*Agricultural* Plow	*Advanced agricultural* Iron	*Industrial* Harnessing of inanimate sources of power

this general view would agree with the statement: "Necessity is the mother of invention."

Some Examples of Population-Push Theories

Herbert Spencer (1892) argued that true progress is measured by human happiness, which is obtained from the increasing living standard. Level of living, in turn, improved because of increases in technology and division of labor, which themselves resulted from a growing population *and* competition with other societies.

Competition ultimately ceases to instigate technological and structural changes as society changes from a military to a commercial type; once technology and an increasing division of labor have created a high degree of rationality among the societal members, fertility is voluntarily curtailed. When these two necessary causes of technological and structural change stabilize, the entire process ceases. By this time, according to Spencer, a utopian condition of sorts is reached.

Spencer stated little about food production or consumption, and his description of technology and its change focuses primarily on military technology, but food is implied in both his level of living and competition concepts. Spencer's thought had a certain currency, flamboyantly represented by Julian Simon (1977). Simon, an economist, argued that while technological change creates higher standards of living, this change was driven by necessity. Simon (1977) proposed a theory and provided a partial test of it; he also entered the public policy debates regarding population growth and immigration. He is opposed to growth controls (fertility limiting programs, for example) both in the more and less developed countries, arguing both will stagnate without population growth.

Durkheim (1933) [1893] also argued that competition for scarce resources under conditions of increased "moral density" leads to a more complex and increasingly interdependent society. Durkheim (1933) [1893] made no explicit mention of food production or consumption; again these appear implicit.

Food Stress and Population-Push

In 1965, Ester Boserup published her path breaking book, *The Condition of Agricultural Growth*, in which she argued that human societies innovate only out of desperation: when their population growth caused "crises of subsistence" (Cohen, 1990). Minnis (1985) has argued that other means of escaping food stress, such as migration or increasing stratification to permit the survival of some, make it possible to avoid such change. In many instances, however, farmers intensified their efforts, bringing under cultivation more land (much of it marginal), establishing irrigation where none existed, etc. Some of their efforts required new technology; all of these, according to Boserup, involved a greater application of the agriculturists' time to their new production. She went as far as to suggest that in early agriculture, the production return increased less rapidly than the labor input. Or in other words, labor was utilized less efficiently. However, as labor was the factor of production most available, its increased use was not surprising. Boserup (1983:208) herself argued that without population pressure, the "positive effects" of infrastructural and technological change would not have occurred.

Minnis (1985) presented further evidence, based on "prehistoric" Southwestern agricultural groups, that suggested during periods of periodic food stress, one technique of survival was to increase interdependence with others, particularly other societies, through trade relations. Similarly, many historians concerned with the links between population, food scarcity, famine, and mortality in Europe have observed that famines there became a thing of the past once sufficient economic interdependence and agriculture development occurred (Gould, 1987; Walter, 1989).

No single convincing set of empirical evidence has appeared to demonstrate the superiority of population-push arguments, but numerous historical periods evidenced population pressure followed by technological changes, especially in agricultural production. However, the heavy plow was propelled across Europe by the economic advantages it offered rather than by the necessity to feed an ever increasing number of mouths (Jones, 1981:50–51).

Demographic conditions create other kinds of pressures as well. Underpopulation can bring societies to the state of economic collapse, stimulating change. In a compelling picture painted by Wallerstein (1974), thirteenth-century Europe, thanks to repeated wars, crop failure, and plague, experienced population shortages. This resulted in lowered food production and then a food crisis. The Western European response was to utilize recent innovations in navigation and shipbuilding in order to explore the world in search of cheap carbohydrates (Wallerstein, 1974).

As convincing as the cases of demographic pressure appear, there exist historical periods in which technological change occurs in the absence of demographic pressures (e.g., twentieth-century U.S. agriculture, which has undergone a tremendous revolution during a time of steady-state population dynamics) and periods in which high population growth stimulates little in the way of agricultural improvement (e.g., twentieth-century Third World countries).

Technological-Pull Models of Evolution

Societies evolve because of conditions that promote inventiveness, according to some evolutionary theorists. One branch suggests that a given society produces innovations to the degree in which it has a large base of knowledge with which to work and encourages innovation by rewarding experimentation and reducing risk (Lenski & Lenski, 1987; Ogburn, 1950).

Furthermore, Ogburn and Lenski and Lenski argued that new knowledge creation is an accumulative process, based on the combination and recombination of existing ideas. From this perspective, discoveries do not exist: A new idea cannot come "out of the blue."

Lenski and Lenski (1987) provided a number of interesting illustrations of how the recombination of existing ideas came to revolutionize food production. Hunters and gatherers discovered, largely by accident, the secret of seeds. They may have even begun to broadcast seeds to make gathering more predictable before they began to engage in actual sedentary agriculture (Cohen, 1990). Seeds were planted through the means of a digging stick, developed initially from a hunting spear (Lenski & Lenski, 1987).

Other technological changes have no bearing on production nor do they necessarily involve material objects. Instead, social organizational changes may take place that affect distribution of resources, particularly food. Service (1975) has made the most compelling case for this, arguing that small bands of individuals, well-adapted to various niches in a local environment, found that seasonal scarcities could be avoided by storing collectively what they extracted or produced from their respective microenvironments. These materials were then redistributed among the bands when needed. A "chief" represented the organizational innovation that allowed this survival mechanism to work, in that the communities involved turn over to this role control of the storage and redistribution of this food.

Furthermore, Post (1985) demonstrated that those countries of Europe that developed laws and organizations designed to deal with subsistence crises experienced lower mortality rates during the morality peak of the 1740s. Parish poor laws in both England and Scotland and public granaries in Denmark and Prussia insulated these countries from the worst effect of the crisis.

Other Applications to Food

Most evolutionary theories have ignored changes in consumption other than in terms of necessity. Lifestyle changes were either ignored or given only passing attention. For instance, the Lenskis (1987) argued that living standards improve as a by-product of technological changes. Better living standards occurred from the differentiation-specialization that surplus production of food supplies permits. Occupational specialization led to craftsmanship and a series of innovations instigated by both the craftsmen and their patrons. Cuisine (as opposed to cooking) may have evolved in this manner (see Goody, 1982).

Furthermore, the evolution of lifestyles opens up a realm of differing possibilities regarding the explanation of technological change, for evolutionary theory ordinarily focuses on technology that directly bears on basic necessities. Once "nonnecessity" types of change are included, "necessity is the mother of invention" represents a less compelling argument. Ideational theories, explored in some detail in Chapter 3, may account for such change.

EQUILIBRIUM THEORIES

The Malthusian Model

Population growth and its consequences have inspired both equilibrium and evolutionary theories and have provided a counterpoint to Marxian theories of social change. Population theories began with Malthus's *Population: The First Essay* (1959) [1798]. The 1959 edition's foreword, written by Kenneth Boulding, described the essay as "almost like a modern Book of Job" (p. viii). Malthus (1959) [1798] believed that (1) population growth would always out-strip the growth in food supply, (2) when such disparities reached a certain point, they were adjusted by mortalities caused by famine, disease, warfare, and (3) that human actions, either in the realm of agricultural increase or fertility decrease, were not possible. According to Malthus (1959) [1798], a population equilibrium was achieved, largely through "misery and vice."

The role of food scarcity or famine in Malthusian theory is of interest. Malthus viewed famine as a check on population growth, along with disease and warfare. The relative importance of famine in the Malthusian model has recently received new attention. Using available wheat prices and mortality data in England during two famines (1597 and 1623), Appleby (1978) found some evidence for a relationship between high grain prices (indicating shortage) and high mortality, but the relationship was not uniform by region of the country. In a study of demographic rates and wheat prices, Lee (cited in Walter & Schofield, 1989:38–39) found that wheat prices explained 16 percent of the variation in short-term mortality rates, and explained 41 and 64 percent, respectively, in the short-term marriage and fertility rates. Walter and Schofield (1989:41) concluded that "the relationship between mortality and food prices was always very weak" and "was entirely broken by the mid-18th century." Watkins and van de Walle (1983:28) drew a similar inference, arguing that "dramatic mortality" appeared to have been "relatively rare, and, because populations could recuperate rather rapidly from a crisis, it appeared that famine was not a major mechanism by which the balance between population and resources was maintained in the past." These analyses suggested that food scarcities led populations to undergo self-adjustments.

Agricultural Involution

Human ecologists have proposed the view that an equilibrium exists between populations and their environments. The balance is maintained largely by controlling population through fertility and mortality. Imbalance usually resulted from interventions external to the ecological system. Geertz (1963) utilized this framework to explain impoverishment of both the population and the environment of Java. He argued that the colonizers of Indonesia (Holland and Great Britain) created a dual economy by developing only the export sector of Indonesia's agriculture. In this sector, plantations were introduced to increase the production of export crops, and these changes were followed by the industrialization of agricultural processing. Other extractive industries such as mining and petroleum were also developed. A small, modern economy was thus created in the midst of a larger, traditional one.

The impact of the modern sector was sufficient to raise Indonesian per capita income, which, in turn, lowered mortality and increased the population size (Geertz, 1963). None of the fertility checks associated with demographic transition emerged, however, and the population thus grew at a rapid rate.

Without a corresponding expansion of nonagricultural opportunities, the ever-increasing population endeavored to intensify agricultural activities (Geertz, 1963). This increased pressure on the land (reducing fallowing periods, etc.), and caused it to ultimately degrade. Once the limits to marginal improvements from labor intensification were reached, unemployment and underemployment increased.

Empirical Tests of the Equilibrium Model

Like many treatises of evolution, equilibrium approaches rely on historical and prehistorical materials for case study and comparative analyses. Quantitative studies are rare. Meadows et al. (1974) in *The Limits to Growth* used quantitative data to *project* future disasters. Population size and growth, agricultural production, and pollution production data form the basis of future outcomes using sophisticated modeling under varying sets of assumptions. One assumption, similar to that of Malthus, is that technological breakthroughs, which might raise the environmental carrying capacity to some new high, will not occur. Thus, the model predicts a worldwide increase in mortality resulting from widespread famine and pollution. Others using similar data, but different assumptions, have attempted to demonstrate that an "abundant future" follows from population growth (Simon, 1977; Simon & Kahn, 1984). In other words, with existing resources and technological innovation, increases in population will not lead to famine but a rather more comfortable living standard.

Some interesting historical tests also exist that pit the Malthusian model against others (abundant earth, induced innovation, science, and stages) (see Kellman, 1987). The abundant earth model is one based on the perception that utilizing existing technology and extensification of effort will compensate for any growth in population; induced innovation is a generalization of the Boserup hypothesis;

the science model stands for technological-pull; stages represent the historical sequences experienced by Western societies.

Using demographic, agricultural, and other available data from the period 1885–1968, Kellman (1987) tested each model. He did so by crop, by region, and by combinations of crops and regions. For the developed world, as well as the Third World, the tests supported both the induced and science models and to a certain extent, the abundant earth model. None of the world's regions, crops, or time periods (except for short periods of time) fit the Malthusian model well. Kellman's (1987) analysis, however, cannot be accepted with any sense of finality regarding Malthusian and competing hypotheses, given the absence of valid and reliable data for many of the key concepts in these hypotheses. As the discussion in the section that follows suggests, the crudeness of existing data as well as choices of indicators of food intake and nutritional status render any attempts at closure premature.

Food and Demographic Change

Critics have ridiculed Malthusian models for their sweeping yet superficial nature. They have pointed out these models' questionable assumptions regarding human nature and their simplistic view of the interconnections between demographic processes such as nuptiality, fertility, and mortality. Recent work by demographers incorporated a more systematic view of demographic processes, additional factors such as climatic change and urbanization, and a greater willingness to consider that the very nature of the interrelationships between demographic and other factors may vary over time and space.

The work by Livi-Bacci (1991), Floud et al. (1990), and Wrigley and Schofield (1981) suggest a greater degree of complexity than heretofore imagined. Livi-Bacci (1991) set out to alter the Malthusian model, particularly the relationship between food and population. Malthus's model claimed that improvement in food supply always lags behind population growth, resulting in famine and increased mortality. Livi-Bacci (1991) argued that only in the most extreme of cases did famine occur and thus, under "normal" circumstances of food shortages, morality rates remained below crisis levels. Populations adjusted to the harsher circumstances through reductions in both nuptiality and fertility. His case for this lack of association is based on the observation that other factors are involved that cloud the issue and that the nutrition-infection relationship is more complex than supposed.

According to Livi-Bacci (1991:34), "malnutrition is always associated with poverty, ignorance, unfavorable environmental and hygiene conditions, all factors which have an influence, whether direct or indirect, on the incidence, spread, and outcome of many diseases." Thus the role of malnutrition in the development of illness remained unclear. Furthermore, as infection lessened the absorption of nutrients, malnutrition might actually be an effect of illness rather than one of its causes.

Even when malnutrition was associated with disease, its influence and whether it increased the chances of death varied by disease (Livi-Bacci, 1991:38; see also Lunn, 1991; Post, 1985). Thus, an immune system weakened by malnutrition enhanced the risk of developing tuberculosis; once TB was contracted, the chance of death increased. The same could not be said for yellow fever, malaria, or plague (Lunn, 1991:137).

Finally, the human body could adapt to shortfalls in food supply through weight loss as well as stunted height (in children and early adolescents) and reduced physical activities. Thus, both reduced basal metabolism requirements and diminished activities permitted physical adaptation to reduced food intake and thus a decreased risk of infection (Livi-Bacci, 1991). As Floud et al. (1990) noted, however, shortened stature has consequences for productivity, which, in turn, may further reduce access to income and/or food.

Livi-Bacci (1991) generally was critical of theories of technological change, and he attempted to demonstrate with his overview of the fourteenth through twentieth centuries that technological change (primarily agricultural in nature) (1) only recently eliminated famine, (2) had little direct impact on the adequacy of diets (in normal times), and (3) had little consequence for demographic expansion and mortality. In fact, he noted that agricultural technologies that increased the quantity of available food resulted in diets of lower nutritional quality, which parallels an argument made by Cohen (1989) regarding the consequences of the transition from hunting and gathering to horticulture. Weak data undercut Livi-Bacci's (1991) otherwise impressive case; he relied on aggregate food supplies to estimate per capita food availability. Since such data are notoriously unreliable and because they provide no clue as to the amount of food physically consumed by individual members of the population, they are considered invalid as well (Evers & McIntosh, 1977).

McKeown (1976) focused on population growth in the "modern" period (nineteenth and twentieth centuries), arguing that improvement in the diet led to decreased mortality and that the decline of mortality was the consequence of improved agricultural practices. This reduction was achieved, according to McKeown (1976), not through a decline in the presence of infectious diseases such as TB but as a result of better diets. Neither modern medicine nor improved sanitation played a role in the decline of mortality. One problem with McKeown's analysis is that the conclusion that improved food supply decreased mortality was accomplished indirectly. McKeown (1976) attempted to eliminate rival explanations (interventions through medicine and sanitation) and then argued that the only factor left is nutrition. McKeown's (1976) case appeared less strong even than Livi-Bacci's (1991), in that McKeown lacked the data required to test his hypothesis.

The strongest case was made by Floud et al. (1990), who analyzed height data originally collected by a number of European countries for the purpose of ascertaining fitness for conscription. Height or stature reflects long-term nutritional status and is considered an excellent indicator of the standard of living (Komlos, 1994; Tanner, 1994). Livi-Bacci's (1991) intent was to explain the "long-term development" (growth) of Europe's population. The work by Floud et al. (1990) examined a more recent period (1740–1980) to argue that (1) improvements in nutrition, as reflected by stature, resulted in declining mortality, particularly when dietary change occurred with improved sanitary conditions, and (2) that improved nutrition resulted from increases in real wages (income relative to food prices). Thus, Floud et al. (1990) supported the general McKeown argument, although they showed that it greatly oversimplified the relationships among changing social and biological factors. However, the maldistribution of resources that sometimes accompanies development and unhealthy conditions brought about by rapid urbanization lessened the impact of these improvements on mortality. Others have found that rapid economic growth frequently exacerbated income inequality, leading to decline in stature and increases in mortality for some groups (Komlos, 1994).

While Floud et al. (1990) appeared well aware of the limitations of their study, it is important to highlight some of them. Height data reflect both childhood experiences of malnutrition and infection; thus their validity as indicators of nutritional status is somewhat questionable. Second, while height data are far more accurate than food budget or food balance sheet data, the reliability of height measures obtained across a wide variety of settings is also questionable. Such measurement error, however, is probably random and is ironed out by virtue of large sample sizes. Third, such height data are restricted to young males, given the circumstances under which they were collected.

Before moving on to other social change perspectives, it is worth assessing the theories just discussed with existing information. The World Bank data provide the means to examine some of the hypotheses discussed in this chapter. Population growth during the time period 1980–90 had a weak but positive effect on both the percentage of pregnant women with anemia and percentage of children with moderate/severe stunting. Increases in population density during this same time period resulted in an increase in the percentage of children with malnutrition. Urban growth was positively related to the percentage of pregnant women who suffered from anemia and percentage of children under age five who had moderate to severe stunting. Increases in population density were positively associated with higher percentages of children under age five with severe underweight. Development of the sort discussed by McKeown and others also received some support. Increases in food production were associated with lower percentages of pregnant women with anemia; increases in food supply per capita were negatively correlated with the percentage of children under age five with malnutrition. Improvements in transportation, as measured by the increase in automobiles per capita (insufficient data were available for miles of road per capita), were associated with lower percentages of all measures of malnutrition.

CONFLICT THEORIES OF SOCIAL CHANGE AND FOOD

Social conflict is defined as the struggle between groups over scarce resources, which can include material objects such as food, land, water, and so on as well as the nonmaterial such as status or prestige. Such struggles involve nonviolent competition as well as violent conflict. We have already discussed social class differences as well as competition in earlier chapters but only in a static sense. Here we are concerned with, among other things, how class competition is both the cause as well as the consequence of change, using food as a focal point.

Marxism and Food

Marx discussed the vital nature of food in terms of its role as a means of production as well as a product of a given means and mode of production (Cohen, 1978:53). It appeared particularly important in terms of his concepts of labor and labor power.

Labor is important in his framework because only labor produces surplus value. Labor *power* includes "strength, skill, knowledge, inventiveness, etc." (Cohen, 1978:32). It (1) helps achieve given levels of economic development (2) shapes the character of economic structure, and (3) affects the output of that structure. Labor power, furthermore, "conditions the character of the production relations" (Cohen, 1978:41). The value of labor power equals the value of those commodities necessary for a worker's existence. Such commodities include those for subsistence, socialization, and training, and for actual work itself (Blane, 1987). Subsistence needs, according to Blane (1987:10), "are neither fixed nor tied to a physiological minimum" but instead are produced by specific historical circumstances. Even within such a "relativist constraint," it is still possible to argue that each stage of history has its own characteristic form of labor power and thus its own characteristic subsistence need. Thus, each stage exhibits its own set of subsistence minimums of health. Aggregate nutritional health thus has a particular impact on labor power, depending on the "strength, skill, knowledge, and inventiveness" needs of that stage.

Human capital theorists of economic development, while not adhering to Marx's stage theories or needs relativism have also argued that only those societies whose labor force, including agriculture, has achieved certain levels of health, education, and other forms of well-being can advance developmentally. As described previously, Call and Longhurst (1971) and others have attempted to demonstrate the link between worker's health and the state of the economy by linking malnutrition to working productivity, on the one hand, and workers aggregate productivity and GNP growth, on the other. Improvements in nutrition thus led to increases in economic growth. From Marx's point of view, however, improving nutrition to increase productivity and gross national product left unaltered the fundamentally exploitive character of labor in nonsocialist systems.

Change of Productive Forces

As discussed in Chapters 4 and 5, Marx argued that the key to a society's character was found in its productive forces. The forces of production included the means of production (i.e., tools, raw materials, etc.) and labor power (strength, skills, etc.) (Cohen, 1978). The level of development of these forces determined the nature of society. Thus, the extent of the division of labor, nature of ownership of the means of production, and method of extracting value from labor depended on the state of the development of the forces of production, land ownership, and treatment of labor (Cohen, 1978; Winner, 1977).

Technological development continued within each mode of production until it exhausted its capacity to increase production (Cohen, 1978). Once this occurs, new technological development led to new modes of production. Thus capitalism replaced feudalism as a mode of production, after all possible productive gains from the technological improvement of this stage's agriculture occurred (Cohen, 1978). Each stage of development has an inherent capacity to develop and increase production. Thus the advantage of capitalism, according to Marx, was found in its ability to extract the enormous amount of surplus value needed to make socialism possible.

Some interpreters of Marx argued that it is economic and political relationships, primarily competitive in nature rather than the technological base, that serve as the engine of change (Miller, 1981). Thus Cohen (1978) would assert, for example, that the knowledge of planting sugarcane and processing it for sugar determines the mode of production (plantations) and the relations of production (slavery). Miller (1981), on the other hand, would argue that slavery and plantations are not simply selected for their efficiency but because of the profits they offer owners. For Miller (1981), new forms of economic production appear not through technological change but from economic competition.

Food production is only important for Marx in that it serves as examples of stages characterized by slavery and serfdom. Marx as well as Engles and Lenin paid considerable attention to agriculture in capitalist countries but belittled its importance for either capitalist development or in the transition from capitalism to communism.

More recently Friedmann (1978a, 1978b, 1980), Mann (1990), and Friedland et al. (1981) have examined agricultural labor under capitalism. Friedland

and his colleagues (1981) began their study of changes in the California lettuce industry by arguing that agriculture is a form of industrial production, and, therefore, changes in economic organization, technology, and labor and in the interrelations between these would provide useful insights into such changes in industry generally.

As in Marx's analysis of change in industrial capitalism, Friedland et al. (1981) noted that labor problems in labor-intensive agriculture, such as tomato and lettuce production, were frequently resolved through the introduction of labor-saving technology. In the tomato industry, this meant not only designing a machine that picked tomatoes but also developing a variety of tomato that could be picked by machine without suffering damage (Friedland & Barton, 1975). Labor costs in the lettuce industry, a labor-intensive harvesting system, were considered highly efficient. However, as much of the supply of labor was dependent on documented as well as undocumented laborers from Mexico, changes in U.S. immigration policy and enforcement practices might have adversely affected both the number and timeliness of the appearance of these harvesters. The greatest threat, according to Friedland et al. (1981), was unionization, which would lead to increased production costs. These authors concluded that further mechanization in the lettuce industry would largely be determined by the industry's ability to continue to control labor, and secondarily, by the economic structure of the industry itself.

Growth of Capitalism and Agrarian Change

Marx argued that only the transition from capitalism to socialism would require revolutionary means. However, students of revolution note that most occur in agricultural rather than industrial societies. Among the primary causes of revolution, according to these observers, were the effects of the penetration of capitalism into traditional agriculture (Paige, 1975; Wolf, 1969).

Eric Wolf (1969) examined six "peasant wars" that have occurred in the twentieth century. In each case, the peasant war can be traced back to the imposition of cash cropping by a colonial or otherwise intruding capitalist country. The intruding force required peasants not only to shift production toward cash crops but also to grow these crops in certain proportions, regardless of the potential effects this might have on subsistence. Thus, poorer peasants were pushed toward destitution. Wolf (1969) argued, however, that the so-called middle peasants experienced the greatest pressures, for not only were they expected to produce for the market, but their traditional obligations to provide aid for kin and clients in time of need grew because of these very pressures.

Paige (1975) essentially built on this argument, but forcefully demonstrated that the simple insertion of capitalism into a peasant society did not automatically trigger a revolution. Revolutions occurred only under circumstances in which agriculturists worked for wages rather than owned land, and where owners of the means of production owned the land but not food-processing facilities and thus could only earn more profits through squeezes on wages (Paige, 1975). These situations characterized sharecropping and migratory labor-style agriculture and led to conflict over land. Since land was scarce and was the only means of capitalist expansion by owners, no basis existed for compromise. Most peasant landowners avoided participation in conflicts because, if their side lost, they likely lost their land as well (Paige, 1975). Agricultural laborers with no land had less to fear during a conflict situation and were thus less conservative in their goals than peasants. In addition, their work placed them in close contact with one another, which facilitated their organizing and setting revolutionary goals.

In the hacienda situation, by contrast, owners had the same stake in land that their counterparts in sharecropping and migratory agriculture did, but hacienda workers had access to their own plots of land (Paige, 1975). Paige argued that workers under this circumstance desired an expansion of their holdings, but not necessarily an overthrow of the entire system. In addition, owning their own land separated their labor activity from one another and it also lent itself to a more competitive orientation regarding potentially available farm land. Gains by others might reduce the amount they owned. These situations led to what Paige (1975) described as revolts, which did not change the system appreciably but more or less successfully redistributed resources.

Theorists of social revolution have tended to insist on developing a single model to explain all revolutions (Goldstone, 1991). Some have found that in order to do so, they had to restrict the number of revolutions they examine (Paige, 1975; Skocpol, 1979). While it was a laudable goal to seek a unifying model for all revolutions, the complexity of radical change may elude the effort. Despite the critique of Skocpol (1979) and others of so-called deprivation models, the evidence collected by scholars regarding the diversity of time periods and settings in which revolutions have taken place indicate that food deprivation figured as a major cause. It was not a sufficient cause nor did its extent appear to have an impact on the success of revolt. Fear of deprivation lurked in the background of the French, Russian, Chinese, and Vietnamese revolutions, and it played a part in peasant uprisings as far back in time as there is recorded history.

Many theories seem to assume destitution as a starting point but focus on the structural conditions that affect wages as well as access to land and other resources. Wolf (1969), Paige (1975), and Skocpol (1979) take deprivation for granted. Others, such as Scott (1976) and Berce (1990), described in great detail food deprivation prior to peasant revolts. Regardless of the role of deprivation, these theories go on to consider (1) international conditions—pressure and competition from other states (Skocpol, 1979), (2) urban conditions (Walton, 1984), (3) the interests of the upper classes (Goldstone, 1991), (4) the involvement of the military (Johnson, 1966), (5) the organizational capabilities of oppositional groups (Tilly et al., 1975), and (6) state failure in ameliorating fiscal crises (Goldstone, 1991). Each of these factors may have connections to food not only in terms of its supply, but also in the nutrition this food produces. This possibility will be examined, in part, in the chapter on food and the state.

Furthermore, part of the inconsistency food deprivation seems to play in societal disruption may have to do with the superficial way theorists have treated food. In their work, food supply and perceptions of that food supply (relative deprivation) are the only food-related variables examined. None of these writers have attempted to examine how nutritional factors might impact on situations of social disruption.

Prolonged food shortages are associated with various forms and degrees of malnutrition. These, in turn, affect the ability to think clearly and to perform hard work or work that requires physical dexterity (McIntosh, 1975; Livi-Bacci, 1991). How effective as revolutionaries are individuals who are malnourished?

Revolutions are often not short-term affairs but rather of a protracted nature. An army made up of the malnourished is likely not to be an effective fighting force. In fact, with sufficient levels of malnutrition, the motivational energy to join dissident groups is likely lacking.

Unfortunately, these speculations will remain as such until students of revolution delve further into food and nutrition issues.

FOOD AND PROGRESS

A major debate rages over whether intensification of food production necessarily decreases the amount of leisure and reduces the efficiency of labor input (the Boserup hypothesis). Intensification from some points of view (Harris, 1974, 1979) was never undertaken voluntarily for it involves risk, less leisure, and less efficient return. Holders of this view provide ample evidence that indeed hunters and gatherers spend less time making a living than horticulturists and that longer hours frequently accompany innovations such as irrigation. More contemporary examples indicated that adopting innovations such as "miracle rice" (e.g., IR-8) involved adopting a new set of practices that are not only initially risky but also costly in terms of time expenditures (Caliendo, 1979; Dahlberg, 1979). At the same time, the history of Western agriculture clearly demonstrates that an increasingly smaller proportion of the economically active portion of the population can feed a greater number of persons.

A second objection made to the progressive nature of evolution lies in the concern for leisure. Humans are said to be worse off because they have less time to devote to nonlabor pursuits. Frequently, this critique has been made by those who find fault with standard versions of evolutionary theory for containing value judgments (e.g., Harris, 1979; Sanderson, 1990). The desirability of leisure, however, is in itself a value judgment.

Those who condemn modern societies for stealing the leisure found in earlier societal states are ideologically of the same camp as those who argue about the inauthenticity of modern societies or their preoccupation with worthless consumer goods, including the proliferation of "new foods," which many times are old foods in new packages. Questions may certainly be raised about the quality of the moral climate in modern societies given their suicide rates and high levels of deviance—attributes said to be largely absent from the idyllic life of hunters and gatherers. But we would do well to recall that these tribal societies experienced high rates of infant mortality and shorter life spans. Is it preferable to die from malaria or cholera than coronary heart disease or lung cancer?

Many of those who made such critiques consider themselves historical materialists. Marx was no defender of earlier, simpler times. The historical process led not to some final state that recapitulated the nostalgic past. In particular, Marx argued that the stages of history were necessary to achieve communism—in particular, capitalism was fundamentally important for it was the only system capable of producing the amount of surplus (including food) necessary to sustain people in a communist society (Cohen, 1978). As we shall see in the chapter on the state and food, neither socialist nor communist regimes had generated sufficient food surpluses to provide for "each according to his needs."

CONCLUSION

As we have seen, food production and consumption hold an important but often overlooked place in theories of social change. Food plays a vital role in evolutionary, equilibrium, and conflict theories, but the role goes unacknowledged by many writers. Economic development theories continue to argue for the special role that agricultural development is said to play in societal advancement. In world systems and dependency theories, it represents a fundamental tool for exploitation of the periphery by core states.

Having made a case for the relevance of food and nutrition in existing theories of social change, we should reflect on whether food and nutrition will continue to influence change in the future. Will food resources and the nutrition-impacted capabilities of societal populations continue to affect development?

I believe the answer is a qualified "yes." Invention of new agricultural technology continues unabated. Production of an increasing supply of food occurs on an increasingly smaller number of farms, particularly in the states of the core and the semiperiphery. A number of these changes involve innovations in biotechnology, rendering many financially beyond the reach of all but a few farmers, particularly those in countries of the periphery. In addition, a number of the innovations render agriculture irrelevant: that is, biotechnological substitutes for products such as sugar may eventually eliminate the need for many kinds of agricultural producers. Ownership of patent rights ensures that a company tightly controls the technology in question.

So what will diffuse? The answer lies with firms and lifestyles. Increasingly, as large-scale companies control food processing and its technology, the technology diffuses and becomes encased in branch offices of the corporation. Companies locate plants in countries that offer a combination of cheap labor and a ready market. The combination is, of course, potentially contradictory. A society made up of largely low-wage workers cannot generate much effective demand. Many companies seeking cheap labor require an educated labor force, rendering countries such as Thailand, with a relatively well-educated population, more attractive than countries such as Kampuchea where the literacy and school attendance rates remain quite low.

Food will perhaps continue as a relevant factor in revolutions in the next century. As Walton and Seddon (1994) have demonstrated, food price riots have once again become a prominent feature in developing countries. These may lead to revolutions as the economic pressures from the restructuring of Third World debt continues. In addition, the diffusion of lifestyles, and the products associated with them, has occurred at a rate previously unimaginable. These will continue to make significant material and symbolic changes in the semiperiphery and periphery and may lead to mortality situations that result from a combination of the diseases of poverty as well as the diseases of affluence. Social changes of these sorts may result from resource accumulations quite different from those of the past. In the past, new production technology created resource accumulations that permitted a few to live with more greatly differentiated lifestyles, but with time these lifestyle benefits were increasingly enjoyed by an increasingly greater portion of the societal population. If surplus accumulation increasingly occurs within countries of the core rather than the periphery, will the latter undergo the same or any recognizable developmental sequence? What form will social differentiation take?

In the process of societal development, food has proved a vital resource. Even late developers such as Japan depended on increases in agricultural production to fuel its growth (Murdoch, 1980). Future development may also rest heavily on technological change in food, but these changes may free food production from agriculture as food becomes increasingly a matter of biotechnological processes. In addition, much of food development will take place in processing and distribution. Advanced countries of the core will likely maintain their lead in these areas given the high degree of core penetration of the poor countries' economies.

Furthermore, do hypotheses such as Boserup's have a future? Will continued population pressures in the Third World spur technological change and foster social differentiation in such a highly interconnected world? We have every indication that population growth under conditions of societal interdependencies such as those created by membership in the world system lead not to induced development but to further impoverishment.

Finally, we still have little strong evidence that population growth leads to permanent food shortages, alleviated only by starvation or mass migration. There has thus been a tendency to reject Malthusian and neo-Malthusian conclusions regarding the consequences of continued population growth. Perhaps technology will remain a half step in front of population growth, averting a global Malthusian catastrophe. The consequences of population growth, at the very least, seem to guarantee continued poverty for vast segments of the world's population. Population growth may eventually lead to such levels of population density that when new rounds of infectious disease evolve, spread, and perhaps interact with lessened nutritional health that usually accompanies poverty, Malthusian checks may visit much of the globe. It is not clear that such growth will eventually come to a halt, as has been the case historically for Europe has developed out of high mortality through industrialization or its equivalent in agriculture. At the same time, societal populations have shown the ability to adjust to hard times by reducing nuptiality and fertility. Presumably, there are additional changes that people can and do make in response to deprivation.

9

THE STATE AND FOOD AND NUTRITION

INTRODUCTION

States play a major role in the production of food and in its distribution and cope with the outcome of food shortages. The state has used food to increase its power and to control the behavior of its citizens. Furthermore, social welfare has always centered on fundamentals such as food, and as the state has preempted local authorities, it has inherited social welfare responsibilities. Dealing with these responsibilities always occurs within a class context. Thus food and food-related health policies arise from the interaction of state and class interests. This chapter focuses on these and other issues.

VIEWS OF THE STATE

The state generally is seen as the governing unit within nation-states. Scholars conceptualize the state in a number of ways. Parsons's systems theory and general systems theorists considered the state as a servomechanism: a unit, monitoring the condition of the system and making necessary adjustments. Threats to the societal population, such as from food shortages, were anticipated and handled. Modern polities thus kept close watch on stocks and flows of grain to maintain adequate domestic supply, farmers' income to maintain political support, and imports and exports to maintain an acceptable balance of payments (Timmer, Falcon, & Pearson, 1983). The state may also make adjustments for market failures and attempt to sustain a "cheap food" policy.

Marxists view the state as the tool of the capitalist class; thus government policies further profit making and shield capitalists from adversity. Government health food programs placate members of the noncapitalist classes for the purpose of maintaining order. Such programs also serve to legitimize the general social order as well as the state itself. Others have argued that certain social welfare policies are also necessary for "production" and "reproduction" (Mann, 1990; Pierson 1991).

Several scholars have argued that because of the peculiar nature of agriculture and the need to reproduce labor, the state has intervened in the agricultural sector to an unprecedented degree (Mann, 1990; Mann & Dickinson, 1978, 1980). Human beings require daily infusions of food if they are both to survive and to function adequately on the job. Short-sighted capitalists in both the production and processing sectors of agriculture might elect to maximize profits by raising prices, but this would surely eliminate the ability of many to purchase adequate amounts of food. Such action would likely affect those segments of the labor force upon which food producers and processors depend.

Still others—some Marxist, some not—perceived the state as relatively autonomous from economic interests (Block, 1987; Skocpol, 1985; Tilly, 1992). States directly competed with economic and other political entities for resources. This potentially leads to pressures that might result in social revolutions in which groups fought for control of the state, not for its disappearance (Skocpol, 1985). States, from this point of view, demonstrate welfare concerns for those groups that side with the state and those that need co-opting. In addition, states may adopt policies that favor supportive interest groups (e.g., farm organizations). Finally, states engage in actions designed to control their populations. These may include coercion, surveillance, and behavioral regulation. In this chapter, these issues will be explored relative to food and nutrition and those groups most affected by governmental food and nutrition policies. This discussion is prefaced by an examination of the part that food plays in the rise of the state and the nature of social welfare and the state's role in providing it.

WHAT ARE STATES?

The state is the principal form of territorial governance (above the community level) in the world. Where it has yet to take hold, movement is in its direction. Thus, the former colonies of Western nation-states work toward this same status. At the same time, the imposition of "nation" as a collective orientation is not always successful or permanent, as present conditions in Eastern Europe illustrate. To avoid this problem, I will focus on national states, which Tilly described as relatively "centralized, differentiated, and autonomous organizations claiming a priority in the use of force within large, contiguous, and clearly bounded territories" (Tilly, 1992:43). The state maintained a degree of political autonomy greater than most other political organizations and functions as the guarantor of territorial integrity, public order, economic exchange, and social welfare.

The Appearance and Growth of the State

As discussed in the chapter on social change, states become possible after two conditions appear. First, surplus food sufficient to support state leaders and their entourage must develop; second, would-be leaders must have both coercive means and ideological justification at their disposal to extract this surplus from its producers. Furthermore, state power waxes and wanes, depending on the food resources within state boundaries and/or the food resources within other jurisdictional boundaries into which the state has the ability to intrude.

States first appeared during the period in which the largest, most powerful societies were agrarian. Only such societies had the resources to maintain such an organization. Functionalists like Parsons (1966) have argued that the administrative bureaucracy of the state was necessary to solve certain developmental problems encountered during the process of societal evolution. Mann (1986:26) described the state as that aspect of power exercised as "centralized, institutionalized, and territorialized regulation of many aspects of social relations." Others, however, argued that states were the by-product of a common set of cultural, political, and economic conditions (Tilly, 1975a). In one sense, autonomous states occurred and remained because no one state became sufficiently powerful to eliminate others and thus form an empire (Jones, 1981; Tilly, 1992; Wallerstein, 1974).

Words such as "rise" or "occurrence" mislead when used with reference to state origins. Building states occurs at the expense of others, wresting autonomy and resources from some and taking power from others. Tilly (1975a, 1975b, 1992) has devoted considerable attention to state building in Europe. Tilly's (1992) most recent work considers carefully the role of military development. Warfare appears endemic during early periods of state building (Carnerio, 1970; Giddens, 1985; Tilly, 1992). Armed conflict, however, places a sizable drain on the treasury and so more resources must be drawn into the treasury. In some places, state building relies on taxing merchant cities; in others, agricultural products serve as the fundamental resource. In the latter case taxes and food are increasingly extracted (Tilly, 1992). The state must tighten its considerable grip to successfully obtain these resources; thus local government and local military autonomy give way to trends of centralization and incorporation into the state. In fact, states that unsuccessfully pursue these resources likely experience incorporation by other states (Tilly, 1992).

Tilly (1975a, 1975b) and his colleagues suggested that the process involved (1) organization of a national military, (2) creation of an effective system of taxation, (3) formation of a police force sufficiently competent to maintain public order, (4) control over the food supply, and (5) creation of a bureaucracy made up of technical experts. All of these represented threats to the autonomy and resources (money, food) of the peasantry and to the authority and control of more localized political forces (magistrates), and it was these groups who resisted state formation. Resistance, at a minimal level, involved noncooperation. More extreme forms included riots and rebellions over the drafting of locals into the military, the imposition and increase of state taxes, and the shipment of food out of the local area. Such resistance and the state's response affected the form that the state took (Tilly, 1975a). Food riots, while not the most serious challenge to state building, represented the most frequent kind of protest (Berce, 1990; Tilly, 1975a, 1975b).

The food riot is of interest. European peasants operated on the basis of what Thompson (1971: 78–79) has characterized as a "moral economy," which included notions about the right to subsist as well as "what were legitimate and what were illegitimate practices in marketing, milling, and baking bread." The market and state were not simply abstractions opposed on ideological grounds but represented concrete threats to local survival. Food riots to lower the price of bread or prevent the shipment of grain from the local areas were viewed by participants and local officials alike as morally defensible acts (Berce, 1990; Kaplan, 1976; Thompson, 1971).

The ideological justification for such action was partially based on "paternalism": Markets should be as direct as possible, involving few if any middlemen; farmers should not hoard their products in anticipation of higher prices; the poor should have the first opportunity to buy these products; and markets were neither natural nor inevitable and thus not to be trusted (Thompson, 1971:83–86). Similarly, locals expected their magistrate to use influence to roll back prices.

The ideology of the "moral economy" has come under closer scrutiny during the past decade. Calhoun (1982) contends that the notion of a moral economy represented an "idealization" of the past: one that varied, depending on the group that drew on it as justification for protest. For example, outworkers and urban artisans, "whose prosperity was of recent origin," confronted higher prices for consumer goods with arguments that suggested that their prosperity represented a long-standing tradition and ought to be protected (Calhoun, 1982:43). Thus, their concern centered on higher wages. Rural peasants and artisans, by contrast, found their well-being directly threatened by the availability of goods and thus as consumers attacked those bent on exporting food to other regions.

Bohstedt (1983) observed that the occurrence and frequency of food riots correlated poorly with increases in the price of wheat; hence while rioters might have utilized a moral economy as justifications for their actions, other factors must be found to explain the unrest. These changes and refinements to the explanation of community protest and resistance take little away from the argument that a strengthening state benefited enormously from decreases in market controls and felt sufficiently strong to deal with any risk posed by local protests.

In most cases, the state's purposes were served by the operation of the market: it made food available to the army, members of the bureaucracy, and urban dwellers. The state was willing to provide some degree of famine relief in exchange for public order (reflecting the limitations of state coercive powers) but was increasingly less tolerant toward food riots, which came to represent sedition (Thompson, 1971). The market, and thus the state, won this struggle. Food riots themselves became less necessary as economic growth and the market made food more widely available (Berce, 1990).

Food riots remain a form of protest in Third World countries, occurring mostly among urban dwellers. These states have felt sufficiently vulnerable to coups d'etat and revolution that they have maintained cheap food and other welfare polices designed to placate urban residents, regardless of the impact on agriculture or other aspects of development. Recent food riots, in fact, represent a response to the elimination of such policies and their replacement by free markets. The shift, however, reflects less the increase in state strength and more the state's vulnerability in the face of external force. In return for the restructuring of external debt, the International Monetary Fund (IMF) has forced these countries to cut expenditures, including those that maintained urban living standards (Walton & Seddon, 1994). Even weakened national states, such as elements of the old Soviet Union, have recently experienced food riots over price and availability issues. They reflect both a weak state and an economy in the difficult transition between command and open status.

Social Welfare and the Growth of the National State

Many, if not all societal communities, maintain some sort of system to deal with food shortages. In some, responsibility lies in the hands of central authorities; in others, local authorities take charge (Garnsey, 1990; Yates, 1990). In ancient Greece, families had to rely on their own resources, social networks, and communal organizations for relief during famine (Gallant, 1991). Few city-states established granaries, although military garrisons apparently maintained the capacity to store food supplies. However, communities did develop arrangements to come to one another's aid during times of dearth (Gallant, 1991). By contrast, famines occurred frequently in both the Tokagowan and Meiji periods in Japan in which millions starved, yet the Japanese state, as well as local lords, made no effort to alleviate conditions (Hane, 1982). While peasants responded to such hardship with mass demonstrations and rioting, the Chinese emperors perceived famine as a threat to continued rule and so established granaries as resources for famine relief (Stavis, 1981).

In the period prior to the rise of European national states, social welfare remained a local affair. In the early Middle Ages market exchange was far less common than at present. During that period resource transfers were unilateral in nature and consisted of charity, gifts, dowry, and plundering (Cipolla, 1980). Charity included gifts to the poor and donations to the church. The well-to-do might give somewhere between 1 and 5 percent of their income to charitable activities; total contributions approximated 1 percent of the societal GDP (Cipolla, 1980:19). Much of what was considered charity consisted of donations to the church; English monasteries converted less than 3 percent of these funds into aid for the poor. The church was thus able to convert ideological power into considerable economic power (Mann, 1986).

The ideology of the church had a great deal to say concerning both poverty and charity (Lindberg, 1993). Briefly, the church's problem was not the poor but rather the rich, whose salvation was endangered because wealth was associated with the worst of sins, pride, and coveting the possessions of others. Humility and alms giving were considered major virtues. Furthermore, salvation lay through pilgrimage, renunciation, alienation, and asceticism (Lindberg, 1993:23). In response to the development of a money-based economy, greater emphasis was placed on renunciation, and pilgrimage receded in importance. A symbiotic relationship grew between the rich and the poor in that the poor offered a means by which the wealthy could work toward salvation through charitable acts (Lindberg, 1993). As the commercial revolution continued, however, sin was redefined again so that wealth no longer posed a threat to salvation (Hirschman, 1976).

Local efforts to ameliorate poverty included devotional confraternities and guilds. Alms giving and charity by members "not only accumulated merit for their members but also expressed a sense of brotherhood and mutual responsibility to their class" (Lindberg, 1993:43). The poor themselves organized on their own behalf: the handicapped and beggars also formed guilds. Paternalism and communalism had their limits, however. To begin with, only the communities' own poor could legitimately receive aid; others were driven away (Post, 1985). Distinctions were often made between the able-bodied poor, who were assigned to workhouses, and the more deserving poor (children, persons over 80 years old, those who were sent to hospitals or almshouses) (Lindberg, 1993). State protections were given with an eye to social stability.

The development of the state's welfare functions involves many factors. First, states established juridical functions regarding the resolution of local disputes, redressing wrongs, and restoring "rightful customs and privileges" (Mann, 1986:419). They included intervening in cases of inflated prices or adulterated foods. The state's primary duties remained largely territorial defense and domestic order. These increased expectations for the fostering of safe conditions for trade (Mann, 1986; Tilly, 1992). The commercial revolution, in the meantime, began to erode guilds, and with this erosion came the disappearance of an important source of social welfare. Similarly, these and other changes lessened the power of the church, and, once more, a traditional source of social welfare declined in significance. With the church's decline, its ideological power weakened, and was replaced by ideologies that ultimately formed the basis for the notion of so-called natural rights. These and other ideologies reduced the importance of charity as a duty (Mann, 1986).

Improvements in the supply and distribution of food are said to have laid to rest Europeans' fears of dearth and their attention then turned to wages and working conditions. These shifts, however, were slow and incomplete. Through the eighteenth century, the king of France was considered the "victualer of last resort" (Kaplan, 1982:72; see also, S. Kaplan, 1990), and even after the French Revolution various groups continued to call for strict governmental controls over the price of food to preserve the natural right to subsist (Sewell, 1980:107). In many states, however, the issues of food prices and access to food remained out of sight until the twentieth century. The study of these issues, the conditions under which they arose, and the response to them involves a different set of perspectives.

THE STRUGGLE FOR RIGHTS UNDER THE NEW STATES

Several competing theoretical approaches have attempted to shed light on the origin of both the modern welfare state's food and health policies. These approaches emphasize material interests over evolving ideology concerning human rights. So-called society-centered approaches emphasize capitalist class influences on policies that potentially provide them with benefits (or reduce their costs) (Boies, 1994). In their interests are policies that reduce competition, subsidize their operations, or exempt them from regulations. Along these latter lines, agricultural and other types of business have found it in their interest to resist health and safety policies that might cost them resources. State-centered approaches argue that policy-making reflects state interests that do not always coincide with capitalist class interests. State managers seek power and resources often at the expense of class interests (Boies, 1994).

State-Centered Arguments

As the state grew in power, removing autonomy, power, and resources from local sources, demands for rights and protection from market excesses grew. Only through struggle were protections similar to those experienced in the community retrieved.

Skocpol and Orloff (1986) argued that social welfare programs tended to go hand in hand with growing state power. However, the nature and strength of social welfare programs depended a great deal on how the state forms. In instances where "state bureaucratization precedes the emergence of electoral democracy, 'spoils of office' are not available to politicians" (Skocpol & Orloff, 1986:243–244). Instead, general ideological appeals and approaches to organized groups such as labor were made in exchange for electoral support. This scenario characterized many European societies. Where elections and political parties grew in strength more rapidly than bureaucratization, as in the United States, spoils systems are more likely the case. The outputs involved "politically discretionary distributional policies, such as financial subsidies or grants of land, tariff advantages, special regulations or regulatory exception, in construction contracts and public works jobs, not general welfare programs such as unemployment insurance" (Skocpol & Orloff, 1986:247).

Skocpol and Amenta (1986) have asserted that the broadest forms of social welfare occurred in societies in which, early in the state-building process, workers organized effective unions and social democratic parties to control the state. This characterization has been used to differentiate those European states that have more complete welfare states from the United States, a relatively underdeveloped welfare state.

The perspective taken by Skocpol and Amenta (1986) focused on relative state autonomy in which welfare policies were crafted by technical experts in the state bureaucracy. The New Deal has received attention, using this approach, and Skocpol and Finegold (1982) argued that the New Deal legislation pertaining to welfare provisions for farmers and consumers resulted not from the influence of consumer or producer groups but rather from university-trained agricultural economists in the United States Department of Agriculture (USDA).

Society-Centered Arguments

As Gilbert and Howe (1991) noted, the Agricultural Adjustment Act protected neither consumers, agricultural workers, nor small farms. Instead, price supports, favoring large-scale farmers, was the major policy outcome. Poppendieck's (1986) *Breadlines Knee-Deep in Wheat* suggested the irony of the situation that faced both farmers and consumers: prices too low to make a profit, incomes too low to purchase farm products. Like Gilbert and Howe (1991), Poppendieck (1986) viewed the New Deal's agricultural policies as the outcome of pressure by groups such as the Farm Bureau, promoting the interests of various commodity producers. She argued that large-scale farmers benefited most at the same time that agricultural labor suffered under policies that encouraged lower production.

Furthermore, Poppendieck's (1986) careful research on the origins of the Agricultural Adjustment Act and Agricultural Adjustment Administration (AAA), as well as the Federal Surplus Relief Corporation (FSRC), made it clear that the main thrust of agricultural legislation during the Great Depression was to support farm prices and only secondarily to provide food for the needy. The AAA was designed to increase the price of food to make agriculture profitable once more; the FSRC was indeed established to provide food relief, but its unpopularity among food producers and manufacturers led to its incorporation into USDA. There it received a new name, the Federal Surplus Commodities Corporation, and a new mission bolstering price support programs. Relief became a lesser priority.

John Mark Hansen (1991) used rational choice theory to explain the conditions under which lobbies affect the enactment of laws in the United States. His
case study involved the farm lobby during the period 1919 to 1981. Laws are not
always written by members of Congress, but their passage depends on Congressional support. Hansen (1991:5) argued that members of Congress seek reelection,
and they find that lobbies "provide political intelligence about the preferences of
congressional constituents, and political propaganda about [their] performances."
However, many more interest groups existed than lawmakers can pay attention to,
and this access was granted on the basis of a demonstration that the interest group
could provide more intelligence and propaganda than rivals and whose issues
were likely to recur. Hansen (1991) observed that the farm lobby had its greatest
influence for legislation during the period 1930 to 1945, when agricultural interests were united and when low farm prices represented a recurring crisis.

This competitive edge began to disappear as the constituency of the farm
lobby declined in numbers. While the farm lobby no longer exists as a single entity, commodity groups have their representatives engage in activities similar to
the earlier farm lobby. Commodity bills are grouped into an overall farm bill in
order to muster sufficient broad-based support. Congressmen who represent farm
districts have had to increasingly rely on coalitions with urban representatives,
who have provided the necessary votes in exchange for support for food stamp and
poverty legislation.

Producer groups may attempt to influence food policies by lobbying either
for or against proposed legislation. Their impact, however, is felt in other ways
as well. In a study of the food stamp program legislation, Berry (1984) traced
how producers' interests became involved in the actual mechanics of policy making. He argued that federal legislation was frequently vague because of disagreements and uncertainties among those crafting the legislation. Many of the
difficulties and uncertainties resulted from clashes between producer and consumer interests. This opened the door for administrative initiatives. The USDA,
the agency in charge of fleshing out rules and administering the food stamp program, developed their approach with producers in mind; "top officials in USDA
considered their primary constituency to be farmers; the clientele for food stamps
was of peripheral interest to them" (Berry, 1984:37). Berry (1984) evaluated the
food stamp program, noting that it was born out of the failure of the commodities
distribution program to make a real dent in eliminating hunger and was, in large
part, supported by Congress because it promised to increase demand for agricultural products.

The Decline of Agriculture's Influence

We can estimate the ability of agriculture to influence public policy by esti-
mating its economic and political power, although this can be accomplished only

in an indirect manner. Agriculture has maintained small but constant contribution to GDP since the 1970s. Its contribution to national income has declined slightly since 1970 (U.S. Bureau of the Census, 1988).

Agriculture's contribution to the dollar value of U.S. exports has steadily declined relative to other goods since 1970. However, these figures are misleading since the food industry contributes eight times that when farming and ranching are included (Browne & Ciglar, 1990:xiii).

Employment by the federal government increased by 7 percent from 1980 to 1992, yet the Department of Agriculture employed 1 percent fewer persons during the same period. However, the Department of Health and Human Services (HHS) lost 16 percent and the Department of Labor lost 26 percent of their personnel during this period. Total federal outlays increased by 151 percent from 1980 to 1992 in expenditures, but expenditures by USDA increased by only 86 percent, and outlays for the Farm Income Stabilization Program increased by only 90 percent. During this period, the HHS budget increased by 316 percent.

As previously discussed, the "Farm Block" no longer dominates the crafting of agricultural legislation, and the decline in political power has continued as rural areas have steadily lost population during the past several decades. While agriculture's influence on production and consumption policies may have waned, efforts to influence public perceptions and expenditures may offset some of the consequences of policies less friendly to the agriculture sector. Senauer et al. (1991) reported that agricultural commodity groups have increased their promotional activities, stressing by means of advertising, for example, the healthfulness of milk, pork, and beef consumption. Of greater significance, the economically powerful food processing sector has multiplied the number of groups attempting to influence agricultural legislation. While the decline in the number of farms continues, the number of interest groups with concerns related to agricultural production, processing, distribution, and consumption has continued to rise. More than 150 groups commented on the Food and Agricultural Act of 1965; by 1985, 215 organizations "expressed concern" during consideration of the 1985 farm bill (Browne & Ciglar, 1990:xxii).

Consumer Interests

Citizen interests have frequently received representation through social movements. The 1960s spawned a number of such movements, beginning with those promoting civil rights and those opposed to the Vietnam War. This activism and the success it seemed to enjoy led to further activism (Belasco, 1993). Some of it was directed at the food industry, whose response, once it was clear the criticism would not abate, was co-optation. Rather than deny that one's food was unhealthy, by repackaging and advertising differently, criticized products were redefined as health foods. A number of new groups appeared dedicated to doing something about poverty and especially about hunger. These included the Center on Budget and Policy Priorities, Food Research and Action Center, Community Nutrition Institute, and Children's Defense Fund (Maney, 1989). Such groups helped develop programs like WIC (Special Supplemental Feeding Program for Women, Infants, and Children). These activities have never had the same impact as those promulgated by producer and industry groups, who have achieved power by making substantial campaign contributions to individual candidates as well as the two major political parties.

Consumer groups generally have had smaller budgets than producer and industry groups and have achieved their aims through mobilizing public opinion and the legal system (Guither, 1980). Thus, in order for programs like WIC to receive congressional approval, the support of farm state congressmen was required. It was only when these congressmen needed the support of their non–farm belt counterparts for legislation benefiting farmers did such programs have a chance of passage. The continued decline of rural and increase in urban population, coupled with reapportionment of Congressional districts, have led to a weakening of farm interests' political power. For example, Browne and Ciglar (1990) found that as early as 1973, commodity groups no longer "reigned absolutely supreme" in the formulation and passage of agricultural legislation. More accommodation and the inclusion of new groups such as those representing environmentalists, labor, consumers, and others were required. Furthermore, the influence on national health policy remained: complaints by producer groups led USDA to delay for a year the promulgation of the "food pyramid"—an educational chart designed to illustrate a healthy diet. Beef and dairy groups apparently viewed the pyramid as a threat to the consumption of their products. To counter this threat, the Beef Council developed a poster for schools that unpacks the pyramid, placing the various food groups in a simple descending order. The poster suggested that those foods at the top are of highest nutritional value. A piece of red meat sits atop the list.

Hansen's (1991) analysis of the effectiveness of consumer as well as producer interest group pressure indicates that consumer groups have failed to consistently mobilize the public behind such issues of food safety, nutrition, and food product labeling, and thus remain largely excluded from the policy-making process. Consumer representation reached its peak briefly during the Carter administration with the appointment of consumer activists to prominent positions in the areas of food assistance and consumer and marketing affairs (Berry, 1982).

A Synthetic Approach to Food and Health Policies

In examining the origins of food, health, and nutrition policies, it becomes clear that no single theory nor recourse to ideological explanation accounts for their diversity. Block (1987) and Staples (1990) have criticized both "state centered" and "society-centered" approaches for oversimplifying the relationship between the state and society. States have reflected class interests, but those interests frequently have failed to coalesce into monolithic blocks (Goldstone, 1991; Mann, 1993). Government actions designed to aid some capitalists have harmed others. Even agricultural policies differentially helped certain kinds of producers: set-aside programs that benefited wheat, cotton, and corn farmers actually hurt bean and feed farmers (Bovard, 1991).

Contending interests of agriculture (some of which can be described as capitalist, others not), consumers and their "representatives" (public interest groups, voluntary organizations), and competing government agencies (USDA, USHHS, State Department, Office of the President) struggle for control over the direction of such policy and the resources needed to engage this policy. The outcome of such struggles depends on the state of the economy, the fiscal policies promoted by the Office of the President, political competition with other states, the interests represented by agencies, and agency interests themselves.

Histories of U.S. food policies indicate these processes. Changes in food policy have occurred during changes in the economy. The momentous initiatives of 1930's agricultural policy occurred because of the Depression. After the Second World War, a period of competitive world food prices led to a return to more "free market" food policies.

During the 1960s food policies were designed to (1) maintain farm prices insuring profitability for farmers, (2) dispose of surpluses generated by price-maintaining policies, (3) deal with domestic hunger, (4) deal with hunger in foreign countries, (5) enhance national security and international political influence, and (6) promote world order and stability (Maney, 1989; M. Wallerstein, 1980). Furthermore, by targeting policies various groups/countries could receive greater benefits or be made more amiable to influence. The Johnson administration utilized the PL-480 program to put pressure on the Indian government to force that government to change its developmental policies from an emphasis on industry to an emphasis on agriculture and to demonstrate unhappiness with India's general socialist orientation. During the Vietnam War, the Nixon administration targeted PL-480 food aid to South Vietnam, Cambodia, and South Korea, choosing to "place strategic political considerations ahead of humanitarianism in its food aid policy" (M. Wallerstein, 1980:194).

As Paarlberg (1985) observes, "food as a weapon" in foreign policy was limited and faced a great deal of opposition by producer groups. Ronald Reagan's first campaign for the presidency was based, in part, on a promise never to use food as an instrument of foreign policy. However, later the Reagan administration was found to have used food aid as a noncontroversial smoke screen for funneling additional military assistance to the Iraqi government.

Thus, differing political and economic interests drive food policies, leading to lopsided compromises in some cases (the food stamp program, Food for Peace policy) and weakened solutions in others (WIC). Food stamps were developed largely to deal with the general problem of commodity surpluses and secondarily to meet nutritional needs. Commodity distribution programs, while targeted at the needy, still largely function to reduce surpluses. Food for Peace aid has been used to reward allies and punish enemies, again with little regard to the most needy. The WIC program, while linked to surpluses, has never had a high level of political (or economic) support. While every county in the country is required to make food stamps available, participation in WIC is voluntary. Thus, in the late 1980s fewer than 100 of the 254 counties in Texas participated.

Health concerns that generate widespread public profits for the medical industry (Light, 1989) or receive organized scientific support (certain forms of cancer) have been those that got attention. Currently, prenatal care, including nutrition, has created neither the public outcry, potential profits, nor sufficient interest group concern to increase funding for research and programs to alleviate the problems. Widespread public interest in and support for consumer issues involving food have occurred only in those times in which inflation made food prices an issue affecting the middle class (Hansen, 1991) or when there was a "food scare" such as the concern exhibited over Alar residues, an insecticide used on apples.

STATE SOLUTIONS TO FOOD PROBLEMS

In addition to examining the role of food in state growth and development and how state food policies evolve, an assessment of the *effectiveness* of state food policies in alleviating problems is in order. This is particularly germane at a time in which the appropriateness of state solutions relative to market solutions to problems is once again under discussion.

The food stamp program has received considerable attention from conservative critics who consider it counterproductive welfare for individuals and unnecessary welfare for farm interests (Bovard, 1991; Maney, 1989). A more charitable view has asserted that the program works well because while it leads to little improvement in the diets of the poor, it releases money for other necessities that otherwise would have been spent on food (MacDonald, 1977). Still others argue that food stamps have improved the diets of selected subgroups in particular ways. At the same time, if success is measured by the degree to which a program reaches the eligible, food stamps must be declared only a partial success at best; many states reach less than 60 percent of those eligible. WIC has a demonstrable positive effect on infant nutrition but reaches even lower percentages of the eligible. Similar comments regarding reasonable impact on the targeted population can be made regarding Meals on Wheels and Nutrition Sites.

Foreign aid in the form of food has also had mixed results. In some cases, famine relief in the Third World has shown success, in others, failure (Varnis, 1990). Promoting agricultural development in countries such as India has had success. India no longer experiences famine and, in some years, exports more food than it imports. Evidence exists, however, that indicates a widening income gap between the rural poor and others thanks to the very success of the Green Revolution (Warnock, 1987). Indian food policy largely has operated to maintain food price stability and food stock levels for use during emergencies (Paarlberg, 1985). Others have noted that food aid actually increased food dependency (M. Wallerstein, 1980).

Many of the problems described above represent "state failures" in terms of ineptness or inappropriateness. Evidence of such failure, however, does not at the same time make a case for market solutions as the chapter on food and social class describes. Markets have made hash of similar situations. At the same time, state solutions to certain food problems have succeeded. Some of these have occurred within state socialist frameworks. Cuba, China, and Nicaragua frequently serve as positive examples for those who support strong state intervention. Data, when available, tend to be used descriptively by those defending these governmental efforts at improving health and nutrition and food production.

Work by Piazza (1986) offered a rigorous data analysis on land reform, food production, and changing health and nutrition. From the standpoint of food supplies and anthropometric measures of nutritional status, the Chinese are clearly better off than they were in 1949. Progress has been uneven across regions and a major setback was suffered during the famine of the late 1950s: millions died because of it (Piazza, 1986). Piazza (1986) argued the severity of the famine can be blamed on governmental ineptness. This particular study represents one of the best of such analyses available, but it has several important weaknesses. The regression analysis carried out to predict nutritional status examines current nutritional status, not its changes. Furthermore, none of the independent variables measure government programs directly. Instead, aggregate (province level) data on income, education, health, and agricultural productivity serve as predictors. Each of these may in fact be the result of government intervention, but Piazza (1986) did not demonstrate this. It is certainly arguable that without state investments, improvements in health and education might not have occurred, but Piazza (1986) himself noted that increases in agricultural productivity are due to decentralized decision making and strengthened work incentives permitting profit making by individuals through the "Production Responsibility System."

Similar problems with state solutions can be found in other countries. The current Nicaraguan government has found itself in a situation in which to earn money for foreign exchange, it has had to allow food prices to remain high and land to remain concentrated in the hands of large landholders (Frenkel, 1991). These two factors have long been associated with extreme levels of Nicaraguan poverty for a sizable portion of that country's population.to alleviate problems without decreasing production and exports, food aid has been made available. The government has thus performed more like a welfare than a socialist state.

A recent review of available evidence on the "nutriture of Cubans" indicates that while Cubans are better off than residents in most Third World countries, there is little evidence to support the hypothesis that credit should go to the revolution. It appears that Cubans are no better off today than they were under the Batista regime (Gordon, 1983). In fairness, countries such as Cuba and Nicaragua have attempted to develop under economic blockade and/or counterrevolutionary activities. These have led to the inability to export crops, disrupted harvests of coffee, and undermined other external sources of currency (Enriquez, 1991).

However, the evidence for state intervention is by no means entirely negative. Sri Lanka and the State of Kerela in India provide excellent examples of utility of state actions. Both Sri Lanka and Kerela had low GNP per capita and, given the usual state of affairs under such conditions, would have low life expectancy and high fertility rates (Mosley & Cowley, 1991). Both rates are in fact similar to those found in economically more advanced countries. This strong performance has resulted largely from state-created public health and education programs, which gave widespread access to both health care and schools (Mosley & Cowley, 1991).

Nor is criticism of state solutions to food problems meant as an indication that market solutions always work better. Radical change from state to market solutions lacks a strong track record. Hakim and Solimano (1978) observed that demand for food increased during the Allende years in Chile but declined under Pinochet. While the economy did not prosper under Allende, it experienced additional problems during the early years of the military dictatorship. Nutritional status and food consumption declined significantly, particularly among low income families (Hakim & Solimano, 1978). Many of the nutritional problems experienced by Third World inhabitants originate from the imposition of market forces from the outside (Whiteford, 1991; Whiteford & Ferguson, 1991).

Finally, the state has played a positive role in dealing with food problems. In spite of the emphasis on market solutions popular today, Dreze and Sen (1989) documented cases in which public action had eliminated famine and reduced deprivation. While local, community-based security systems were a vital part of public action, state "strategies of entitlement protection based on employment creation particularly in the form of public works programs" represent a highly successful intervention (Dreze & Sen, 1989:15). This practice not only reentitles individuals, but the payment of wages provides a market stimulus, avoiding the inefficiencies of government food distribution programs. Another state-established measure comes in the form of public food stocks. These not only supplement the market but also reduce the possibility of oligopolistic practices by traders, prevent price increases resulting from panics created by dearth, and fill the gap while additional food is imported (Dreze & Sen, 1989:265).

THE STATE AS A MEANS OF SOCIAL CONTROL

Modern states represent advanced forms of social organization. "They combine three sets of capacities: surveillance and supervision, specialization in intellectual labor, and military and police sanctions" (Jessop, 1989:107). These capacities have permitted the state great power over individuals, for it could "manipulate the settings in which human activities occur and thereby control their timing and spacing to a greater or lesser extent" (Jessop, 1989:107).

The state comes to rely less on violence and more on surveillance as a mode of control, where surveillance constitutes control of information and the monitoring of activities. The idea of surveillance as a mechanism for social control parallels Foucault's concern about the monitoring of institutionalized "disciplines" (Said, 1988). For Foucault, it is decentralized disciplines such as medicine and social sciences, rather than the state, that have provided social control. Interestingly, Lasch (1977) made a similar argument but suggests that the social sciences have introduced into the family the same rationalizing process found in modern capitalism, making it more fit for an industrial society.

In Giddens's theory, the state and cooperating institutions conduct this form of control. What Giddens has in mind pertains to vast accounting efforts conducted by state agencies, to obtain population information regarding agriculture, crime, health, and a huge variety of economic data. The themes developed in the novels *1984* and *Fahrenheit 451* suggest that states can enjoy a significant increase in their power relative to citizens directly through the increase in surveillance capacity offered by data linking. Various civil libertarian groups have warned of the dangers of seemingly innocuous video telecommunications. Others regard with alarm the potential mischief involved in tying census and tax data together. From such a perspective, the population census and National Health and Nutrition Examination Survey (NHANES) threaten rather than enlighten. The Foucaultian extension of the governmental uses of such data suggests that information about health and health habits can be used to formulate policies and laws designed to alter health habits in order to create a more productive labor force.

Turner (1984) drew on Hobbes's conception of politics as the control of bodies in time and space. He suggested a typology, based partially on Hobbes but also on Malthus, Weber, Rousseau, and Goffman. Turner deduced "four problems of order" posed by Hobbes's geometry of bodies. Two problems exist at the population level. These concern (1) *reproduction*: the problem of reproducing societal members or that of fertility control; and (2) *regulation*: the problem of controlling bodies in physical space (Turner, 1984). The other two problems operate at the individual level and concern: (3) *restraint*: the problem of controlling sexual desire; and (4) *representation*: the problem of expressing one's identity (Turner, 1984).

State interests also include maintenance of the *means* of social control, which, in some instances, require certain kinds of bodies. The quality of human capital in uniform may make a decisive difference in the waging of war. Floud et al. (1990) noted that the very real possibility of recruiting an insufficient number of fit troops led to the measurement of the stature of all volunteers and conscripts in nineteenth-century Europe. During the Second World War, as many as one-third of all draftees were rejected by the U.S. military for unfitness. Much of this was due to childhood experiences of deficiency diseases. After the war, the federal government embarked on a fortification program that included adding nutrients to milk, bread, and salt in the School Lunch Program. Recently, the Food and Drug Administration examined the results of NHANES and other studies in order to determine whether iron deficiency anemia was sufficiently prevalent to warrant the iron fortification of foods.

Of the four "problems of order" described by Turner (1984), the state played the greatest role in reproduction, although the modern state effected some degree of control over the other three. This perspective is consistent with what some view as state paternalism, or what recently has been described as the therapeutic state (Polsky, 1991). Furthermore, the therapeutic state is strengthened by attacks on traditional seats of authority such as community and family.

Policymakers in the therapeutic state percieved misery in terms of the personal failure to adhere to the values and rules of everyday life. Social workers were employed to identify marginal individuals, diagnose their troubles, win their confidence, provide them with new values and behavior patterns, and monitor them to insure against slippage (Polsky, 1991). These efforts included interventions into personal health care practices (e.g., smoking and consuming fats), which some characterize as "health fascism" (Edgley & Brissett, 1990).

State actions have, on occasion, achieved "nannyism." Furthermore, state solutions ultimately mean bureaucratic solutions (as are corporate solutions as well). Bureaucracy eliminated nepotism, cronyism, dishonesty, and incompetence; bureaucratic solutions lessened the inequity associated with traditionalism. However, the very characteristics associated with the salubriousness of bureaucratic action are now thought to increase inefficiency and dehumanization. (Traditional solutions might not be efficient, yet their dispensers are neither nameless nor faceless, but rather are communal/familial members.) Recognizing that state solutions have major problems or that the state has "gone too far" should not blind us from history. The history I have examined in this chapter is that of the state. I have ignored family and community history. Let us briefly examine these.

Much of the work on state and social control history have utilized "madness" as a case demonstrating that as modern social life and its attendant problems grew, the state and the human sciences were offered ever fresh opportunities to increase power and control by dealing with the increasing numbers of unemployed and mad (Clark & Dear, 1984; Foucault, 1973; Staples, 1990).

Perhaps state power and human science control benefited from these growing problems, but at the same time are we willing to carry the argument forward with Foucault by suggesting that these "problems" are nothing more than opportunities to exercise power? Unemployment, insanity, and the physical abuse of human beings are not voluntarily undertaken lifestyle choices, nor have they been especially amenable to communal and family solutions. Often families and communities have caused these very problems. Nor has market performance shown much promise in reducing mental illness, abuse, or even unemployment. (In fact, economists have long accepted "structural unemployment" as a natural element in a "healthy" economy.) Simply reducing state and professional power will not lead to the ultimate disappearance of unemployment, abuse, madness, food maldistribution, or the power of producer interest groups.

The contribution that the "human sciences" (I include both sociology and nutrition here) make to the growth of state power, particularly in the social control sense, has received little attention. The human sciences have increased state power, if through no other reason than their assault on families and communities, and have done so in exchange for state legitimization and resources. In the tenth chapter of this book, I present a critical review of the transformation of certain food habits and nutritional status into social problems and the potential disempowerment this process has had for social groups.

CONCLUSION

The development of the state depends on food. So-called new states of the Third World still depend on this resource, but the contemporary world condition makes it more difficult for these nascent organizations to derive the same benefits from their resources. At the same time, states increase their power by withholding food from ethnic and other groups within their borders, as in the recent cases of Bosnia, Somalia, and the Sudan.

Several centuries ago, the international marketing of food was at a low enough level so that indigenous supplies served as a valuable resource. The more open world market of today, with vast amounts of raw as well as finished food products available at low prices, renders indigenous sources less likely to develop unless other resources not widely available on the world market can be drawn upon. An increasing dependence on the international market for food may, however, render states more vulnerable. The embargo on imports to Iraq as punishment for nonadherence to United Nations' resolutions following the former's unsuccessful invasion of Kuwait indicates that an alliance of powerful states can prevent another state from obtaining food.

The state continues to rely on the market, under most circumstances. Only a few cases of command economies remain. In these cases, agriculture may be manipulated for various reasons without attempts at modernizing this sector. Modern states have greater power than their predecessors and have amassed regulations regarding many aspects of food production and food consumption. Yet the market relative to the state appears even stronger today than in the past. State reliance on large-scale oligopolies has lessened the abilities of the state to restrain economic actors. Economic power has shifted away from producers to processors and marketers. Agricultural producer interests have less effect on national policy than in past times, and this decline will continue as both the number of producers and the contribution to total GNP from agriculture decline.

Worldwide, food processing has become a 1,500 billion dollar industry (Rama, 1992) and has been a major element in the growth and development of many of the world's largest transnational corporations (Barnett & Cavanagh, 1994). Transnationals have purchased many large food companies (e.g., the purchase of both General Foods and Kraft by the Philip Morris Corporation) because of the food industries' countercyclical tendencies. That is, during an economic downturn when consumers reduce purchases of other goods, they continue to buy food (Rama, 1992).

Mann (1993) observed that while a state's power depends on its ability to concentrate forces within given territories, market power comes from its very ability to diffuse across borders and for long distances. Transnational corporations have the ability to concentrate power by virtue of absorbing many companies so that the market is controlled by a small number of very large companies. This further extends the reach of the market across not only space but also season. Because of the increasing power of the transnationals, a number of observers have suggested the state's relevance has declined significantly; it can no longer so readily control economic activities within its borders (McMichael, 1994). Bonnano (1994) argued that while the state may become a less significant actor in the economy, its role as preserver of social order will not likely decline. In addition, Evans's (1979) case study of the tripartite relationship between the state, indigenous capital, and transnationals suggested that the state can control, to a certain extent, the activities of even the largest of transnationals.

State responsibility for social welfare, including food, has grown. Recent budgetary constraints have brought about a temporary halt to the expansion of existing programs and the creation of new ones, but the growth in the number of homeless and of hungry persons suggests political pressure will mount to alleviate these problems.

State paternalism might be expected to grow unabated. An ever-increasing number of health related surveys, made possible by expanding National Institutes of Health budgets, increases the state's surveillance capabilities. State preparation of the population for service in the economy and military will likely continue. Evidence for this is found in the widening ban on smoking, new regulations regarding the provision of nutrition information on labels attached to food products, and the continued campaign to reduce dietary fat.

Yet recent challenges by the Republican party and by regional governments suggest expansion may have limits; national states may be autonomous, but societal interests establish boundaries to further growth.

10

FOOD AND NUTRITION AS SOCIAL PROBLEMS

INTRODUCTION

Social problems are "troubles" that befall individuals or groups and are said to be caused by social conditions. Furthermore, social problems are generally troubles identified by groups or institutions as such; thus they have a subjective dimension (Best, 1989). Troubles often become identified as social problems after a great deal of effort to persuade others that a problem exists. Definers of social problems include social activists, scientists, and moralists. While these statements regarding social problems might be acceptable to most sociologists, students of social problems have recently revived the debate over whether the objective or the social part of social problems should take priority in their studies. Objectivists and positivists tend to take seriously the objective nature of a problem and search for causes in the manner of a social epidemiologist. Social constructionists, by contrast, argue that the objective nature of the problem is beyond the scope of sociology. The sociological aspects of social problems concern the identification of groups that successfully define a situation as a social problem worthy of attention and the rhetorical tools these groups use to persuade others of the problem's existence and importance.

Food and nutrition offer both the objectivist and the social constructionist a wealth of "problems" worthy of analysis. Many of these problems have an objective base, involving the failure to meet some of human beings' most basic needs (McIntosh, 1995). Furthermore, these problems clearly have both social origins and social consequences. At the same time, consensus regarding the problematic nature of many of these objective conditions, when first identified, was slow to develop. It was not immediately obvious to all that a problem existed. Kwashiorkor was not recognized as a deficiency disease until over a decade after its first identification by Dr. Cicely Williams (Williams, 1933), the first female to serve in the British Colonial Medical Corps. Her gender status apparently had a great deal to do with the resistance to her diagnosis by fellow health officials (Latham, 1973; McLaren, 1976b). The objective status of eating disorders remains the subject of considerable debate, and activists and scientists alike have begun to contest obesity, once thought to have a clearly established objective status (see Sobal, 1995).

This chapter illustrates that the study of social problems has included issues involving food and nutrition, but their potential for widening the scope of inquiry has yet to be exhausted. Various theoretical approaches used to study social problems can be extended to food and nutrition issues. Furthermore, distinct approaches that have arisen regarding the latter have considerable value for the study of other kinds of social problems. As previously stated, many of these examples come from extant social problems literature, including a recent volume devoted to food and nutrition as social problems (see Maurer & Sobal, 1995). These include some seemingly self-evident problems such as: hunger, malnutrition, and famine; obesity and eating disorders; and unsafe foods. Other social problems include the less obvious, such as vegetarianism; red meat avoidance; vitamin supplement usage; working conditions on farms and in food-processing plants; and a number of others. These problems will be discussed first in terms of their objective nature, then in terms of their social constructedness. The chapter begins, however, by discussing several of the theoretical orientations utilized in social problems studies.

ORIENTATIONS TO SOCIAL PROBLEMS

Sociologists use a variety of approaches in dealing with social problems, sometimes drawing simultaneously on several perspectives to elucidate a problem. These orientations include the functionalist or, more recently, the human capital approach, as well as the normative, Marxist, and social constructionist approaches.

Functionalism

Functionalists view social problems in several different ways. First, they argue that inequalities are a normal and necessary feature of social systems, for functioning social systems require a division of labor. A division of labor, in turn, requires individuals with differing levels and types of education and skills. Some positions in the division of labor require a longer period of either apprenticeship or schooling than others. In order to motivate individuals to forego immediate rewards and undergo longer periods of training, greater rewards must accrue to those positions requiring more training. Second, functionalists assume that a problem represents a dysfunction or deviation in the system. This dysfunction could result from several things. One of these is a negative change in another part of the social system. For example, a functionalist account of hunger would argue that a downturn in the economy might result in hunger for some. However, hunger itself would not threaten the integrity of the social system; social systems naturally generate inequalities, and hunger here results from a lack of access to resources. As Parsons (1951) noted, conditions such as hunger become dysfunctional only when they affect the capacities of a large portion of the societal population to a degree sufficient to undermine the functioning of the social system. Dysfunctions suggest imperfections; systems operate imperfectly; not all needs can be fully met.

Functionalists would also argue that social systems respond to dysfunctions. The polity might move to stimulate the economy; elements in the societal community would attempt to ameliorate hunger by establishing emergency feeding programs. From a functionalist perspective, this might be understood as an attempt to reintegrate those excluded from societal roles and benefits. Critics of the functionalist approach argue that the inequalities associated with differing positions in the division of labor exceed those required to motivate some to undergo the costs and difficulties associated with greater amounts of education. Others have often relied on a Marxist perspective, arguing that surplus or exchange value can be increased by inflating the exchange value or by restricting the amount of use value returned to labor. Piven and Cloward (1993) argued, for instance, that to motivate people to work under capitalism, resources necessary for survival must be connected to that work. In the words of Sen (1981), for many, entitlement to food required that they either work directly to produce it or pay for it with their wages.

The Human Capital Approach

A clear descendant of the functionalist approach can be found in the so-called human capital approach, developed by Gary Becker (1965) and applied to nutrition by Alan Berg in his book *The Nutrition Factor* (1973). From this perspective, malnutrition constitutes a social problem because it represents an inefficient use of resources. Human beings are resources in which investments can be made to increase their productive capacities. Thus, an individual in which society has invested resources represents human capital investment. Should that person become temporarily or permanently incapacitated because of disease or malnutrition, then resources have been wasted. Earlier work by Kallen (1973) and others characterized malnutrition in a similar light by examining its consequences for role competence and role performance. McIntosh (1975) extended this perspective by applying it to the individual, group, and societal levels, arguing that malnutrition has negative consequences for performance at each of these levels. Malnutrition threatens the individual's well-being through damage to mental capacity, group well-being by reducing role performance, and societal well-being through the cumulative effects of poor performance in school and at work.

The human capital approach measures this poor performance in terms of inefficiencies. Cook (1971) exemplifies this approach through his development of the term "child wastage." Wastage refers to the resources invested in a child by a family and community that were lost when the child died and was given monetary significance by calculating the total amount of money spent on that child's food, clothing, school supplies, and so on. The death of a Jamaican child under two years of age represented "wastage," on average, of $1,200. Other studies undertaken to calculate the costs of malnutrition have focused on school performance (Popkin & Lim-Ybanez, 1982) or work output (Immink & Viteri, 1981; Straus, 1986; Viteri, 1982).

Related to the human capital approach are cost-benefit analyses of the health risks associated with food technologies such as irradiation. Similarly, the costs of diseases are often estimated to make the case that prevention would be less expensive. For example, the total cost of obesity was estimated by Graham Colditz of Harvard Medical School as $39.3 billion annually (Berg, 1991a, 1991b). This estimate included both direct and indirect costs from obesity-caused ailments such as coronary heart disease, gallbladder disease, noninsulin diabetes, and hypertension.

In sum, the human capital model has proved a powerful tool in both research and policy-making. At the same time, however, its limitation ought to be obvious: it considers human health and well-being solely in economic terms. A child's worth is based entirely on his or her costs relative to future economic contributions; a spouse's career is judged in terms of the economic value of his or her time. Surely, the worth of human beings constitutes more than an economic value. In fact, as a means of generating sympathy and relief, the normative approach to social problems such as hunger is perhaps even more powerful than the human capital approach.

The Normative Approach

The normative approach regards social problems as instances of social injustice. Many who focus on famine and hunger find both conditions horrifying and in need of intervention. Whit (1995:193) began his chapter on world hunger with a lengthy quote that compared the consequences of the holocaust with the annual death rate due to starvation, and he follows with the question: "How can the world tolerate this in the midst of plenty?" Poppendieck (1986:xvii), an academic as well as a self-described activist, ended her book's introduction with: "More specifically, it [her book] is an attempt to understand how high-minded, well-intentioned, and hardworking reformers produced so inadequate a set of programs in the face of so remarkable an opportunity."

The normative approach may serve as the basis for social action aimed at alleviating the problem. Many of the food programs developed by the U.S. government in the 1960s were the result of political pressure by activists whose depictions of the plight of hungry children generated public outrage. Sen. George

Aiken (R-VT) and Rep. Leonore Sullivan (D-MO) had raised the hunger issue repeatedly on the floors of their respective legislative bodies during the 1950s but were unable to generate much interest (Maney, 1989). Activists apparently focused on a different set of problems during this period.

Rural sociologists have had a history of concern for social problems that affect both farms and rural communities (Christenson & Garkovich, 1985). These include the disappearance of family farms, the population decline, and their negative effects on small businesses and school systems. A number of problems associated with farming, such as treatment of farm labor, have received serious attention (Friedland et al., 1981). Rural sociologists have not been alone in this regard. The mass media shows occasional interest in the conditions under which farm workers and their families live and work. Sustainable agriculture has caught the attention of scientists and populists alike. Wes Jackson has established the Land Institute in Nebraska to develop and disseminate agricultural practices that sustain the land.

In 1987, the State Legislature of Iowa founded the Leopold Institute at Iowa State University with a mandate "to identify negative impacts of agricultural practices, contribute to the development of profitable farming systems that conserve natural resources, and cooperate with Iowa State University Extension to inform the public of new research findings" (Leopold Center, 1993:inside cover page). Concerns regarding sustainability originate from earlier worries about the demise of the family farm and damage to the environment. Rural sociologists have been troubled by the increasing lack of viability of family operated farms since the Depression (Christenson & Garkovich, 1985).

This interest was revitalized in the 1980s as agriculture underwent what has come to be known as the "farm crisis." The crisis was essentially financial in origin; namely, a substantial increase in farm debt (Leistritz & Murdock, 1988). The debt grew so large that many families had to abandon farms that had been owned for several generations or more. This was thought to threaten not only family farming as a way of life, but also the viability of many rural communities that depend on farmers for economic resources (Albrecht, Murdock, Hamm, & Shifflett, 1987). The crisis extended well beyond economics, however, as rural sociologists began to observe that the financial crisis led to both family and personal problems (Armstrong & Schulman, 1990; Lorenz, Conger, & Montague, 1994). This has led to a greatly increased interest in rural mental health and social stability.

Environmental sociology has strong roots in rural sociology and involves sociologists who focus on the adoption, diffusion, and impact of soil conservation practices. Unlike other social problems, advocates of soil conservation are far less public. Perhaps this is because—unlike the case of hungry children—advocates of soil conservation have no central values on which to enjoin depictions of eroding soil. A number of private foundations and groups, such as the Soil Conservation Association of America, have worked with the academic community and USDA officials rather than attempting to generate public pressure to accomplish policy changes in agriculture.

Merton and others have criticized the normative approach because of its consensual basis. The normative approach implies that members of society are able to readily agree on what constitutes a social problem. Such consensus appears never fully realized. There are few problems that all persons readily accept as social problems. At the same time, there may exist a small number of conditions that capture universal concern. These deal with health conditions that are frequently described in terms of "basic human needs" and that are said, because of their biological nature, to transcend culture and social circumstance (Dasgupta, 1993; Moon, 1991).

Researchers such as Moon (1991) and Firebaugh and Beck (1994) have used mortality rates to reflect lack of human well-being. Philosophers and others have argued that, in addition, certain conditions can be considered universal because they fall either within the domain of "charity" (and charity is said to be a characteristic of all known ethical systems) or within the domain of the Kantian notion of humanity, which argues that to be human both body and mind must be physically capable or competent (Doyal & Gough, 1991; Dreze & Sen, 1989). These arguments lend reasonable credibility to a limited normative approach (McIntosh, 1995).

The Marxist Approach

The Marxist approach is drawn upon by a number of students of social problems. This perspective argues that social problems largely result from various contradictions of capitalism. Hunger, famine, and even anorexia are laid at the doorstep of the capitalist system. This perspective is also used to analyze agricultural labor and problems experienced by family farms. Famine and hunger thus result from the maldistribution of resources caused by the drive of capitalists to accumulate capital, which results in lower wages and higher prices. This is illustrated by the commercialization of agriculture in the Third World in which peasants are forced to grow cash crops. Stonich (1991) described the consequences of the expansion of commercial agriculture in southern Honduras. This move has resulted in an emphasis on certain cash crops for which only large, commercial farms are in a financial position to pursue. The expansion of such farms occurred at the expense of both small holders and the environment. As a result, while the Honduran economy grew, the peasant class grew substantially poorer. These declining fortunes have exacerbated the risk of undernutrition.

A second example that takes Marxism as an approach is found in the recent exposé of labor conditions in a major meat packing company, now part of a transnational corporation (Andreas, 1994). A third involves very recent studies describing the impact of investment and debt dependency on children's health. Burns et al. (1994) found that children under five years of age living in countries in which external debt (relative to export earnings) was high experienced a greater likelihood of wasting (severe underweight), a lower chance of receiving immunization for diphtheria, and a greater chance of death.

A number of rural sociologists have argued that the industrialization of agriculture lies at the root of many rural problems. Some asserted that family farms are being replaced by corporate versions; others have focused on the food-processing and retailing industries that have had negative consequences for both producers and consumers. DeLind and Speilberg-Benetiz (1990) described the "reindustrialization" of agriculture in Michigan through a series of policies promoted by state government. These included further development of "value-added" technologies intended to increase the economic worth of the products. Second, new financial institutions such as the "Capital Access Program" were introduced to increase the amount of credit available for investments in agriculture. Finally, commercial strategies to place Michigan's agricultural products on the world market were expanded. DeLind and Speilberg-Benetiz (1990) argued that such policies had contributed to Michigan's continued loss of 1,000 farms per year, will further commodify agricultural labor and products, and make it more difficult to promote sustainable agricultural practices.

Buttell and Swanson (1986) argued that farm survival strategies include growth in size. While some have claimed that such growth fosters "corporatization," larger farms have engaged in more soil conservation practices than smaller ones. However, survival also has depended on capitalization and labor-saving technologies, which tend to contribute to both soil and water degradation (Buttell & Swanson, 1986). The rhetoric surrounding the increase in the scale of farming has indiscriminately argued that large-scale farms are detrimental because they are neither owned nor managed as family businesses and thus damage the agrarian way of life. Critics also have charged that labor exploitation more likely occurs on corporate rather than family farms. These same critics often have confused the size of farms with particular ownership and management practices (Browne et al., 1992). As research by Heffernan (1972) suggested, the negative effects on rural communities and farm labor resulted not from large-scale farms but from farms that operate in more of an industrial mode.

One need not espouse Marxism to find value in this approach. It focuses on the same sorts of problems as does the normative approach, but it draws attention to causes located in both the economic and political systems. It also overlaps in interesting ways with the human capital approach in which Pierson (1991) and others have argued that state intervention into agriculture and social welfare concern reduction of contradictions in both production and reproduction. First, the production of food is risky and uncertain and thus agriculture has not experienced a transition to capitalism to the same degree as other sectors of the economy

(Mann, 1990). Second, the reproduction of the labor force requires a relatively cheap supply of food (Mann, 1990).

The Social Constructionist

The approaches discussed thus far take an objectivist stance relative to social problems. Essentially, this means that proponents assume that social problems are real and have social antecedents. From this perspective, poverty represents a real state of deprivation; AIDS, a real disease. This perspective calls for sociologists to act as social epidemiologists in a search of social causes. There is little question regarding the objective status of the condition, rather the concern is for adequate measurement to ascertain the magnitude of the problem. The final perspective under consideration here is the so-called social constructionist which side steps the issue of whether what is described as a problem is a "real" condition and instead focuses on the following: (1) of the many social conditions said to exist, why are some accorded more importance than others; (2) what social mechanisms are used to successfully draw attention to a problem; and (3) what kinds of individuals successfully draw attention to problems? Problems associated with both food and nutrition provide a great number of case materials with which to demonstrate the diversity of answers available to these questions.

Social constructionists have asserted that sociologists should focus on social problems by identifying the actors involved in drawing attention to the problem (claims-makers), the kinds of arguments they use to draw attention (claims), the kinds of evidence utilized in claims (often "official statistics"), and cycles in claims-making (Best, 1989). Ibarra and Kitsuse (1993:27) have argued that social problems should be studied by means of an ethnomethodological approach that involves an examination of the "vernacular of the constituents of moral discourse" as social problems like abortion are semantically ambiguous categories. This involves a dissection of the rhetoric of social problems and includes "rhetorical idioms" (statements of definition, classifying conditions in terms of moral universes: loss, unreason, calamity), counterrhetorics utilized by opponents, motifs or figures of speech that provide shorthand descriptors of conditions (e.g., calamity, crisis, tragedy, plague), and claims-making styles or the bearing and tone of the claim (e.g., legalistic, journalistic, civic, comic).

The Rhetoric of Social Problems

The current debate over the healthfulness of red meat provides an excellent example of the discourse surrounding a social problem. Maurer (1995) described the rhetorical idioms and dominant discourse of claims-making about meat as a "problem." One set of idioms emphasized "dangers" of meat to health. A second set drew on a "rights" rhetoric, arguing that humans and animals have similar rights, and thus animals have the same right to life and protection from torture as do human beings. When these two sets are combined, a moral high ground was achieved in that by eschewing meat for reasons of personal health, an individual took a moral stance with regard to animals (Maurer, 1995).

Others in this camp, however, have attempted to separate the animal rights/ personal health issues, perhaps believing that the rhetoric of personal health would reach more people than will that of animal rights. Thus, the Physicians Committee for Responsible Medicine (1990:3) has downplayed its connection to the animal rights movement and argued, "Generally speaking, the closer you are to a diet that is free of animal foods, the better off you are." Some nutritionists and most animal scientists attempted to counter these claims by using a scientific claims-making style. The rhetoric here is less moral, at least on the surface.

Counterclaims were made, suggesting that the findings from scientific nutrition demonstrate that certain nutrients were more easily attained in suitable quantities by consuming red meat. "With regard to the positive contribution of red meat to the diet, it is widely recognized and generally accepted that red meat provides significant amounts of B-vitamins, minerals, and nutritionally complete protein" (Breidenstein & Williams, n.d.:ii). While acknowledging that the fat content of red meat may increase the risk of certain chronic illnesses, the claim was made that these risks are minimal when red meat was eaten in moderation. Others have avoided a confrontation with the health risk claims and stress the low fat and cholesterol content of meat. "For those who have been advised by a qualified health care professional to control dietary cholesterol, it is important to note that such an ingestion level [2,000 kcal] supplies only about 89 mg of cholesterol" (Breidenstein & Williams, n.d.:ii).

Similarly, the stand taken by the professional communities of nutrition and dietetics on vegetarianism has generally decried some of the practices as potentially unhealthy. Todhunter (1973) described the beliefs of many vegetarians as faddish (an interest pursued with exaggerated zeal and devotion for a short period of time) and described vegetarians as "cult-like" in their practices. He illustrated the point using the Zen macrobiotic diet which "typifies some of the very serious dangers to health when adherents follow a regimen that has been shown to cause irreversible health damage and ultimately leads to death" (Todhunter, 1973:313). The macrobiotic diet represents an extreme form of vegetarianism practiced by few persons. Dietitians generally consider more mainstream versions of vegetarianism as safe. Defenders have described vegetarians in terms of their desire to develop greater harmony with nature, "vegetarians reject meat because we are one with nature and thus to do so [eat meat] is to be cannibalistic and horrible" (Twigg, 1979:21).

Heick (1991) described the rhetorical context of the debate over the merits of margarine versus butter. Margarine was invented to give disadvantaged groups access to fats. The dairy industry, however, viewed margarine as a threat to its entire market and began a rhetorical offensive to prevent its manufacture and sale. Around the turn of the last century, the dairy industry fired its first salvo, taking aim at the mechanical basis of margarine production. The dairy industry argued that while butter was a natural product, produced as a part of the "natural rural lifestyle," margarine came from factories and represented the less attractive urban way of life.

In this context specific claims were made to secure margarine's banning. These include the product's "unhealthfulness" (because some imported versions contained adulterations) and its lower vitamin content compared to butter. Later, proponents of butter argued that, unlike margarine, butter was a "perfect" source of protein (Heick, 1991), an argument similar to that made by current defenders of red meats (see Breidenstein & Williams, n.d.). More recently, defenders of butter returned to the differences in the social nature of production. Sounding a bit like social critics, representatives of the dairy industry portray margarine as the product of large corporations, whereas butter is the product of small, family operations (since butter is now produced by creameries, some of which are large scale, this rhetoric is no longer used).

Debunkers use rhetoric in an attempt to persuade others that a particular condition is not a problem. For example, some have claimed that desertification represents one of the world's most important environmental problems. Critics have depicted this claim as a "myth," arguing that much of the environmental "damage" blamed on sightless human intervention is, in fact, the result of "natural cyclic change" (Thomas & Middleton, 1994). While the Green Revolution creators of IR-8, a high-yielding type of rice, labeled it a "miracle variety," others have use the term "violence" in conjunction with the social disruptions associated with the spread of such seeds (Shiva, 1991).

Some have attempted to redefine problems. McLaren (1974) described as a "fiasco" the mistaken conventional wisdom that protein-calorie malnutrition (PCM) resulted from a protein rather than calorie shortage. He argued that PCM was indeed as serious as others have argued, but that much time had been wasted solving the "wrong" problem. Fingarette (1988) utilized a strictly scientific style in his attempt to persuade researchers to substitute the term "heavy drinking" for "alcoholism," arguing that symptoms such as "loss of control" and "addiction" that supposedly characterize this malady simply did not occur. Instead, heavy drinking connoted the way of life in which alcohol "becomes the central activity in the drinker's life, it shapes his or her daily schedule, friendships, domestic life, and occupational choices" (Fingarette, 1988:102–103). At times the redefinition of problems involved shifting interpretations to benefit differing groups. The efforts to develop food relief programs in both the 1930s and 1960s in the United States became "commodity relief" programs as the emphasis changed towards alleviating the surplus commodity problem to increase prices (DeVault & Pitts, 1984; Poppendieck, 1986).

Critical analyses of social movements not only may utilize the rhetoric associated with the field of social problems but may also create moralistic rhetorics of their own. For example, Edgley and Brissett (1990:259) in an effort to make health "both an individual responsibility and a public duty," described those involved in the health movement, as "health nazis." They argued that for the original Nazis, restoration of the physical body was equivalent to restoration of the social body. The so-called health nazis took aim at "sinful" behaviors, dictating changes that would lead not only to better physical health but also better social health as well. The totalitarian aspect of this lay in the "public surveillance and monitoring" of what were once "personal and private" matters (Edgley & Brissett, 1990:260). Participants in this movement were referred to as part of the "no generation"; the positive outcomes they expected were known as the "wages of virtue" and attainment of the "garden of Eden of health."

Social Organizations

Entrepreneurial activity often leads to the formation of groups around a particular issue. The abortion question has spawned groups on both sides of the issue: the various "pro-choice" and "pro-life" entities that engage in protest and lobbying attempting not only to influence public opinion but also to change law. Hunger has led to the formation of over 100 groups in the United States alone that deal with this issue as their principal focus or as one of many issues. Examples include the Food and Research Action Center, the National Committee for World Food Day, the Hunger Coalition, the Interfaith Hunger Appeal, Community Nutrition Institute, and the Institute for Food and Development. Some of these groups solicit funds; others obtain grants. Some engage solely in educating the public and lobbying the federal government, others provide emergency relief in times of crises, others stimulate local self-help development projects in order to lessen the risk of hunger or famine, while still others conduct a combination of these efforts. A small number conduct research, with the aim of pinpointing the causes of hunger and famine.

Other food-related problems have spawned groups as well. For example, concerns about obesity not only have resulted in major research centers but also have generated weight loss groups of various sorts. Hunger is less amenable to profit making than weight problems; thus, while there are no hunger groups that exist clearly to make money, profit making has combined with group therapy in the area of weight loss (e.g., Weight Watchers). While there are no "hunger pride" organizations, some of those who take issue with weight as a problem founded Fat Pride.

To the degree that groups pursue a national agenda, they can be described as part of a social movement. Thus, Kandel and Pelto (1980:332–333) found that the health food movement had an ideology, members with deep personal commitment, a real or perceived opposition, recruitment through both personal networks and various institutions of the mass media, and a "segmented, polycephalous, cellular" organizational form. Participants of the health food movement attempted to "revitalize" their lives not only to achieve improved personal health, but also to change the way in which food is produced, to relieve environmental pressures caused by the food system, or to fight for animal rights. With regard to hunger, it appeared that movement membership drew from the well educated, socially and politically liberal, and those involved organizationally in dealing with other social issues (Cohn, Barkan, & Whitaker, 1993).

Groups of Professionals

Among claimants are academics whose attention to troubles lends credibility to their status as social problems. Academics often disagree considerably over the status of a condition as well as its causes. Thus, famine has become the subject matter of public health, nutrition, economics, geography, anthropology, and sociology, to name a few (McIntosh, 1995). Similarly, eating disorders have attracted an increasingly wide array of disciplines, and with them, competing explanations. The medical community has become to view bulimia as a lack of neural control of the appetite or a neurological disorder (Bolo, 1993). Psychologists have speculated that eating disorders result from an affective disorder, such as depression (Marx, 1993).

Sociologists and feminists have located causes in the so-called culture of slimness, patriarchy, or capitalism (Blumberg, 1988; Gordon 1990; Thompson, 1994; Way, 1993; Whit, 1995). Some have claimed that in periods in which women were encouraged to compete with men as equals, women strove to look more like men. During such periods, eating disorders were most prevalent (Gordon, 1990). Others argued that the culture of slimness represented male backlash to female demands for equality (Thompson, 1994). Social psychologists and others have tended to treat eating disorders as a result of dysfunctional relations between adolescents and young women and one of their parents. A recent variant of this theme found a significant relationship between eating disorders and incest (Goodwin & Attias, 1994; Thompson, 1994). In addition, sociologists have begun to treat eating disorders as a response to the stresses created by racism, sexism, and pressures for upward mobility (Thompson, 1994).

The example of disorders reflects the entrepreneurial aspect of social problems. The troubles of some represent opportunities for others. Eating disorders represent an opportunity for a discipline to make claims about its ability to explain and deal with the designated problem. Success brings acclaim to the discipline; a record of failure regarding a number of problems may threaten that discipline's status. As Abbott (1988) has argued, professions maintain legitimacy by means of their apparent successes. In the case of eating disorders, many disciplinary claimants have stepped forward. Perhaps the fact that no "cure" for this disorder is in sight has protected these disciplines from suffering the consequences of their individual lack of success.

A final example suggests that, on occasion, academics from various disciplines work together in the formation of a problem definition. This might be thought of as another form of entrepreneurship. USDA sponsors numerous "regional projects" that are multidisciplinary efforts to deal with particular problems related to agricultural production and consumption. Recent projects have dealt with the socioeconomic dimensions of soil conservation, the career experiences of graduates from agricultural colleges, and changes in the dairy industry.[1] The latter project involves determining the effects of technological change in the dairy industry on the survivability of smaller farms and the impact of these changes on farm family life.

These projects allow scientists to begin to broaden and redefine problems, thus creating more work for their respective disciplines. Soil conservation becomes more than just a problem of topsoil loss and is also seen as an issue of economic and social sustainability. Similarly, technological change in the dairy industry, aimed at improving the milk production of cows, has the attention of agricultural economists ("adopt BST, it will increase your competitiveness") and rural sociologists ("stop the spread of BST before it puts more family farms out of business"). Because many issues in agriculture involve fundamental disagreements regarding both causes and solutions, a regional project to deal with them is either never established or it is unable to produce anything of use.

The so-called Green Revolution was the result of the efforts of interdisciplinary teams of plant and soil scientists located in international agricultural research centers. Many of those participating in this effort firmly believed that their work would enable poor farmers to improve their conditions. Agricultural economists have generally supported such work in that they argue it results in greater levels of production for a given bundle of inputs (Mellor, 1966). Organizations like IFSAT, who produce Green Revolution technology such as fertilizer, have employed rural sociologists to design programs for its diffusion.

Sociologists and political scientists have focused on the role technological change in agriculture plays in redistribution of societal resources. With regard to technologies such as those associated with the Green Revolution and with recent changes in the dairy industry, they have observed that these increase inequality and drive some of the poorest farmers out of business altogether (Dahlberg, 1979; Lipton, 1989; Shiva, 1991). For example, Shiva (1991:72) argues that the "only miracle that seems to have been achieved by the Green Revolution is the creation

---

[1] The title of this USDA regional project is "Structural and Organizational Change in the Dairy Industry" (NE-177), with participating scientists from California, Kentucky, Maryland, Minnesota, Michigan, New York, Pennsylvania, Texas, Vermont, and Wisconsin.

of new pests and diseases, and with them the ever increasing demand for pesticides." Furthermore, many of India's the poorer farmers have had to leave agriculture because, in order to remain competitive, farmers had to invest in the Green Revolution's technology and many simply could not afford to do so.

Group Conflict

Finally, "successful" social problems are those that come to be accepted by the public as such. The health food movement has had limited success; the co-op movement has struggled. Differential success resulted from a number of factors associated with the groups or "departments" involved in defining the problems (Hilgartner & Bosk, 1988). Competing groups may be unable to establish the agenda and definitions. In other cases, however, competing groups, such as those involved on both sides of the environmental issue, "generate work for one another." In the meantime, their activities "raise the prominence of the environment as a source of social problems" (Hilgartner & Bosk, 1988:69). Conflict, however, can also lead to the destruction of the groups involved. This may result from struggle within a group as its members attempted to redefine the nature of the problem. For example, Cox (1994) revealed that conflict ultimately destroyed the network of food co-ops in the Minneapolis–St. Paul area as a new generation of members, inexperienced in the radicalism of the 1960s, joined and began to redefine the purpose of the network in terms of personal rather than social liberation.

Within the discipline of nutrition, there exists considerable disagreement over what advice the public should be given relative to their eating habits. For example, while a number of national bodies have argued that an individual's health will likely improve if she or he reduces the percentage energy from fat to under 30 percent of total calories (Center for Science in the Public Interest), others have argued that only a select few would actually benefit from this change in eating habits. Furthermore, when the public discovers that their efforts in fat reduction will have little likelihood of affecting them, they will become disenchanted with all of the advice from the nutrition community (Harper, 1987). These concerns are not only for the public's welfare but also for the well-being of nutrition as a profession.

Conflict can involve the various scientific disciplines as well. For example, sociologist Szasz (1974) has attacked psychiatry, claiming that mental illness is a myth created by a discipline seeking legitimacy and status (see also Scull, 1993). The debate over whether population growth constitutes a problem or an opportunity continues to rage, largely across disciplinary lines. A similar claim could be made about the desertification issue.

Finally, groups compete for clients and resources. Even during famines, relief organizations position themselves differentially relative to U.S. foreign policy and host country politics to gain access to resources and clientele. Nor are groups reluctant to criticize another's efforts. The Bread for the World Institute and RE-SULTS Educational Funds (1995) joint report on the U.S. Agency for Internation-al Development's child survival programs argued that too many bureaucratic rules and political goals have come to characterize this aid, reducing its effectiveness.

Communicating Social Problems

The mass media has played a major role in the social construction of various social problems involving food and nutrition. Hunger has waxed and waned as a target of public concern, but this discomfort reflects the content of news reporting. Reporters themselves, however, are concerned with what constitutes "good" news. For example, some of the more recent famines in Africa went practically unreported because journalists and/or editors decided that the public would not be interested in another African famine (McIntosh, 1995). Interest and awareness in eating disorders has received a major boost not only by news stories but by the ap-pearance of victims on talk shows. Similarly, widespread coverage of recent food poisonings contracted in commercial establishments has heightened public inter-est and concern, prompting the crafting of legislation that would profoundly alter the food system as well as potentially increase the cost of food by significant amounts. Such legislation will likely be significantly changed before it ever leaves committee level. The fate of food safety legislation is much in doubt, since it will likely be opposed by those lobbies representing both food companies and farmers. Of equal interest, however, was the ability of large fast-food chains to keep earlier food poisonings out of the news altogether. News stories on food safety and envi-ronmental impacts of food companies are more common that in previous years. Recent stories have begun to tie these problems to politics. For example, a recent Associated Press release describes accusations of conflict of interest in the race for Texas governor with regard to a lawsuit filed against Pilgrim's Pride, the largest chicken producer in the state ("State Investigates," 1994). Ann Richards's camp has claimed that her challenger, George W. Bush, "doesn't see a problem in taking money from this man [Bo Pilgrim, owner of the corporation] and chumming around with him" while the company has "hundreds of thousands of dollars in pending fines against the state of Texas"; Pilgrim labeled the comments as "sour grapes" ("State Investigates," 1994:A7).

A variety of groups publish newsletters. For example, the Center for Science in the Public Interest puts out the *Nutrition Action Newsletter*. A number of the issues published in 1994 contained exposés of the fat and sodium content of com-mon dishes served in Chinese, Italian, and Mexican restaurants. The newsletter contains several regular sections, one of which is called "Just Desserts" which has two subsections. The first, titled the "Right Stuff," provides information on foods considered healthy, and the second, "Food Porn," focuses on food products with high fat or sodium contents. *Consumer Reports* is published monthly by the Consumers Union and includes a yearly assessment of the dietary quality of fast-food entrées as well as special features such as "The Vitamin Pushers," which criticizes the pharmaceutical profession for promoting "unnecessary supplements," the Food and Drug Administration for failing to investigate questionable claims regarding the efficacy of supplements, and the Federal Trade Commission for permitting misleading advertising. The food industry is frequently defended in the newsletter *Priorities*, published by the American Council on Science and Health. Several major universities, such as Harvard, Berkeley, and Tufts, have created health or nutrition newsletters. These tend to be more middle of the road ideologically. Other university research centers, however, may take stronger advocacy stands, such as that of the Agricultural Technology and Family Farm Institute (Department of Rural Sociology, University of Wisconsin), which favors sustainable agricultural technologies. Its newsletter is called *As You Sow...Social Issues in Agriculture*.

In addition, many of these problems have journals devoted to them. *The Journal of the American Dietetic Association* and the *American Journal of Clinical Nutrition*, for example, deal with the gamut of problems associated with nutrition; others such as the *International Journal of Obesity*, the *International Journal of Eating Disorders*, and *Agriculture, Food and Human Values* have a more narrow focus.

The proliferation of research reports and groups promoting various interests and points of view results in public confusion. A Gallup poll conducted in December 1993 for the American Dietetic Association and the International Food Council found that when adults were confronted with conflicting information about nutrition and health, only 33 percent felt confident in making decisions about what to eat (Evers & Mason, 1994).

Numbers, We Got Numbers

Numbers give social problems an appearance of reality. If it can be counted, it must be true. Furthermore, it would appear that the greater the number of victims, the more significant the problem. However, the severity of consequence is a necessary condition for social problem formation. In these circumstances, numbers give way to description. For example, millions catch the common cold, but as its consequences are so negligible, it is not perceived as a national problem in the same way as is coronary heart disease. Thus, no organization similar to the American Heart Association has emerged for the cold.

Hunger, however, has great salience, even though it affects far fewer persons in the United States than in the Third World. Hunger has potentially serious consequences, and the numbers are thought to be sufficiently great to cause embarrassment in a country of great wealth. Hunger afflicted as many as 20 million persons (Brown & Pitzer, 1987). Others, using alternative means of estimation, claimed that as many as 28 million children suffer or risk suffering hunger (Food Research and Action Center [FRAC], 1991). Malnutrition, reflected by many deficiency diseases, was estimated to afflict as many as 177 million children under the age of five in the Third World (Grant, 1991). Obesity struck one in five adolescents and up to 33 percent of adults in the United States ("Feds," 1994:A7). Eating disorders have caused the death of 150,000 women in the United States each year (Thompson, 1994). The weight loss industry earned 33 billion dollars a year (Wolf, 1991:17).

Such figures describe existing conditions; at the same time, their presenters often mean to shock and persuade others of the need for action, for the allocation of resources. The greater the number of individuals afflicted with a problem accompanied by severe consequences, the easier it is to make a case for action and resource generation. The numbers themselves, however, are often problematic. Measuring malnutrition is both expensive and imprecise. Various indicators used for such purposes have problems of validity, reliability, and precision. Hunger is a poorly defined concept and is thus difficult to measure. It stands for famine, inadequate dietary intake, malnutrition, sensations of tension and emptiness, and desire (Baudrillard, 1993; Brown & Pitzer, 1987; DeWaal, 1989; Keys et al., 1950; Millman & Kates, 1990). Recent hunger studies measured meal skipping and the inability to afford enough food, but enough is defined by the respondent (FRAC, 1991). Hunger, as so measured, may provide some indication of the risk of malnutrition, but this remains to be demonstrated. Others have relied on the increase in the number of low-wage jobs, the number of persons living at or below the poverty line, or the increase in the number of persons using food banks and emergency centers as estimates of hunger's magnitude. Those who have provided such estimates rarely give any information regarding how the numbers were obtained; thus, their reliability was often suspect (Lochhead, 1991). Figures such as the estimate of the number of malnourished children in the world are estimates that rely on projections from small-scale studies. These studies frequently involve unrepresentative samples and may use differing measurement techniques. The adequacy of estimates based on such studies is rarely questioned, however, despite its apparent weaknesses. Imprecision would seem to lead to overestimates that err on the side of caution—caution in the sense of avoidance of excluding any persons at risk of the malady in question. This caution makes it easier to politicize the issue; as a result the numbers become politicized as well.

Getting Public Attention

An indicator of the success of rhetorical claims about social problems is whether they appear in the mass media. Hunger has successfully garnered attention at various times. The 1960s were a watershed for articles on hunger; by the 1970s, public disenchantment over welfare had grown and the proportion of those who thought that too much money was being spent on welfare grew significantly (Neimi, Mueller, & Smith, 1989). Critics successfully portrayed welfare programs as riddled with fraud and abuse, with many reaching the conclusion that a high proportion of food stamp recipients were able-bodied men (Levenstein, 1993). Hunger was "rediscovered" in the early years of the Reagan administration as activists sought evidence for the negative effects of the budget cutbacks. Thus, a typical article from the latter period stated: "America is not starving. There are, however, millions of Americans who are underfed and there is more to hunger that meets the eye....They go hungry. Their worn faces show the toll of too little food or long hours spent haggling for a handout" ("All Across," 1984). In 1993 the president of OXFAM was quoted in a story regarding the opening of that organization's first office designed to handle hunger in the United States. "You don't have to go overseas to find the Third World. The Third World exists in the United States, and in urban as well as rural areas" (Marcus, 1993). Members of the Reagan administration were quick to publicly claim that they had no evidence of hunger; critics responded with references to specific studies (Marcus, 1993).

Infant feeding became a social problem in the 1970s when Derrick Jelliffe, an internationally prominent nutritionist, wrote an article claiming that the Nestle Corporation's promotion of its infant formula in Third World countries placed infants from those counties at grave risk (Gerber & Short, 1986). The War on Want and Interfaith Center on Corporate Responsibility followed suit with papers and books of their own. The success of the Nestle's boycott in the 1970s resulted not from the initial boycott itself but rather from the publicity the social movement organizations received from the press. Once television and print journalism made the boycott and its reasons into an issue, the boycott became widespread (Gerber & Short, 1986). Nestle's fought back by means of a publicity campaign that championed their version of the situation; at the same time, however, they changed their promotion practices.

Pictures

The case for social problems is more easily made when it can be illustrated by means of photographs or film. Pictures are a success to the extent they must, first, present apprehensible conditions easily and, second, have an emotive quality: they must demonstrate suffering or some other strong normative condition. Problems such as eating disorders, obesity, and hunger, for example, are easy to portray because of the clear physical circumstances that they provide in pictures. Hunger in Africa has been perhaps easier to illustrate because of the high concentration of victims that can be filmed both as a group and as individuals. This has had the consequence of helping transform, almost overnight, problems of which the public was unaware into an issue of great public concern (McIntosh, 1995).

Culprits and Entrepreneurs

In studies of social problems, objectivists present victims and culprits; social constructionists search for entrepreneurs. A culprit is someone who has acted in such a way so as to cause or contribute to a problem. An entrepreneur is an individual or group that seeks to persuade others that a condition constitutes a problem worthy of attention and intervention. Marxists frequently identify the capitalist system itself as the culprit, the implication being that without an end to the system, the problem will persist. Whit (1995), Friedland et al. (1981), and others argued that the capitalist drive for surplus value leads to exploitation of agricultural labor and the creation of unhealthy "industrial foods." Whit (1995) described several unhealthy results from the industrialization of food production. Regarding beef, Whit (1995) has suggested that cattle once freely grazed on pastures left otherwise natural rather than on land that has been transformed by fertilizer and other agro-chemicals. As Cronon (1991) observed, even "natural" pastures are the result of human interference. Whit (1995) also noted that cattle got more exercise in the process, leading to beef higher in muscle and lower in fat.

Others have suggested that oligopolies threaten the food supply. Morgan (1979), in his widely cited *Merchants of Grain*, describes the historical trend in grain toward concentration. By definition, oligopolies use resources inefficiently, but Morgan's concern lay more with power, wielded by a handful of companies over the lives of millions of persons. Zwerdling (1976) stated that concentration in the food industry as a whole has contributed to higher-priced foods. The process of globalization has contributed to trends in concentration of food production, processing, and marketing (Bonnano, 1994; Gereffi, Korzenicwicz, & Korzenicwicz, 1994; McMichael, 1994). This trend suggests that agencies will have increasing difficulty in controlling the quality and safety of food products.

Scientific nutrition was established by a coalition of scientists, industrialists, and philanthropists interested in labor reform, particularly in ways of dealing with unrest (Aronson, 1981, 1982a). Wilbur O. Atwater provided major intellectual grounds for proposed reforms by arguing that labor unrest resulted from underproduction rather than exploitation. This problem could be resolved by workers adopting "scientifically determined diets." Such diets were achievable through improving education rather than raising wages. Congress found this solution sufficiently compelling to provide funding for experiment stations on land grant university campuses (Aronson, 1982a).

The weight loss industry is filled with entrepreneurs who promote ever new means for dietary change and/or exercise. Among the most recent of these included those who promote what Spitzack (1990) calls the "antidiet." Using the antipatriarchy and self-empowerment rhetoric, Jane Fonda has developed a small industry in exercise tapes, equipment, and clothing. On the one hand, her approach, criticized the weight loss industry for its patriarchal emphasis on beauty, while, on the other hand, her approach promoted weight loss/body development as a means of empowerment. Susan Powter has recently entered this lucrative market by promoting a similar message.

CONCLUSION

The purpose of this chapter was to illustrate the range of food and nutrition troubles available to students of social problems. Those concerned with hunger, eating disorders, and obesity, for example, are increasingly interested in social epidemiological explanations that would include sociological variables. New grist for the objectivist mill includes issues of food safety. Some may choose to focus on household level knowledge and practice (see McIntosh et al., 1994b, 1994c), while others may sharpen the attention already paid to food safety problems at the organizational level (see Whit, 1995). The relationship between body image and self-image, on the one hand, and body image and depression, on the other, represents a new link between socially derived images of self and mental health. Those who take a more social constructionist view will have a veritable field day with these same problems, for each has a variety of academic, social movement, and entrepreneurial groups associated with it. The social construction of "oils" ought to provide researchers with insights into the social construction of biochemical entities and medical outcomes (see Jurska & Busch, 1994, for the beginning of such an effort). Similarly, the construction of ethnic foods as at once a preferred lifestyle choice and health risk represents another such topic. A voluminous literature from which to draw examples and case materials abounds. Many of these problems have one or more journals and newsletters written about them. Obesity, famine, and eating disorders, for example, have become major industries of study, debate, and social action. Finally, for those who seek a set of conditions that provides universal criteria for establishing an objective basis for social problems studies, food and nutrition problems present conditions that many consider universal in nature and thus are less subject to the relativistic interpretations associated with culture, social structure, or vested interests (McIntosh, 1995).

11

THE SOCIOLOGY OF FOOD AND NUTRITION
A Sociological Assessment

INTRODUCTION

Sociologists have made few self-conscious efforts in the study of food and nutrition as potential sources of social phenomenon. Founding sociological theorists such as Marx, Simmel, Sorokin, and Mead and contemporary theorists such as Bourdieu, Collins, Lenski, Wallerstein, Goldstone, Tilly, Lamont, and others have used food as a scarce resource or as a symbol of class membership and nutrition as a state of deprivation to develop sociological theories of a general nature. A growing number of rural sociologists have enjoined efforts that contribute to such a subfield, but these largely concern labor and equity issues.

A fully developed sociology of food and nutrition would also encompass such concerns but, additionally, would include cultural, consumption, and health issues as well. Highly visible work by Fischler, Murcott, Bourdieu, and Mennell has established a basis for such developments. Lesser known work by Sobal, Poppendieck, Whit, and McIntosh represents conscious attempts to define a new food and nutrition subfield within sociology. This includes their research as well as their teaching and efforts to formally organize sociologists of food and nutrition. Other sociologists have applied various general frameworks and middle-range theories to study social issues and problems that revolve around, if not directly involve, food, such as women's domestic roles and hunger (Aronson, 1982b; Hochschild, 1989). This work, like that of Bourdieu, has no agenda, hidden or otherwise, regarding the creation of a new field of study within sociology. Some of the authors of this latter work might indeed find such efforts both curious and unnecessary.

This chapter will evaluate the current efforts, conscious or otherwise, as they contribute to the new field or subdiscipline, the sociology of food and nutrition. Tools from the sociology of sociology will serve as the means for this assessment. Such an effort requires several approaches as suggested by both Ritzer (1991) and Diesing (1991). The first few are cognitive in nature. The ontological-epistemological character of existing work can be judged relative to common modes of social ontology and epistemology. General comparisons of this sort by themselves provide an insufficient understanding of how work in a new field compares with that in existing fields, for they are too general but, at the same time, insufficiently inclusive. This necessitates further comparison, based on criteria involving more refined ontological categories.

The final form of cognitive assessment considers the manner in which an emerging field fits a more general pattern of change in a discipline. Therefore, sociological work in food and nutrition can be compared with emerging theoretical trends in sociology as a whole. The second major basis of assessment is social in nature. It involves an examination of the degree to which the field has developed as a community of scholars as well as the degree to which the field has experienced influences from other fields and disciplines. On the basis of these various evaluations, the chapter ends with a discussion of the subdiscipline's future prospects.

SOME APPROACHES FOR ASSESSING THE SOCIOLOGY OF FOOD AND NUTRITION

So-called cognitive approaches in the sociology of science often begin at the metatheoretical level. Metatheory itself undergoes continual evaluation, as recent work by Ritzer (1990, 1991) suggested. Ritzer (1991) argued that one role metatheory plays is in deepening our understanding of existing theory through a thoroughgoing assessment of its underlying philosophical assumptions. This not only permits a deeper understanding of a given theory but also of its relationship with

Table 11.1. Lloyd's (1988) Classification Scheme of Social Ontology

Social ontology	Social epistemology	Representatives
A. Behaviorist individualism	A. Empiricism	
	1. Behaviorism	Sapp
	2. Statistical probabilism	Schafer
B. Phenomenology/Symbolism	B. Interpretism	
	1. Mentalism	Denzin
	2. Hermeneutical interpretism	Shifflett
C. Holism	C. Holism	
	1. Functionalism	Parsons
	2. Symbolic holism	Levi-Straus
D. Structurism	D. Realism	Tilly

other theories. A second role for metatheorizing lies in its potential for aiding in the creation of new theories.

Metatheoretical Assessments

Ritzer (1990, 1991), Martindale (1960), and Hinkle (1980) have provided examples of how metatheoretical evaluations might be done. The recent scheme developed by Lloyd (1988) has, despite its limitations, the greatest utility. Lloyd (1988) had a particular aim in making his excursion into the metatheoretical bases of sociological theory—he was interested in developing a rationale for sociological realism. A modified version of his scheme is displayed in Table 11.1, which classifies work by sociologists in terms of ontological and epistemological assumptions as well as typical methodological approaches.[1] The first two distinctions will be of most use in the assessment that follows.

The first level of ontology is behaviorism. Work here assumes, among other things, that all social action, regardless of its apparent complexity and unit of analysis, can be ultimately reduced to individual behavior. In other words, the actions of aggregates of persons are understandable through an examination of each person's behavior. In addition, explanation comes from direct observations of behavior, rather than inquiries into mental states, motivations, and the like. Thus, proponents stress the necessity of methodological individualism. George Homans's (1974) *Social Behavior: Its Elementary Forms* provides an exemplar of this approach. A number of social psychologists practice behaviorism, including Molm (1990) and Macy (1991), but no such examples exist in the sociologies of food and nutrition. Other ontological categories that deal with individual actors include the phenomenological and the symbolic.

Symbolists such as interactionists argue that humans acquire and utilize symbols through social interaction. Such acquirement facilitates their ability not only to adapt to their surroundings but to form ideas about themselves and others. Symbolic interactionists and phenomenologists such as Berger and Luckmann (1966) posited the existence of social institutions in the form of more regularized aspects of social interaction and argued that these were maintained, to a certain degree, through everyday interactions. Some phenomenologists and ethnomethodologists are less concerned with how order is created and maintained than with how the sense of a common reality and orderliness come into being. From this perspec-

---

[1] In his review of this chapter Paul Thompson reminded me that sociologists tend to conflate and simplify a number of complex issues regarding ontology. Nowhere is this more apparent than in the distinction made between realism and idealism. Lloyd's (1988) categories do not do justice to the whole range of idealism's perspectives regarding the nature of the entities that exist in the universe, but Lloyd is merely classifying work done by sociologists.

tive, actors actually share less by way of common frameworks than they assume they share (Turner, 1991).

Both symbolists and phenomenologists have utilized an interpretist epistemology (Lloyd, 1988). However, they differ regarding the extent to which the subjects' interpretations serve as the sole source of explanation. One approach, referred to as mentalism by Lloyd, explains an action by means of an interpretation of what the actors say about their behavior. Mentalists are willing to make generalizations regarding behavior, often based on a prior theoretical concept. Hermeneutical interpretists are much more relativist in their approach, relying on empathy to ascertain the actor's motives and taking into account the particular sociocultural circumstances in which the action is embedded. Concepts and relations among them emerge from the interpretive process (Lloyd, 1988). Many of the studies and approaches reviewed earlier fall into one of these categories. Much of the work on the sociology of the body, particularly Allon's work on obesity, argues that symbolic interactionism represents the proper theoretical approach, and it should rely on a more mentalistic epistemology. Social constructionist examinations of hunger, obesity, anorexia, and other problems tend to combine symbolic interactionism with hermeneutical interpretism.

Peggy Shifflett's (1980) (Shifflett & McIntosh, 1986–87) study of future time perspectives and age-appropriate food habits followed a conceptual framework established by Mead, but she developed her categories using the respondents' own classification of their actions. DeVault (1991), who relied so heavily on Dorothy Smith's theoretical and methodological views, represents a further example. Murcott's (1993b) work on the socially defined conception of infant feeding and infant bowel movements is also of this sort as are many of the papers in her edited volume (Murcott, 1983a). Denzen's work on alcoholism provides the only real application of interactionism to this important area of concern. Thus far, interactionists and phenomenologists have made no real attempts to study body disorders such as anorexia.

Before departing for ontological destinations of a macronature, it should be recognized that many works in sociology, in general as well as in the sociologies of food and nutrition, involve assumptions that differ from behaviorism, phenomenology, and symbolism. For example, much of what occurs in present-day social psychology cannot be classified under any of these headings. One area of particular importance involves the assumption that culture, ethnic heritage, and class background, among others, provide the individual with beliefs, attitudes, norms, and values that determine behavior. Much empirical work is done under this set of assumptions. Although this work has received a great deal of criticism, it remains popular both within sociology and other social sciences and has actually grown in application within the dietetics field. Work in this field either has been atheoretical or has employed perspectives such as the Ajen-Fishbein theory of reasoned action or the health belief model. Sociologists of food and nutrition have contributed substantially, hereby providing a firmer theoretical underpinning to these studies. Examples include much of Robert Schafer's (Schafer, 1978; Schafer & Keith, 1981; Schafer & Schafer, 1989) research and recent research by Sapp and Harrod (1989) and Zey and McIntosh (1992).

The remaining set of ontological categories in Lloyd (1988) involve macro-considerations. Symbolic ontology takes the stance that cultural categories form a deep, often unrecognized set of instructions for organizing social existence. Few sociologists appear to conform to this approach, although Parsons (1966), in what defenders believe was a momentary lapse of judgment, classified himself as a cultural determinist. Sociologists have not adopted the Levi-Straus or Mary Douglas versions of macrosymbolism. Given the criticisms of this form of anthropological theory, this is just as well.

Holism follows macrosymbolism in the typology. Social entities here involve "an irreducible, tightly integrated individual with properties and powers of its own which are not emergent from or reducible to the properties and powers of its parts" (Lloyd, 1988:151). Systemic holism treats society as institutionalized relationships that are observable in fairly static roles and organizations of various levels of complexity. Structural functionalism, much of conflict theory, and exchange structuralism conform to such assumptions. Conceptual work by Sobal (1992) and McIntosh (1975) are examples of its use in the sociologies of food and nutrition. Empirical work utilizing world systems theory also fits into this ontological perspective. A less widely used version of holism in sociology is idealist holism. However, postmodernism and poststructuralism fit best into this category of ontology.

Finally, Lloyd (1988) developed the category that reflects his perspective for studies of social change: structurism. The term is selected, one supposes, to avoid confusion with the ambiguous term of structuralism or Giddens's more recent conception of structuration. Lloyd's term shares much in common with Giddens's claims about social relations. Here roles, groups, organizations, and general institutionalized patterns bear on actual behavior, but individuals through their collective action can deviate from and, ultimately, alter these structures. Giddens's theorizing and Tilly's empirical work on social unrest and food riots provide useful examples. In addition, Bryan S. Turner's (1984, 1992) efforts to develop a sociology of the body through synthesizing ideas about structure from Marx, Weber, and Foucault would appear to follow this particular ontology.

A number of strange bedfellows emerge from this exercise, which has lumped together otherwise incompatible theoretical approaches such as human ecology, functionalism, and conflict theory into a single category. The next step involves taking a more refined look at sociological theories to develop a more discriminating typology. The sociology of sociology literature abounds with methods of assessment at this level; the problem becomes one of identifying those methods that provide the most comprehensive of evaluations. Several approaches converge on similar assessment criteria. Over 10 years ago colleagues at Texas A&M University began to develop criteria for categorizing and judging the sociological content of journal articles. Results of their early work appeared in *Rural Sociology* in the late 1970s (see Picou, Wells, & Nyberg, 1978). Improvements were made in the scheme, which was then applied to 40 years of articles published in the *American Sociological Review* (see Wells, 1980; Wells & Picou, 1981). Recent reassessments of research in rural sociology were published, using this scheme (Falk & Zhao, 1989; Picou, Curry, & Wells, 1990). Essentially, the scheme combines the criteria for identifying the nature of the subject matter, based on Walter Wallace's (1969) taxonomy, Mullins's (1973) classification of groups of sociologists in communication with one another regarding shared research concerns, and Friedrichs's (1970) distinction between sociologists who perform the role of the priest as opposed to that of the prophet.

A More Refined Ontological Assessment

Picou and colleagues draw heavily on the Wallace (1969) taxonomy. This essentially classifies how work in sociology views the subject matter at hand. More specifically, this involves identifying how "the social" is defined; that is, subjective versus objective. The second criterion involves how "the social" is explained; in other words, are materialist versus ideational forces involved? Wallace breaks this down further so as to denote material causes that are largely environmental and those that have to do with the attributes of populations themselves. The ideational involves a split between mind and body. Wallace's scheme is somewhat difficult to follow; perhaps this explains his simplification of the scheme in his 1983 work. However, the simpler scheme appears less complete; thus the earlier scheme will drive the evaluation.

The Wallace taxonomy is sufficiently complex to warrant an extended discussion. As previously mentioned, Wallace argues that sociological theories are distinguishable through how they both define and explain "the social." The chief distinction in social definitions lies in the difference between objective and subjective definitions. Durkheim's social facts constitute an objective definition of the social, while Weber's notion of meaningful social action reflects a subjective approach. Explanations of the social involve the distinction between conditions "imposed" on the social and conditions "created" by members of the social. The distinction here, roughly, is between determinism and voluntarism.

The two primary distinctions of explanation and description create a fourfold space, but Wallace wisely divides the criteria of explanation into four additional categories. The deterministic category can be further differentiated into subcategories: (1) imposed environmental conditions that consist of other human beings (e.g., populations) and (2) deterministic physical attributes of the environment (e.g., food supply, weather). Voluntarism involves characteristics of the participants themselves, which can be subcategorized as involving either the nervous system (mind) (e.g., motives, perceptions, desires, beliefs) or the nonnervous system (body) (e.g., physiological needs, height, weight). These additional distinctions expand the original four cells into sixteen. Half of these cells involve those approaches that begin with subjective definitions of the social (see Table 11.2). Wallace (1969) filled these cells with theoretical segments from Parsonian structural functionalism and action theory, although other theories such as postmodernism and poststructuralism also belong on this side of the divide. It should also be noted that despite Parsons's (1966) self-proclaimed "cultural determinism," his work on social action is clearly dualistic: the constraints of the physical environment operate independently from any particular cultural definitions of resource shortage, pain, or hunger.

There remain eight cells that lie on the objectivist side, and Wallace fills seven of these with existing theoretical approaches. For example, the cell that represents objectively defined social relations, in which explanations are couched in terms of the imposition of physical constraints on social behavior, is represented by theories such as human ecology. In contrast, explanations generated by nervous system (mind) characteristics of the participants are represented by symbolic interactionism. The single empty cell involves nonnervous system (body) characteristics of the participants as causes of behavior.

The examples from the sociologies of food and nutrition provided in the table ought to be reasonably self-explanatory. Demographism would involve those studies of the effects of population variables such as size and density on societal food practices and availability. Similar analyses are found at the family level in which family size, birth order, and birth spacing affect the amount of time devoted to obtaining and preparing food and supervising its consumption. Ecologism would look more closely at resource availability and social relationships that develop around it. Many studies, of course, combine demographism and ecologism, for example, Lenski and Lenski (1987) and Goldstone (1991).

Wallace devotes one cell in his table to various versions of exchange theory. Marcel Mauss, Marshall Sahlins, and others have focused on primitive, nonmonetary exchanges of goods. For some these exchanges represent long-term adaptation patterns which permit those who experience deprivation the chance to survive through drawing on obligations generated through past exchanges. Cheal (1988) examined gift exchanges in modern societies in terms of their instrumental and expressive payoffs. Among the items exchanged are food and food-making utensils. He is particularly interested in those exchanges in which the giver expects little in return. These, he argues, help maintain noninstrumental relationships. The role of specific sorts of gift items is less of a concern here, but one might predict that gifts given for symbolic purposes would likely have less practical value. Thus, jewelry or chocolate would be more appropriate than a new set of pans. This would seem

Table 11.2. Wallace's Theory Classification Scheme, with Additions and Examples

The principal phenomena that explain the social are:

	Imposed on the social				Generated by the social			
	By participants' environment		By participants' characteristics		By participants' environment		By participants' characteristics	
	Not people	People	Body	Mind	Not people	People	Body	Mind
Objective	Ecologism Murdock	Demographism Murdock Floud	Materialism Friedland Sobal Friedmann	Psychologism	Technologism	Social structuralisms: Functional, exchange, conflict McIntosh Sobal	Existential phenomenology Turner Sobal	Symbolic interactionism Denzin Allon Schafer
Subjective	Functionalism, postmodernism, poststructuralism					Social actionism		

Source: Wallace, 1969.

a viable avenue for research regarding the role that food plays in exchange relations. Such investigation need not stop with gift giving. The exchange of food occurs daily in nongift contexts. A family member's efforts in providing family meals day in and day out may follow exchange principles. Breast feeding may represent more than just the instrumental provision of needed sustenance but conform to Cheal's notion of expressive exchange in which repayment is not anticipated. The elderly may survive the potential problems associated with living alone because of exchanges of food, mealtime companionship, and rides to the grocery store (Torres et al., 1992). Food consumed while on a date may also represent an exchange. Some women have complained that if their date takes them out for dinner, he expects sexual favors in return. Is there evidence of this? If so, have men always held this expectation in their exchanges with women? Or is the phenomenon a product of modernism or late modernism?

Other forms of exchange of a structural nature exist, but these generally are handled by means of the conflict perspective. Direct and indirect links exist between farms, sources of agricultural inputs, sources of credit, immediate purchasers of commodities, food processors, and food retailers among others. Unequal exchanges occur at various points in this network, based on differential economic and political resources. It appears that as one moves up this chain of relationships, profits increase (Friedmann, 1988; Heffernan & Constance, 1994).

Work in the sociology of agriculture has taken either a ecologism approach or conflict structuralism approach. Work by Albrecht and Murdock (1990), for example, focuses on county-level differences in resources in its explanation of employment patterns in rural areas. Friedland and his colleagues (1981) have relied on a more Marxist approach in explaining exploitive labor practices in agriculture, and Bonnano's studies of land tenure (1988) and the globalization of food production and consumption (1994) also depended on Marxist interpretation. The work by Busch and Lacy and Buttel is less easy to classify. Given the sources they tend to cite, it would appear that they are critical sociologists.

Wallace's (1969) schema contained an empty cell that disappeared in his 1983 typology. Wallace described this as a viewpoint in which "the explanandum consists chiefly of objective behavior relations and whose explanation is chiefly generated by the social and operates via 'non-nervous system' characteristics of the participants themselves" (1969:34). He argued that such a view might consist of behavior shaped by "socially generated differences in participants' height, weight, brain structure, musculature, or other physiological attributes" (1969:34). Turner's (1992) discussion of the phenomenology of the body described body attributes as outcomes of social processes. Sobal and Stunkard's (1989) review of the research on gender and class differences in weight clearly demonstrated that weight was a social product. Other work by Sobal et al. (1992) showed that differences in weight had an impact on achievement and thus social mobility. Socially generated weight and social position thus interact in complex ways. Evidence regarding social interaction and anthropometric status suggests a similar complexity.

Priests and Prophets

A final means of assessing sociological work utilized effectively by Picou and his colleagues draws on the distinction between prophets and priests developed by Friedrichs (1970). A prophet represents the scientific approach in sociology and views sociology's role as the prediction and explanation of human behavior. Priests, on the other hand, take social criticism as the main task, pointing out the nature of society's ills and the means for their alleviation. Gouldner represents the priests; Merton, the prophets. Sociologists working in food and nutrition, such as Mennell, Murcott, Sobal, and Fischler, appear to adhere to the goals of prediction and explanation; they may not agree regarding the scientific status of sociology but, for the most part, limit their social criticism.

At the other extreme, sociologists such as Whit maintain an activist stance in both their writing and teaching. Whit's 1995 text ardently defended a Marxist–feminist view of society, arguing that prior to the development of property, women's role in food production was of greater importance than men's. In between are those who conduct research for the purposes of both explaining and criticizing the social system. Many in the sociology of agriculture camp have taken this position, including William Friedland, Harriet Friedmann, Fred Buttel, Gill Gillespie, and others. Allon's work with weight loss groups clearly expresses a sense of identification and sympathy with their members. DeVault's studies of the family (1991) and the food stamp program (1985), while theoretically based, took a critical stance regarding the place of women and the poor in society.

CURRENT TRENDS IN SOCIOLOGICAL THEORIZING

Ritzer (1990) has attempted to chart current trends in sociological theorizing and argues that the dominant trend is synthesis of existing frameworks. One example is found in Giddens's efforts at linking phenomenology with macroperspectives of structuralism; another is Bryan Turner's (1992) bridging of the micro–macro gap via phenomenology and ideas from Weber and Marx. Jonathan Turner (1988) has brought together symbolic interactionism, behaviorism, action theory, exchange theory, and conceptions of motives for action to develop a theory of social interaction. Other emerging trends include the revival of theories such as structural-functionalism by Alexander, Munch, Sciulli, and others. Furthermore, long-established theories such as symbolic interactionism continue to find useful employment. Finally, European scholars have provided a series of new developments in the form of poststructuralism, postmodernism, figurational theory, and Bourdieu's approach to culture. Sociologists working on food and nutrition problems have only just begun to apply these perspectives, as evidenced in earlier chapters of this book.

In addition to these trends, there is also an observable renewed interest in so-called economic sociology, picking up where Parsons and Smelser's (1956) *Economy and Society* left off. Stinchcombe's (1983) *Economic Sociology* reflects this renewed interest. This permits sociologists, in general, and sociologists of food, in particular, to argue that when consumption patterns change something more than changes in "price and income" may have occurred. Social problems studies have developed a social definitionist or constructionist branch that argues that the objective basis to the study of social problems has no relevance for sociological examination. Rather, social problems are important to the degree that some process identifies putative conditions that may become successfully labeled as problematic for society.

A whole host of new problems such as homelessness and child abuse have received attention by both more traditional approaches and the constructionist approach to social problems. Obesity is viewed by some to consist of a real problem for real people because of either the health or the stigmatization problems that accompany this condition. Others, such as Allon, while not denying that obesity was stigmatizing, argued that the stigma resulted from the very social construction of obesity (see Sobal, 1984b). Obesity existed only after it was so defined by claimants who successfully persuaded others that such a condition existed and was problematic. As Allon (1979) demonstrated, obesity was defined by insurance companies that persons above a certain weight experienced a probability of premature death greater than those of a lesser weight, thus placing the company at risk of "premature" payment to beneficiaries.

Finally, areas either neglected until recently or ignored altogether by sociologists include culture, consumerism, the body, emotions, and mental health. As previously discussed, the sociology of the body has developed a great deal of interest, thanks to Turner and the postmodernists, poststructuralists, and feminists. The importance of body image in self-development and the phenomenological experience of body disorders suggest a natural link between food, nutrition, and bodies. The recent interest in the sociology of emotions suggests another link. Food, eating, and experiences of the body all have emotional implications. Another recently declared subfield in sociology is mental health. A link between food intake and depression exists; depression generally suppresses appetite; this effect is well-enough established such that loss of appetite is used as one of several indicators of depression in field studies. Cultural sociology has experienced rebirth, again largely due to developments in European social thought. Many postmodern social theorists have expressed the opinion that postmodern culture is consumer culture. Thus, food as cuisine and the commodification of bodies and family meals have taken on an important role in these discussions as illustrated by the work of Symons (1991).

Developments in the sociologies of food and nutrition square nicely with these overall patterns of change and continuity in sociological theory. By nature the sociologies of food and nutrition are the unique, synthetic blending of economics, biology, anthropology, and sociology. The biological aspects of nutritional health, for example, encourage the study of the relationship between personal biology and social interaction in new ways, without having to resort to biological reductionism. These syntheses are possible both at the interaction level via theoretical approaches such as Jonathan Turner's and at a more general action theory level using Parsons, as Sobal (1991a, 1991b) has suggested, or through some latter-day improvement of functionalism. Other syntheses are possible, including the closer linking of present work in the sociology of the body, such as that of Bryan Turner, with various developments underway within the sociologies of nutrition.

The Sociology of Food and Nutrition as Social Organization

Those working in the area of the sociology of science argued that much of the development of a science occurs within its various specialties (Zuckerman, 1988). The growth and development of specialty areas or fields is thus highly relevant for understanding a science. Such change involves not only cognitive entities such as new theories or changing perspectives of relevant subject matters, but also the creation of an increasingly formalized series of communications among those working in the new area. Crane (1969) referred to these as invisible colleges, but Mullins (1973) developed a scheme that traces the stages that new specialty areas generally pass through.

The first stage involved the growth of informal communications among scholars as they discover that others are working on similar problems. So-called founding parents or innovators were easily identifiable. At the end of this stage, articles and books concerning the area's subject matter begin to appear. Mullins described this as the "normal" stage. This was usually followed by the "network" stage, in which concepts were agreed on, students were produced in increasingly formalized programs in the specialty, and informal relations involved as many as 40 persons. A "cluster" stage follows, which involves the appearance of academic positions, journals, and associations representing the new area. Group size ranges from 7 to 20 persons formally organized; the less formal group of interested scientists working in the area, or in closely related areas, may involve several hundred. The final stage was referred to as the "specialty" stage, in which many of the innovators involved in the earliest stages have moved on to other specialties. The area was no longer viewed as new or revolutionary; criticism of the specialty by scientists working in other areas becomes routine; textbooks and overviews of the field such as those published in the *Annual Review of Sociology* appear; the formal organization involves between 20 and 200 scholars.

Mullins (1973) and others relied on a series of secondary sources such as the citation index to trace specialty area development. The citation count provides insights into several things. First, it tells what intellectual and possible social influences from areas and fields outside the specialty have the greatest influence. It can also help identify founders who may not have the same visibility as newcomers to the area. As scientists begin to cite one another, informal organization is said to have developed.[2] Other secondary data include book reviews, histories of associations, and departments that list the area as a specialty in graduate training. Additional data must come from the participants themselves. Only they can easily provide information regarding informal communication patterns in which they have had involvement, when they first began work in the area, and other details. Both primary and secondary data are used here to describe the social organization of the sociology of food and nutrition.

As one might suspect, the development of a specialty area may not follow exactly the same sequence as that described by Mullins. However, his indicators and stages appear sensible enough and so will be utilized. When differences are found between developments in the sociologies of food and nutrition and his scheme, they will be duly noted.

The first step would appear to involve the identification of the specialty's founders, individuals who are among the first to work in an area and who successfully encourage further work. The "sociology of agriculture" group includes founding influences such as Heffernan (1972) and Rodefeld (1978) who began their work in the 1960s. Walter Goldschmidt's (1974) [1946] hypotheses regarding the community-level effects of the development of capitalist agriculture anticipated the rise of this group by a number of years, and its rediscovery helped fuel the effort to redirect rural sociology (Buttel et al., 1990). Sociologists interested in the links between sociology and food and nutrition begin to appear in the 1970s in sociology and rural sociology departments located in land grant universities. Perhaps the earliest work done by a sociologist in the area of nutrition lies in the experience of David Kallen, who found himself involved as an NIH project officer on a study of influences of nutritional status on children's development. Others that followed Kallen's footsteps found this early work a great source of inspiration. Kallen influenced Yvonne Vising and William Whit, who met through the Michigan Sociological Association, and later cofounded the Association for the Study of Food and Society. Ann Murcott began her work on food and family in the early 1980s. Another early influence is Robert Schafer, who began to work with dietitians in the early 1970s at Iowa State University. Schafer has published numerous social psycholog-

---

[2] Because of the enormity of the task, I did not conduct a formal citation count analysis to develop "citation" matrices.

ical studies of food intake and dietary adequacy, the majority of which have appeared in dietetics journals. I became involved, like many, somewhat accidentally. No sudden flash of insight occurred, propelling me into the field. Rather, I was working on a methodological study of indicators of social development for USAID while in graduate school (the project was led principally by Leslie Wilcox and Gerald Klonglan). Part of the project involved extending the general model to the specific area of nutrition. As no one else on the project had either the interest or background, I volunteered to take responsibility for this part of the project. Susan Evers, a graduate student in nutrition (who now holds a Ph.D. in epidemiology and specializes in nutritional epidemiology), was hired to work with me. My work on the USAID project led to a dissertation, further research, the development of courses, and a desire to create a new specialty area. Jeff Sobal, another early contributor, attended health and nutrition conferences as a medical sociologist, and upon hearing papers concerning nutrition, saw connections between sociology and nutrition. Other early influences include Natalie Aronson, Judith Gordon and Natalie Allon, who came at nutrition from a social problems perspective.

LINKS BETWEEN MEMBERS OF THE FIELDS

A questionnaire was mailed to all individuals displaying some degree of prominence in either the sociology of agriculture or the sociologies of food and nutrition. Personal knowledge on the author's part served as the primary mechanism for selection. Apologies are offered to deserving individuals thus excluded. The questionnaire sought information regarding with which of the areas the respondents identified; how long they had worked in the area(s); the names of those sociologists who had the most influence on them; those sociologists with whom they had communicated, collaborated, or coauthored; and the names of students they had produced in the area(s). Just over 50 percent of the 37 individuals who were mailed the questionnaire completed it. These data were used to determine the nature of the network structure in the areas. Of the twenty respondents, nine (39%) described one of their areas as sociology of agriculture, eighteen (78%) chose sociology of food, and six (23%) selected the sociology of nutrition. More than half (56%) of the 23 selected only one of the three specialties; 35 percent picked two out of the three; 9 percent listed all three. The most frequently identified category as a single specialty was the sociology of food followed by the sociology of nutrition. The most common two-specialty combination was the sociology of agriculture coupled with the sociology of food. Three respondents selected the sociology of food/sociology of nutrition combination.

Origins

Land grant universities have produced the largest percentage of the group (52%), with 17 percent having graduated from Cornell University in either rural sociology or developmental sociology. Another 13 percent originated from the Department of Sociology and Anthropology at Iowa State University, which has a strong rural sociology research program. And 9 percent graduated from the Department of Sociology at Texas A&M University, although several of these had research assistantships in the Department of Rural Sociology there. The remainder come from other sociology departments, principally those located at universities with strong liberal arts traditions (Harvard, Berkeley, Penn, Boston College). Of the twenty-three, twelve (52%) currently work at land grant universities including Iowa State, Cornell, Texas A&M, Penn State, and Michigan State. The largest concentrations are found at Cornell (9%) and Michigan State (9%). The remainder are located at small liberal arts colleges. Schools that bridge the three specialty areas are clearly Cornell, Penn State, and Michigan State, in that each of these campuses includes individuals who claim one or more of the specialties. Frequently these individuals work in different academic units on the same campus, but more often than not have little contact with one another.

Influentials and Communications Groups

An examination of those sociologists who have had the greatest influence on their work reveals that a few are sociologists outside the group, including Marx, Weber, Elias, Parsons, Lenski, Howard Becker, Michael Burawoy, and Michael Arrighi. Each of these was identified by a single group member. Several of these influentials were functionalists; others were identified as developmentalists; still others, conflict theorists. Save for Becker, the work of these influentials was lodged firmly at a macrolevel. The remaining influentials are from within the group and can be better understood by dividing the group into the specialties that they represent.

A clear communications group is found among those who primarily identify with the sociology of agriculture and the sociology of food (but not nutrition, for the most part). The influentials or sociometric stars include Fred Buttel and Bill Friedland, and to a slightly lesser extent, William Lacy and Larry Busch. These four tend to list one another as influences, but Friedland is clearly the star in this regard. Once again, a strong Cornell connection is apparent; of all those who identified with the sociology of food and the sociology of agriculture, five have worked at one time or another in a department of that campus. Three graduated in development sociology from Cornell.

Iowa State has served as a primary source of those in the sociology of food/ sociology of nutrition. The stars in the food/nutrition group include McIntosh, Sobal, Whit, Kallen, Mennell, and Murcott, in descending order.[3] Collaboration be-

---

[3] I suspect the fact the since I mailed out the survey had something to do with the frequency with which my name was mentoned by respondents.

tween the European members (Mennell, Murcott, van Otterloo) is nearly as intense as it is between their U.S. counterparts (Sobal, Whit, and McIntosh). The latter group have collaborated to produce a paper (published in *Teaching Sociology*) regarding three approaches that they take to the teaching of the sociology of food and/or nutrition (see Sobal, McIntosh, & Whit, 1993). Both Sobal and Whit, as well as Mennell, have commented on the present work; McIntosh and Sobal gave Whit input on his 1995 book. Sobal and McIntosh are currently working on several papers together. Maurer and Sobal (1995) organized McIntosh, Murcott, Poppendieck, and other scholars for the production of a social problems reader on food and nutrition issues.

FORMAL ARRANGEMENTS

The Sociology of Agriculture subgroup began with a one-day informal meeting held just prior to the 1978 annual meeting of the Rural Sociological Society (RSS) (Friedland, 1991:13). The subgroup now meets formally the day prior to the beginning of every annual RSS meeting. As meetings developed, publications also developed, beginning with Rodefeld et al. *Change in Rural America* (1978) and followed by *The Rural Sociology of the Advanced Societies* (1980) by Buttel and Newby (Friedland, 1991).

While the American Anthropological Association was forming a nutritional anthropology interest group, within the Rural Sociological Society a research interest group developed called the "sociology of human nutrition." This first appeared in the 1978–1979 RSS Membership Directory. Of the 917 active domestic and foreign members listed, eleven, or approximately 2 percent, claimed this specialty. The percentage dropped to less than 2 percent until the 1988–89 edition, at which time it rose back to 2 percent; the 1990–92 edition reports the percentage at 2.7 (25 out of 918 active members). Over the eight editions published since 1979, the identity of the participants has fluctuated as well. John Ballweg, McIntosh, Virginia Purtle, Robert Moxley, Peggy Shifflett, Jacques Viaene, and Mervin Yetley are the only rural sociologists to appear on the list five or more times. The group has no elected leadership, nor is it assigned sessions to organize at the annual meetings. Members of the RSS, such as Rex Warland, who currently conduct research in the sociologies of food and nutrition have appeared only once. The American Sociological Association has no such specialty area, although papers on nutrition have been read in the medical sociology sessions and papers regarding cuisine were presented in culture sessions at the annual meeting.

More formal efforts at organization have occurred outside existing sociological associations. A group of rural sociologists, ethicists, nutritionists, and others from various agricultural sciences began to meet in 1986 at the Agriculture, Food, and Human Values Conference (AFHV). A journal, *Food, Agriculture, and Hu-*

man Values, had already begun in 1984. It was not until 1990 that this group formalized by means of a charter. A second group, the Association for the Study of Food and Society (ASFS), was formed in 1985 by William Whit and Yvonne Vising, who in their own words "sought to increase interest in the study of the social aspects of food and nutrition." The first meeting was held at Aquinas College, Grand Rapids, Michigan, in 1987; meetings have occurred every year since then, the most recent at Tuskegee University in 1995. Membership was 29 persons at the end of the 1986 meeting; slightly more than half of these were sociologists. Membership now is approximately 80 persons, slightly less than half of whom are sociologists.

Nonsociologist members have largely come from nutrition science and dietetics, with a few food scientists who have joined more recently. A handful of philosophers and other social scientists make up the remainder. Annual meeting attendance has fluctuated between 70–120 registered participants. In 1991, ASFS and AFHV began to hold their annual meetings jointly because of the overlap in subject matter and disciplines and the desire to increase conference attendance. Discussions continue as to the desirability of a formal merger of the two groups.

ASFS has had a newsletter, published twice a year, since 1987. AFHV began a newsletter in 1991. ASFS plans publication of its first issue of *Food and Society*, a refereed journal, in the Spring of 1996. The journal *Food, Agriculture, and Human Values* publishes issues quarterly and currently has over 600 subscribers. In addition to these, several other journals oriented toward food or nutrition issues have made page space available to a number of sociologists in the sociologies of food and nutrition. These include *Rural Sociology*, *Appetite*, *Food and Foodways*, the *International Journal of Sociology of Agriculture*, and the *Ecology of Food and Nutrition*.

Critical reviews by those involved in the emerging field have begun to appear, beginning with Ann Murcott's (1988) review of cultural approaches to food and the special issue of *American Behavioral Scientist* edited by George Peters and Leon Rappaport (1988). These were followed by Mennell, Murcott, and van Otterloo (1992), who have attempted to provide a review that links various sociological theories, concepts, and interest areas found in writings about food and nutrition. At some points, they provide critical assessments; at others, the effort reflects more of a cataloguing.

Mullins (1973) noted that at the cluster stage texts began to emerge for teaching purposes. William Whit (1995) has produced such a text, and others have expressed interest in writing such works that place greater stress either on nutrition as a health issue or on sociological theory. Whit and Lockwood (1990) produced a syllabus collection of folklore, anthropology, nutrition, and sociology courses that focuses on the social aspects of food and nutrition. More recently, Sobal, McIntosh, and Whit (1993) published a paper on teaching the sociology of food and nutrition. The point is, however, that such texts have begun to appear. Interest has also grown in the social problems aspects of food and nutrition; thus, recently Sobal and Maurer were approached by Aldine De Gruyter, a publishing company that specializes in social problems studies, regarding the editing of a social problems work organized around food and nutrition (see Maurer & Sobal, 1995).

PROSPECTS

There is cause for optimism. The numbers of sociologists and publications in the sociologies of food and nutrition, although small in number, have both increased. In addition, an increasing number of sociologists have called for the formation of a formally recognized specialty area (Calasanti & Hendricks, 1986; DeVault, 1991; Peters & Rappaport, 1988). The new journal sponsored by ASFS increases to four the number of refereed journals that provide a specific outlet to social scientists working on food and nutrition issues.

Furthermore, and more importantly, the sociologies of agriculture, food, and nutrition possess a number of characteristics that favor their growth. First, they represent new opportunities for scientific work. As Zuckerman (1988) observed, science grows through the establishment of new areas of work. These represent new fields of endeavor for established scholars who have exhausted the potential of the older specialties and provide openings for career-building by young scholars. However, as Zuckerman (1988) and Diesing (1991) suggested, new ideas, while necessary, are not sufficient for the establishment of a specialty. Without the creation of new roles in the specialty, and faculty positions for them, the subdiscipline will never grow and develop. At present, few rural sociology (Iowa State, Washington State) and no sociology departments have advertised for applicants for sociology of food or nutrition positions. Some departments have explicitly sought and hired sociology of agriculture and consumer sociology specialists. Many of the sociologists working in the sociology of food or nutrition were hired as specialists in culture, social organization, or other well-established areas and have pursued their food and nutrition interests through these older specialties.

A perusal of the *Rural Sociologist* indicates that over the past five years, rural sociology departments have not sought agricultural, food, or nutrition specialists. Fewer than 10 openings occur each year, and the plurality have sought either environmental or community sociologists. The demand for nutritional sociology has come from departments of nutrition; however, these entities have sought social scientists with interests and expertise in nutrition rather than sociologists per se. This demand has been neither steady nor strong. Jeff Sobal was hired by the Division of Nutrition at Cornell several years ago; in the early 1980s, the Department of Nutrition at UC Davis interviewed six candidates for an opening, including two sociologists. Ultimately, an anthropologist was hired. Agencies and foundations interested in research on development have sought social scientists with interdisciplinary training and experience in such areas as nutrition.

Some research opportunities are available for sociologists in agriculture, food, or nutrition. The Competitive Grants program within USDA established a behavioral science category in the late 1970s, and, for several years, sociologists received these grants (including Robert Schafer and Peggy Shifflett). However, a project funded under this category received a "Golden Fleece" award from then Sen. William Proxmire, and the category was eliminated. Only in 1991 was this category resuscitated. Rex Warland and Robert Hermann received a grant from the behavioral science category in the same year. The National Institutes of Health (NIH) have included human nutrition in their calls for proposals (e.g., National Institute on Aging, National Institute on Child Health and Human Development). In some cases these requests have included interest in "human" or "behavioral" factors. Maridee Davis, Jeff Sobal, and McIntosh have received such grants. One difficulty reported by both sociologists and anthropologists who have sought NIH funding for studies involving social factors and nutrition lies in the "epidemiological" bias that undergirds the review process. This has meant that the research design has had to follow epidemiological standards and the research team includes epidemiologists and biostatisticians. Thus, sociologists who have attempted to write such proposals have had to develop relationships not only with dietitians and nutritionists but also epidemiologists and biostatisticians. This likely means bringing together individuals who have had little interdisciplinary experience in general and no previous history of working together. Finding and bringing together such individuals is often complicated by the organizational setting: such individuals work not only in different academic departments but also in different colleges on a university campus. Building such teams represents a major investment of time and attention, and there is no guarantee that a given campus will contain the requisite personnel or interests. My optimism is thus guarded; opportunities abound, but the new field must compete with attractive alternatives. Its fate depends on the persuasiveness of the work of my colleagues and me.

REFERENCES

Abbott, A. (1988). *The systems of professions: An essay on the division of expert labor.* Chicago: University of Chicago Press.

Adorno, T. W. (1975). Culture industry reconsidered. *New German Critique*, 6, 12–19.

Agueros, J. (1993). Beyond the crust. In K. Aguero (Ed.), *Daily fare: Essays from the multicultural experience* (pp. 216–227). Athens: University of Georgia Press.

Ahrne, G. (1990). *Agency and organization: Towards an organizational theory of society.* Newbury Park: Sage.

Aiken, M., & Hage, J. (1968). Organizational interdependence and interorganizational structure. *American Sociological Review*, 33, 912–930.

Aiken, M., & Hage, J. (1971). The organic organization and innovation. *Sociology*, 5, 63–82.

Alamgir, M. (1981). An approach towards a theory of famine. In J. R. K. Robson (Ed.), *Famine: Its causes, effects, and management* (pp. 19–40). New York: Gordon/Breach.

Alasuutari, P. (1992). *Desire and craving: A cultural theory of alcoholism.* Albany: State University of New York Press.

Alba, R. (1990). *Ethnic identity: The transformation of white America.* New Haven: Yale University Press.

Albrecht, D. E., & Murdock, S. H. (1984). Toward a human ecological perspective on parttime farming. *Rural Sociology*, 49, 389–411.

Albrecht, D. E., & Murdock, S. H. (1990). *The sociology of U.S. agriculture.* Ames: Iowa State University.

Albrecht, D. E., Murdock, S. H., Hamm, R. R., & Shifflett, K. L. (1987). *Farm crisis: Impact on producers and rural communities in Texas (Departmental Tech. Rep. No. 87–5).* College Station: Texas A&M University, Department of Rural Sociology.

All across America, it's feast and famine. (1984, October 14). *Chicago Tribune*, pp. 1, 22–23, section 1.

Allan, G. (1985). *Family life: Domestic roles and social organization.* New York: Basil Blackwell.

Allen, P. (1993). Connecting the social and the ecological in sustainable agriculture. In P. Allen (Ed.), *Food for the future: Conditions and contradictions of sustainability* (pp. 1–16). New York: John Wiley.

Allon, N. (1973). The stigma of overweight in everyday life. In G. A. Bray (Ed.), *Obesity in perspective: Fogarty International Series in Preventive Medicine.* Vol. 2, part 2 (pp. 83–102). Washington DC: U.S. Government Printing Office.

Allon, N. (1979). Group dieting. In N. Allon (Ed.), *Urban lifestyles* (pp. 29–81). Dubuque: W. C. Brown.

American Medical Association. (1992). *Physician characteristics and distribution in the United States.* Chicago: AMA.

Anderson, E. N. (1988). *The food of China.* New Haven: Yale University Press.

Andreas, C. (1994). *Meatpackers and beef barons: Company town in a global economy.* Niwot: University of Colorado Press.

Angel, R. (1989). The health of the Mexican origin population. In P. Brown (Ed.), *Perspectives in medical sociology* (pp. 82–94). Belmont: Wadsworth.

Antonovosky, A. (1987). *Unraveling the mystery of health.* San Francisco: Jossey-Bass.

Appadurai, A. (1988). How to make a national cuisine: Cookbooks in contemporary India. *Comparative Studies in History and Culture, 30,* 3–24.

Applebaum, R. (1972). *Theories of social change.* Chicago: Markham.

Appleby, A. B. (1978). *Famine in Tudor and Stuart, England.* Stanford: Stanford University Press.

Armstrong, P. S., & Schulman, M. D. (1990). Financial strain and depression among farm operators: The role of perceived economic hardship and personal control. *Rural Sociology, 55,* 475–493.

Arnold, D. (1988). *Famine: Social crisis and historical change.* New York: Basil Blackwell.

Aronson, N. (1981, August). *Vitamins: The social construction of a scientific concept.* Paper presented at the annual meeting of the American Sociological Association, Toronto, Canada.

Aronson, N. (1982a). Nutrition as a social problem: A case study of entrepreneurial strategy in science. *Social Problems, 29,* 473–487.

Aronson, N. (1982b). Social definitions of entitlement: Food needs, 1885–1920. *Media, Culture, and Society, 4,* 51–61.

Arrighi, G., & Drangel, J. (1986). Stratification of the world system-economy: An explanation of the semi-peripheral zone. *Review, 10,* 9–74.

Ashkenazi, M. (1991). From Tachi Soba to Naorai: Cultural implications of the Japanese meal. *Social Science Information, 30,* 287–304.

Ayalah, D., & Weinstock, I. J. (1979). *Breasts: Women speak about their breasts and their lives.* New York: Summit.

Baird, P., & Schutz, H. (1980). Life style correlations of dietary and biochemical measures of nutrition. *Journal of the American Dietary Association, 76,* 228–235.

Barkin, D. (1985). Global proletarianization. In S. Sanderson (Ed.), *The Americas in the new international division of labor* (pp. 26–45). New York: Holmes/Meier.

Barnett, R. J., & Cavanagh, J. (1994). *Global dreams: Imperial corporations and the New World order.* New York: Simon/Schuster.

Baron, J. N., & Beilby, W. T. (1985). Organizational barriers to gender equality: Sex segregation of jobs and opportunities. In A. S. Rossi (Ed.), *Gender and the life course* (pp. 23–51). New York: Aldine.

Barrett, D. F., & Frank, D. A. (1987). *The effects of undernutrition on children's behavior.* New York: Gordon/ Breach.

Barthel, D. (1989). Modernism and marketing: The chocolate box revisited. *Theory, Culture & Society, 6,* 429–438.

Barthes, R. (1972a). *Critical essays* (Richard Howard, trans.). Evanston: Northwestern University Press.

Barthes, R. (1972b). *Semiology.* St. Albans: Paladin.

Barthes, R. (1973). *Mythologies.* St. Albans: Paladin.

Barthes, R. (1982). *Empire of the signs.* New York: Hill/Wang.

Basta, S. S., & Churchill, A. (1974). *Iron deficiency anemia and the productivity of adult males in Indonesia.* World Bank Staff Working Paper No. 175. Washington, DC: International Bank for Reconstruction and Development (IBRD).

Bateman, R., & McIntosh, W. A. (1994, August). *Development versus women's empowerment in children's nutritional status.* Paper presented at the annual meeting of the Rural Sociological Society, Portland, OR.

Baudrillard, J. (1981). *For a critique of the political economy of the sign.* St. Louis: Telos.

Baudrillard, J. (1988). *Jean Baudrillard: Selected writing.* Cambridge: Polity Press.

Baudrillard, J. (1989). The anorexic ruins. In D. Kamper & C. Wulf (Eds.), *Looking back at the end of the world* (pp. 29–45). New York: Semiotext(e).

Baudrillard, J. (1993). *Symbolic exchange and death*. Thousand Oaks: Sage.

Bayley, S. (1991). *Taste: The secret meaning of things*. New York: Pantheon Books.

Beck, U. (1992). From industrial society to risk society. *Theory, Culture, and Society*, 9, 97–123.

Becker, G. S. (1965). A theory of the allocation of time. *Economic Journal*, 75, 493–517.

Becker, H. (1963). Becoming a marijuana smoker. In H. Becker (Ed.), *Outsiders: Studies in the sociology of deviance* (pp. 41–58). New York: Free Press.

Behrman, M. (1988). *All that is solid melts into air: The experience of modernity*. New York: Penguin.

Belasco, W. J. (1993). *Appetite for change: How the counterculture took on the food industry, 1966–1988* (rev. ed.). Ithaca: Cornell University Press.

Bell, D. (1976). *The cultural contradictions of capitalism*. New York: Basic Books.

Berce, Y. M. (1990). *History of peasant revolts: The social origins of rebellion in early modern France*. Ithaca: Cornell University Press.

Berg, A. (1969). Priorities of nutrition in national development. In N. S. Scrimshaw & A. S. Altschul (Eds.), *Amino acid fortification of protein foods* (pp. 12–25). Boston: MIT Press.

Berg, A. (1973). *The nutrition factor: Its role in national development*. Washington, DC: Brookings Institute.

Berg, A. (1987). *Malnutrition: What can be done? Lessons from the World Bank experience*. Baltimore: Johns Hopkins University Press.

Berg, A. & Muscat, R. (1971). Macronutrition. In P. L. White & N Selvey (Eds.), *Proceedings of the 3rd Western Hemisphere Nutrition Congress*, (pp. 318–323). Acton: Publishing Sciences Group.

Berg, F. (1991a). Obesity costs reach $39.3 billion. In C. C. Cook-Fuller (Ed.), *Annual editions, nutrition, 92/93* (pp. 118–119). Guilford: Dushkin.

Berg, F. (1991b). Obesity: Year 2000 crisis? In C. C. Cook-Fuller (Ed.), *Annual editions, nutrition, 92/93* (pp. 114–116). Guilford: Dushkin.

Berger, P. L., & Luckman, T. (1966). *The social construction of reality*. Garden City: Doubleday.

Berkman, L. A., & Syme, L. S. (1979). Social network, host resistance, and mortality: A nine-year follow-up study of Alameda county residents. *American Journal of Epidemiology*, 190, 186–204.

Berry, J. M. (1982). Consumers and the hunger lobby. In D. F. Hadwiger & R. B. Talbot (Eds.), *Food policy and farm programs*. Proceedings of the Academy of Political Science (Vol. 34, No. 3, pp. 68–78). Montpelier: Capital City Press.

Berry, J. M. (1984). *Feeding hungry people: Rule making in the foodstamp program*. New Brunswick: Rutgers University Press.

Berry, W. (1990). *What are people for?* San Francisco: North Point Press.

Bertaux, D. (1982). The life course approaches as a challenge to the social sciences. In T. K. Hareven & K. J. Adams (Eds.), *Aging and life course transitions: An interdisciplinary perspective* (pp. 127–150). New York: Guilford Press.

Best, J. (1989). Introduction: Typification and social problems construction. In J. Best (Ed.), *Images of issues: Typifying contemporary social problems* (pp. xv–xiv). New York: Aldine De Gruyter.

Biagi, H. (1992, June). *The school lunch program in America: The politics of child nutrition*. Paper presented at the annual meeting of the Association for the Study of Food and Society and the Agriculture, Food, and Human Values Society, East Lansing, MI.

Birch, L. L. (1990). The control of food intake by young children: The role of learning. In E. D. Capaldi & L. Powley (Eds.), *Taste, experience, and feeding* (pp. 116–135). Washington, DC: American Psychological Association.

Bishop-Tramm, A. D. (1995). *Content analysis of the 1995 national fluid milk processor promotion board advertisements*. Unpublished manuscript, Texas A&M University, Department of Sociology, College Station.

Blake, J. (1981). Family size and the quality of children. *Demography*, 18, 421–428.

Blane, D. (1987). The value of labour-power and health. In G. Scambler (Ed.), *Sociological theory and medical sociology* (pp. 8–36). London: Tavistock.

Blaxter, M. (1990). *Health and lifestyles*. New York: Tavistock/Routledge.

Block, F. L. (1987). *Revisiting state theory: Essays in politics and postmodernism*. Philadelphia: Temple University Press.

Blood, R. O., & Wolfe, D. M. (1960). *Husbands and wives*. New York: Free Press.

Blumberg, R. L. (1988). Income under female versus male control. *Journal of Family Issues*, 9, 51–84.

Boakes, R. A., Popplewell, D. A., & Burton, M. J. (1987). *Eating habits: Food, physiology, and learned behavior*. Chichester: John Wiley.

Bogue, D. J. (1969). *Principles of demography*. New York: John Wiley.

Bohstedt, J. (1983). *Riots and community politics in England and Wales 1790–1810*. Cambridge: Harvard University Press.

Boies, J. L. (1994). *Buying for Armageddon: Business, society, and military spending since the Cuban missile crisis*. New Brunswick: Rutgers University Press.

Boisseau, C. (1992, March 23). Mexican staple creates a multibillion-dollar business. *Houston Chronicle*, p. C1.

Bokemeir, J. L., Sachs, C., & Keith, V. (1983). Labor force participation of metropolitan, nonmetropolitan, and farm women: A comparative study. *Rural Sociology*, 48, 515–539.

Bolo, P. M. (1993). The biological basis for bulimia. In A. J. Giannini & A. E. Slaby (Eds.), *The eating disorders* (pp. 45–62). New York: Springer-Verlag.

Bonnano, A. (1988). Theories of the state: The case of land reform in Italy, 1944–1961. *Sociological Quarterly*, 29, 131–147.

Bonnano, A. (1994). The locus of polity action in a global setting. In A. Bonnano, L. Busch, W. Friedland, L. Gouvia, & E. Mingione (Eds.), *From Columbus to ConAgra: The globalization of agriculture and food* (pp. 251–264). Lawrence: University Presses of Kansas.

Bordo, S. (1993). *Unbearable weight: Feminism, Western culture, and the body*. Berkeley: University of California Press.

Bose, C. (1980). Social status of the homemaker. In S. Fenstermaker Berk (Ed.), *Women and household labor* (pp. 69–87). Beverly Hills: Sage.

Boserup, E. (1965). *The conditions of agricultural growth*. Chicago: Aldine.

Boserup, E. (1970). *Women's role in economic development*. New York: St. Martin's Press.

Boserup, E. (1983). The impact of scarcity and plenty on development. In R. I. Rotberg & T. K. Rabb (Eds.), *Hunger and history: The impact of changing food production and consumption on society* (pp. 185–210). Cambridge: Cambridge University Press.

Bossard, J. H. S., & Boll, E. S. (1950). *Ritual in family living: A contemporary study*. Philadelphia: University of Pennsylvania Press.

Bouis, H. (1994). Consumption effects of commercialization of agriculture. In J. von Braun & E. Kennedy (Eds.), *Agriculture, commercialization, economic development, and nutrition* (pp. 65–78). Baltimore: Johns Hopkins University Press.

Bourdieu, P. (1984). *Distinction: A social critique of the judgment of taste*. Cambridge: Harvard University Press.

Bouton, C. A. (1993). *The flour war: Gender, class, and community in late Ancien Regime French society*. University Park: Penn State University Press.

Bovard, J. (1991). *The farm fiasco*. San Francisco: Institute for Contemporary Studies.

Bradley, C. C., Burton, M. L., & White, D. R. (1990). A cross-cultural historical analysis of subsistence change. *American Anthropologist*, 92, 447–457.

Bradshaw, Y. W., Noonan, R., Gash, L., & Sershen, C. B. (1993). Borrowing against the future: Children and Third World indebtedness. *Social Forces*, 71, 629–656.

Braudel, F. (1979a). *The structures of everyday life: Civilization and capitalism 15th–18th Century.* Vol. I. New York: Harper/Row.

Braudel, F. (1979b). *Civilization and capitalism: The wheels of commerce.* Vol. II. New York: Harper/Row.

Braverman, H. (1974). *Labor and monopoly capital: The degradation of work in the twentieth century.* New York: Monthly Review Press.

Bread for the World Institute and RESULTS Educational Fund. (1995). *Putting children first: A report on the effectiveness of U.S. Agency for International Development Child Survival Programs in Fiscal Year 1991* (Occasional Paper No. 3). Silver Spring: Bread for the World Institute.

Breidenstein, B. C., & Williams, J. C. (n.d.). *Contribution of red meat to the diet.* Chicago: National Live Stock and Meat Board.

Brown, J. L., & Pitzer, H. F. (1987). *Living hungry in America: The Harvard physician task force on hunger in America reports on the face of hunger in a bountiful land.* New York: Macmillan.

Brown, L. A. (1981). *Innovation diffusion: A new perspective.* New York: Methunen.

Browne, W. P., & Ciglar, A. J. (1990). *U. S. Agricultural groups: Institutional profiles.* Westport: Greenwood Press.

Browne, W. P., Skees, J. R., Swanson, L. E., Thompson, P. B., & Unnevehr, L. J. (1992). *Sacred cows and hot potatoes: Agrarian myths in agricultural policy.* Boulder: Westview Press.

Bruch, H. (1988). *Conversations with anorexics.* New York: Basic Books.

Brumberg, J. J. (1988). *Fasting girls: The emergence of anorexia nervosa as a modern disease.* Cambridge: Harvard University Press.

Burawoy, M. (1979). *Manufacturing consent: Changes in the labor process under monopoly capitalism.* Chicago: University of Chicago Press.

Burns, J., McIntosh, W. A., & Zey, M. (1994, August). *Globalization of capital resource dependency and children's nutritional status.* Paper presented at the annual meeting of the Rural Sociological Society, Portland, OR.

Butler, S., & Skipper, J. K., Jr. (1983). Working the circuit: An explanation of employee turnover in the restaurant industry. *Sociological Spectrum, 3,* 19–33.

Buttel, F. H. (1995). *Sustainable agriculture: Beyond self-fulfilling marginality* (Center for Biotechnology Policy and Ethics Discussion Paper CBPE 95–4). College Station: Texas A & M University, Institute of Biosciences and Technology.

Buttel, F. H., & Gillespie, G. W. (1984). The sexual division of farm household labor: An exploratory study of the structure of on-farm and off-farm men and women. *Rural Sociology, 49,* 183–209.

Buttel, F. H., & Newby, H. (1980). *The rural sociology of the advanced societies.* Montclair: Allanheld/Osmun.

Buttel, F. H., & Swanson, L. E. (1986). Soil and water conservation: A farm structural and public policy context. In S. B. Lovejoy & T. L. Napier (Eds.), *Conserving the soil: Insights from socioeconomic research* (pp. 26–39). Ankeny: Soil Conservation of America.

Buttel, F. H., Larson, O., & Gillespie, G. W. (1990). *The sociology of agriculture.* Westport: Greenwood Press.

Calasanti, T. M., & Hendrick, J. (1986). A sociological perspective on nutrition research among the elderly. *Gerontologist, 26,* 232–238.

Caldwell, J. C. (1986). Routes to low mortality in poor countries. *Population and Development Review, 12,* 171–220.

Calhoun, C. (1982). *The question of class struggle: Social foundations of popular radicalism during the industrial revolution.* Chicago: University of Chicago Press.

Caliendo, M. A. (1979). *Nutrition and the world food crisis.* New York: Macmillan.

Call, D. L., & Longhurst, R. (1971). Evaluation of the economic consequences of malnutrition. In P. L. White & N. Selvey (Eds.), *Proceedings of the 3rd Western Hemisphere Nutrition Congress* (pp. 312–317). Acton: Publishing Sciences Group.

Camp, C. (1989). *American foodways: What, when, why, and how we eat in America.* Little Rock: August House.

Campbell, C. (1987). *The romantic ethic and the spirit of modern consumerism.* Oxford: Basil Blackwell.

Campbell, T. C., Chen, T., Parpia, B. B., Yinsheng, Q., Chumming, C., & Geissler, C. (1992). China: From diseases of poverty to diseases of affluence, policy implications of the epidemiological transition. *Ecology of Food and Nutrition,* 27, 133–144.

Camporesi, P. (1989). *Bread of dreams: Food and fantasy in early modern Europe.* Chicago: University of Chicago Press.

Caplow, T., Bahr, H. M., & Chadwick, B. A. (1982). *Middletown families: Fifty years of change and continuity.* Minneapolis: University of Minnesota Press.

Carnerio, R. L. (1970). A theory of state development. *Science,* 169, 733–738

Carroll, G. R., Preisendoefer, P., Swaminathan, A., & Wiedenmeyer, G. (1993). Brewery and brauerei: The organizational ecology of brewing. *Organization Studies,* 14, 155–188.

Cassel, J. (1976). The contribution of the social environment to host resistance. *American Journal of Epidemiology,* 104, 107–123.

Charles, N., & Kerr, M. (1988). *Women, food, and families.* Manchester: Manchester University Press.

Chase, P., & Martin, H. P. (1970). Undernutrition and child development. *New England Journal of Medicine,* 282, 934–939.

Chase-Dunn, C. (1989). *Global formation: Structures of the world economy.* Cambridge: Basil Blackwell.

Chastanet, M. (1992). Survival strategies of a Sahalian society: The case of the Soninke in Senegal from the middle of the 19th century to the present. *Food and Foodways,* 5, 127–149.

Chavas, J. P. (1983). Structural change in U.S. demand for meat. *American Journal of Agricultural Economics,* 65, 148–153.

Cheal, D. (1988). *The gift economy.* New York: Routledge.

Childe, V. G. (1963). *Social evolution* (2nd ed.). Cleveland: Merdian Books.

Christenson, C. (1978). World hunger: A structural approach. *International Organization,* 32, 745–774.

Christenson, J. A., & Garkovich, L. E. (1985). Fifty years of rural sociology: Status, trends. *Rural Sociology,* 50, 503–522.

Cipolla, C. M. (1980). *Before the industrial revolution: European society and economy, 1000–1700.* New York: W. W. Norton.

Clark, G. L., & Dear, M. D. (1984). *State apparatus: Structures and language of legitimacy.* Boston: Allen/Unwin.

Clegg, S. R. (1990). *Modern organizations: Organizational studies in the postmodern world.* London: Sage.

Cobble, D. S. (1991). *Dishing it out: Waitresses and their unions in the twentieth century.* Urbana: University of Illinois Press.

Cockburn, C., & Ormrod, S. (1993). *Gender and technology in the making.* Thousand Oaks: Sage.

Cohen, G. A. (1978). *Karl Marx's theory of history: A defense.* Princeton: Princeton University Press.

Cohen, M. N. (1989). *Health and the rise of civilization.* New Haven: Yale University Press.

Cohen, M. N. (1990). Prehistoric patterns of hunter. In L. F. Newman, W. Crossgrove, R. W. Kates, R. Matthews, & S. Millman (Eds.), *Hunger in history: Food shortage, poverty, and deprivation* (pp. 56–97). Cambridge: Basil Blackwell.

Cohen, P. T., & Purcal, J. T. (1989). The political economy of primary health care in Southeast Asia: Problems and prospects. In P. Cohen and J. Purcal (Eds.), *The political economy of primary health care in Southeast Asia* (pp. 1–22). Canberra: Australian Development Studies Network, ASEAN Training Centre for Primary Health Care Development.

Cohn, S. F., Barkan, S. E., & Whitaker, W. H. (1993). Activists against hunger: Membership characteristics of a national social movement organization. *Sociological Focus*, 35, 113–131.

Collins, R. (1975). *Conflict sociology*. New York: Academic Press.

Collins, R. (1988). *Theoretical sociology*. San Diego: Harcourt/Brace/Jovanovich.

Collins, R. (1994). Women and the production of status culture. In M. Lamont & M. Fournier (Eds.),
Symbolic boundaries and the making of inequality (pp. 231–231). Chicago: University of Chicago Press.

Colson, E. (1980). In good years and in bad: Food strategies of self-reliant societies. *Journal of Anthropological Research*, 92, 447–457.

Conquest, R. (1986). *Harvest of sorrow: Soviet collectivization and the terror-famine*. New York: Oxford University Press.

Cook, J., Altman, D. J., Moore, D. M. C., Topp, S. G., Holland, W. N., & Elliott, A. (1973). A survey
of the nutritional status of schoolchildren: Relation between nutrient intake and socio-econom-
ic factors. *British Journal of Preventative Social Medicine*, 27, 91–99.

Cook, R. (1971). The primary costs of malnutrition and its impacts on society. In P. L. White & N
Selvey (Eds.), *Proceedings of the 3rd Western Hemisphere Nutrition Congress* (pp. 324–327).
Acton: Publishing Sciences Group.

Cooley, C. H. (1962) [1909]. *Social organization: A study of a larger mind*. New York: Schocken
Books.

Copp, J. H. (1972). Rural sociology and rural development. *Rural Sociology*, 37, 515–533.

Coppock, M. L., & McIntosh, W. A. (1991, March). *The relationship of family mealtime to family satisfaction and cohesion*. Paper presented at the annual meeting of the Southwest Social Science
Association, San Antonio, TX.

Corporate support to dietitians group is called unhealthy. (1995, November 15). *New York Times*, p.
B1.

Correa, H. (1963). *The economics of human resources*. Amsterdam: New Holland.

Correa, H. (1969). Nutrition, working capacity, productivity, and development. In P. L. White & N
Selvey (Eds.), *Proceedings of the 2nd Western Hemisphere Nutrition Congress* (pp. 188–192).
Acton: Publishing Sciences Group.

Correa, H., & Cummins, G. (1970). Contributions of nutrition to economic growth. *American Journal
of Clinical Nutrition*, 23, 560–565.

Coser, R. L. (1987). Power lost and gained: A step in the direction of sex equality. *Kolner Zeitschrift
für Soziologie und Soziolpsychologie*, 39, 23–41.

Cowan, R. S. (1983). *More work for mothers: The ironies of household technology from the open
hearth to the microwave*. New York: Basic Books.

Cox, B. D., Huppert, F. A., & Whichelow, M. J. (1993). *The health and lifestyle survey: Seven years
on*. Broookfield: Dartmouth.

Cox, C. (1994). *Storefront co-ops and the counterculture*. New Brunswick: Rutgers University Press.

Cox, G. W. (1981). The ecology of famine: An overview. In J. Robson (Ed.), *Famine: Its causes, effects, and management* (pp. 5–18). New York: Gordon/Beach.

Crane, D. (1969). Social structure in a group of scientists: A test of the "invisible college" hypothesis.
American Sociological Review, 34, 335–352.

Cravioto, J., & DeLicardie, E. R. (1972). Environmental correlates of severe clinical malnutrition and
language development in survivors from kwashiorkor or marasmus. In Pan American Health
Organization (Pan American Sanitary Bureau) (Ed.), *Nutrition, the nervous system, and behavior* (Scientific Publication No. 251, pp. 73–94). Washington, DC: Pan American Health Organization.

Creighton, H. (1982). Tied by double apron strings: Female work culture and organization in a restaurant. *Insurgent Sociologist*, 11, 59–64.

Crimmins, E. M., Saito, Y., & Inegneri, D. (1989). Changes in life expectancy and disability-free life expectancy in the United States. *Population and Development Review*, 15, 235–267.

Cronon, W. (1991). *Nature's metropolis: Chicago and the great West*. New York: W. W. Norton.

Crook, S., Pakulski, J. S., & Waters, M. (1992). *Postmodernism: Change in advanced society*. Newbury Park: Sage.

Crosby, A. W. (1986). *Ecological imperialism: The biological expansion of Europe, 900–1900*. New York: Cambridge University Press.

Dahlberg, K. A. (1979). *Beyond the Green Revolution: The ecology and politics of global agricultural development*. New York: Plenum Press.

Dasgupta, P. (1993). *An inquiry into well-being and destitution*. New York: Oxford University Press.

Davidson, A. (1992). Europeans' wary encounter with tomatoes, potatoes, and other New World foods. In N. Foster & L. S. Cordell (Eds.), *Chilies to chocolate: Food the Americas gave the world* (pp. 1–14). Tucson: University of Arizona Press.

Davis, K. (1958). *Human Society*. New York: Macmillan.

Davis, M. (1992). *City of quartz: Excavating the future of Los Angeles*. New York: Vintage Books.

DeGarine, I. (1972). The socio-cultural aspects of nutrition. *Ecology of Food and Nutrition*, 1, 143–163.

Delacroix, J., Swaminathan, A., & Solt, M. E. (1989). Density dependence versus population dynamics. *American Sociological Review*, 54, 245–262.

del Castillo, G. (1992) Foreign direct investment, capital formation, and the balance of payments of developing countries. In C. R. Lehman & R. M. Moore (Eds.), *Multinational culture: Social impacts of a global economy* (pp.45–60). Westport: Greenwood.

DeLind, L. B., & Spielberg-Benetiz, J. (1990). The re-industrialization of Michigan agriculture: An examination of state agricultural policies. *The Rural Sociologist*, 10, 29–41.

Delphy, C. (1979). Sharing the same table. In C. Harris (Ed.), *The sociology of the family: New directions for Britain*. Sociological Review Monograph (pp. 214–231). Manchester: University of Keele Press.

Denzin, N. K. (1984). *On understanding emotion*. San Francisco: Jossey-Bass.

Denzin, N. K. (1987). *The alcoholic self*. Beverly Hills: Sage.

Derber, C. (1984). *The pursuit of attention: Power and individualism in everyday life*. Boston: G. K. Hall.

DeVault, M. L. (1991). *Feeding the family: The social organization of caring as gendered work*. Chicago: University of Chicago Press.

DeVault, M. L. (1995). Between science and food: Nutrition professionals in the health care hierarchy. *Research in the Sociology of Health Care*, 12, 287–312.

DeVault, M. L., & Pitts, J. P. (1984). Surplus and scarcity: Hunger and the origins of the foodstamp program. *Social Problems*, 31, 545–557.

Devereux, S. (1993). *Theories of famine*. New York: Harvester Wheatsheaf.

DeWaal, A. (1989). *Famine that kills: Darfur, Sudan, 1984–1985*. Oxford: Oxford University Press.

Dewey, K. G. (1979). Agricultural development, diet, and nutrition. *Ecology of Food and Nutrition*, 8, 265–273.

Dewey, K. G. (1980). The impact of agricultural development on child nutrition in Tabasco, Mexico. *Medical Anthropology*, 4, 21–54.

Dewey, K. G. (1981). Nutritional consequences of the transformation from subsistence to commercial agriculture in Tabasco, Mexico. *Human Ecology*, 9, 151–187.

Dicken, P. (1992). *Global shift: Industrial change in a turnabout world (2nd ed.)*. London: Harper/Row.

Diesing, P. (1991). *How does social science work? Reflections on practice*. Pittsburgh: University of Pittsburgh Press.

Dirks, R. (1980). Social response during severe food shortages and famine. *Current Anthropology*, 21, 21–32.

Dirks, R. (1993). Starvation and famine: Cross-cultural codes and some hypothesis tests. *Cross-Cultural Research*, 27, 28–69.

Dolch, N. A., & Heffernan, W. D. (1978). Applicability of complex organization theory to small organizations. *Social Science Quarterly*, 59, 202–209.

Douglas, M. (1971). Deciphering a meal. In C. Geertz (Ed.), *Myth, symbol, and culture* (pp. 61–81). New York: Norton.

Douglas, M. (1973). *Natural symbols: Explorations in cosmology*. Hammondsworth: Penguin.

Douglas, M. (Ed.). (1984). *Food and the social order: Studies of food and festivities in three American communities*. New York: Russell Sage Foundation.

Douglas, M. (1991) [1966]. *Purity and danger*. New York: Routledge.

Douglas, R. R. (1968). Dinnertime dynamics. *The Family Coordinator*, 17, 181–184.

Doyal, L., & Gough, I. (1991). *A theory of human need*. New York: Guilford Press.

Dreze, J., & Sen, A. (1989). *Hunger and public action*. Oxford: Oxford University Press.

Dryer, C. D., & Dryer, A. S. (1973). Family dinnertime as a unique behavior. *Family Process*, 12, 291–301.

Durham, C. A., & Sexton, R. J. (1992). Oligopsony potential in agriculture: Residual supply estimates in California's processing tomato market. *American Journal of Agricultural Economics*, 74, 966–972.

Durkheim, E. (1933) [1893]. *The division of labor in society*. New York: Free Press.

Durkheim, E. (1951) [1897]. *Suicide: A study in sociology*. New York: Free Press.

Dutton, D. B. (1989). Social class, health, and illness. In P. Brown (Ed.), *Perspectives in medical sociology* (pp. 23–45). Belmont: Wadsworth.

Dynes, R. R., & Tierney, K. J. (1994). *Disasters, collective behavior, and social organization*. Newark: University of Delaware Press.

Edgley, C., & Brissett, D. (1990). Health Nazis and the cult of the perfect body: Some polemical observations. *Symbolic Interaction*, 13, 257–279.

Elder, G. H., Jr., & Liker, J. K. (1982). Hard times in women's lives: Historical influences across forty years. *American Journal of Sociology*, 88, 241–269.

Elias, N. (1978) [1939]. *The history of manners. The civilizing process*. Vol. I. New York: Pantheon Books.

Elixhauser, A., Harris, D. R., & Coffey, R. M. (1995). *Trends in hospital diagnoses: Regional variations, 1980–87 (Provider Studies, Research Note 23)*. Washington DC: Center for General Health Services Intramural Research, Agency for Health Care Policy and Research.

Enge, K. I., & Martinez-Enge, P. M. (1991). Land, malnutrition, and health: The dilemmas of development in Guatemala. In S. Whiteford & E. Ferguson (Eds.), *Harvest of want: Hunger and food security in Central America and Mexico* (pp. 75–102). Boulder: Westview Press.

Enriquez, L. J. (1991). *Harvesting change: Labor, and agrarian reform in Nicaragua, 1979–1990*. Chapel Hill: University of North Carolina Press.

Epstein, C. F. (1988). *Deceptive distinctions: Sex, gender, and the social order*. New Haven & New York: Yale University Press/Russell Sage Foundation.

Estes, C. A., Gerard, L. E., Zones, J. A., & Swan, J. H. (1984). *Political economy, health, and aging*. New York: Little Brown.

Evans, P. (1979). *Dependent development: The alliance of multinational, state, and local capital in Brazil*. Princeton: Princeton University Press.

Evers, B., & Mason, S. H. (1994). Survey overview-1994-update. How are Americans making food choices? (Summary of a Gallop Poll conducted for the American Dietetic Association). *Electronic Food Rap*, 4, 1.

Evers, S., & McIntosh, W. A. (1977). Social indicators of human nutrition: Measures of nutritional status. *Social Indicators Research*, 4, 185–205.

Ewen, S. (1988). *All-consuming images: The politics of style in contemporary culture*. New York: Basic Books.

Falese, J. S., & Unnevehr, L. J. (1988). Demand for beef and chicken products: Separability and structural change. *American Journal of Agricultural Economics*, 70, 521–532.

Falk, W. W., & Gilbert, J. (1985). Bringing rural sociology back in. *Rural Sociology*, 50, 561–577.

Falk, W. W., & Zhao, S. (1989). Paradigms, theories, and methods in rural sociology: A partial replication and extension. *Rural Sociology*, 54, 587–600.

Fallon, A. E., & Rozin, P. (1985). Sex differences in perceptions of desirable body shape. *Journal of Abnormal Psychology*, 94, 102–105.

Faurschou, G. (1987). Fashion and the cultural logic of postmodernity. *Canadian Journal of Political and Social Theory*, 11, 8–15.

Feds: 20 percent of U. S. teens overweight. (1994, November 11). *The Eagle*, p. A7.

Ferguson, C. E. (1972). *Micro-economic theory* (3rd ed.). Homewood: Irwin.

Fine, B., & Leopold, E. (1993). *The work of consumption*. New York: Routledge.

Fingarette, H. (1988). *Heavy drinking: The myth of alcoholism as a disease*. Berkeley: University of California Press.

Finklestein, J. (1989). *Dining out: A sociology of modern manners*. Washington Square: New York University Press.

Firebaugh, G. (1992). Growth effects of foreign and domestic investment. *American Journal of Sociology*, 98, 105–130.

Firebaugh, G., & Beck, F. D. (1994). Does economic growth benefit the masses?: Growth, dependence, and welfare in the Third World. *American Sociological Review*, 59, 631–653.

Fischler, C. (1980). Food habits, social change, and the nature/culture dilemma. *Social Science Information*, 19, 937–953.

Fiske, J. (1989). *Understanding popular culture*. Boston: Urwin Hyman.

Fiske, J. (1991). Postmodernism and television. In J. Curran & M. Gurevitch (Eds.), *Mass media and society* (pp. 55–67). New York: Edward Arnold.

Flood, A. B., & Scott, W. R. (1987). *Hospital structure and performance*. Baltimore: John Hopkins University Press.

Floud, R., Wachter, K., & Gregory, A. (1990). *Height, health, and history: Nutritional status in the United Kingdom, 1750–1980*. New York: Cambridge University Press.

Food and Agriculture Organization. (1993). *FAO Yearbook. Trade, 1992* (Statistical Series No. 115, Vol. 46). Rome: Food and Agriculture Organization.

Food and Agriculture Organization. (1994). *FAO Yearbook Production, 1993* (Statistical Series No. 117, Vol. 47). Rome: Food and Agriculture Organization.

Food Research and Action Center (FRAC). (1991). *Community childhood hunger identification project: A survey of childhood hunger in the United States*. Executive Summary, Washington, DC.

Forker, O. D., & Ward, R. W. (1993). *Commodity advertising: The economics and measurement of generic programs*. New York: Lexington Books.

Foucault, M. (1973). *Madness and civilization*. New York: Vintage.

Foucault, M. (1977). *Discipline and punish: The birth of the prison*. New York: Random House.

Foucault, M. (1978). *The history of sexuality Vol. 1: An introduction*. New York: Random House.

Fox, K. D., & Nichols, S. V. (1983). The time crunch: Wife's employment and family work. *Journal of Family Issues*, 4, 61–82.

Frank, A. G. (1978). *Dependent accumulation and underdevelopment*. London: Macmillan.

Franke, R. W., & Chasin, B. N. (1980). *Seeds of famine: Ecological destruction and the development dilemma in the West African Sahel*. Totowa: Rowman/Allanheld.

Freeman, J. H., & Hannan, M. I. (1983). Niche width and the dynamics of organizational populations. *American Journal of Sociology*, 88, 1116–1145.

Freeman, M. (1977). Sung. In K. C. Chang (Ed.), *Food in Chinese culture* (pp. 143–176). New Haven: Yale University Press.

Frenkel, M. V. (1991). The dilemma of food security in a revolutionary context: Nicaragua. In S. A. Whiteford & E. Ferguson (Eds.), *Harvest of want: Hunger and food security in Central America and Mexico* (pp. 141–189). Boulder: Westview Press.

Freudenburg, W. R. (1993). Risk and recreancy: Weber, the division of labor, and the rationality of risk perceptions. *Social Forces*, 71, 909–932.

Freudenburg, W. R., & Pastor, S. K. (1992). Public responses to technological risks: Toward a sociological perspective. *Sociological Quarterly*, 33, 389–412.

Friedland, W. H. (1989). Is rural sociology worth saving? *The Rural Sociologist*, 9, 3–5.

Friedland, W. H. (1991). Introduction: Shaping the new political economy of advanced capitalist agriculture. In W. H. Friedland, L. Busch, F. H. Buttel, & A. P. Rudy (Eds.), *Towards a new political economy of agriculture* (pp. 1–34). Boulder: Westview Press.

Friedland, W. H., & Barton, A. (1975). *Destalking the wily tomato: A case study in social consequences in California agricultural research*. Davis: University of California, Department of Applied Behavioral Sciences.

Friedland, W. H., Barton, A. E., & Thomas, R. J. (1981). *Manufacturing green gold: Capital, labor and technology in the lettuce industry*. Cambridge: Cambridge University Press.

Friedmann, H. (1978a). Simple commodity production and wage labour in the American plains. *Journal of Peasant Studies*, 6, 71–100.

Friedmann, H. (1978b). World market, state, and family farm: Social bases of household production in an era of wage labour. *Comparative Studies in Society and History*, 22, 639–652.

Friedmann, H. (1980). Household production and the national economy: Concepts for the analysis of agrarian formations. *Journal of Peasant Studies*, 7, 158–184.

Friedmann, H. (1988). Form and substance in the analysis of the world economy. In B. Wellman & S. D. Berkowitz (Eds.), *Social structures: A network approach* (pp. 304–325). New York: Cambridge University Press.

Friedmann, H. (1990). The origins of Third World food dependence. In H. Bernstein, B. Crow, M. Mackintosh, & C. Martin (Eds.), *The food question: Profits vs. people* (pp. 13–31). New York: Monthly Review Press.

Friedmann, H. (1991). Changes in the international division of labor: Agri-food complexes and export agriculture. In W. H. Friedland, L. Busch, F. H. Buttel, & A. P. Rudy (Eds.), *Towards a new political economy of agriculture* (pp. 65–93). Boulder: Westview Press.

Friedmann, H. (1994). The international relations of food: The unfolding crisis of national regulation. In B. Harriss-White & R. Hoffenberg (Eds.), *Food: Multidisciplinary perspectives* (pp. 174–204). Cambridge: Basil Blackwell.

Friedrichs, R. W. (1970). *A sociology of sociology*. New York: Free Press.

Friesema, H. P., Caporaso, J., Goldstein, G., Lineberry, R., & McCleary, R. (1979). *Aftermath: Communities after natural disaster*. Beverly Hills: Sage.

Frisbie, W. P, & Poston, D. (1976). The structure of sustenance organization and population change. *Rural Sociology*, 41, 355–370.

Gacitua, E. A., & Bello, R. (1991). Agricultural exports, food production, and food security in Latin America. *Rural Sociology*, 56, 391–405.

Gallant, T. W. (1991). *Risk and survival in ancient Greece*. Stanford: Stanford University Press.

Galtung, J. (1990). The Green Movement: A socio-historical explanation. In M. Albrow & E. King (Eds.), *Globalization, knowledge, and society* (pp. 235–250). Newbury Park: Sage.

Gane, M. (1991). *Baudrillard's bestiary: Baudrillard and culture*. New York: Routledge.

Garner, D., Garfinkel, P. E., & Thompson, J. (1980). Cultural expectations of thinness in women. *Psychological Reports*, 47, 483–491.

Garnham, N., & Willliams, R. (1980). Pierre Bourdieu and the sociology of culture: An introduction. *Media, Culture, and Society*, 2, 209–223.

Garnsey, P. (1990). Responses to food crisis in the ancient Mediterranean world. In L. F. Newman, W. Crossgrove, R. W. Kates, R. Matthews, & S. Millman (Eds.), *Hunger in history: Food shortage, poverty and deprivation* (pp. 126–146). Cambridge: Basil Blackwell.

Gartman, D. (1991). Culture as class symbol or mass reification? A critique of Bourdieu's Distinction. *American Journal of Sociology*, 97, 421–447.

Geertz, C. (1963). *Agricultural involution: The process of ecological change in Indonesia*. Berkeley: University of California Press.

Geertz, C. (1973). The integrative revolution: Primordial sentiments in the new states. In C. Geertz (Ed.), *The interpretation of cultures* (pp. 255–310). New York: Basic Books.

Gerber, J., & Short, J. F., Jr. (1986). Publicity and the control of corporate behavior: The case of infant formula. *Deviant Behavior*, 7, 195–216.

Gereffi, G., Korzenicwicz, M., & Korzenicwicz, R. P. (1994). Introduction: Global commodity chains. In G. Gereffi & M. Korzenicwicz (Eds.), *Commodity chains and global capitalism* (pp. 1–14). Westport: Praeger.

Gerhardt, U. (1989). *Ideas about illness: An intellectual and political history of medical sociology*. Washington Square: New York University Press.

Gerstl, J. E. (1961). Leisure, taste, and occupational milieu. *Social Problems*, 9, 56–68.

Gerth, H. H., & Mills, C. W. (1946). *From Max Weber: Essays in sociology*. New York: Oxford University Press.

Giddens, A. (1973). *The class structure of the advanced societies*. New York: Harper/Row.

Giddens, A. (1984). *The constitution of society*. Berkeley: University of California Press.

Giddens, A. (1985). *The nation-state and violence*. Berkeley: University of California Press.

Giddens, A. (1991). *Modernity and self-identity: Self and society in the late Modern Age*. Stanford: Stanford University Press.

Gilbert, J., & Howe, C. (1991). Beyond 'state and society': Theories of the state and New Deal agricultural policies. *American Sociological Review*, 56, 204–220.

Giuffre, P. A., & Williams, C. L. (1994). Boundary lines: Labeling sexual harassment in restaurants. *Gender and Society*, 8, 378–401.

Glassner, B. (1988). *Bodies: Why we look the way we do (and how we feel about it)*. New York: Putnams' Sons.

Glassner, B. (1990). Fit for postmodern selfhood. In H. S. Becker & M. M. McCall (Eds.), *Symbolic interaction and cultural studies* (pp. 215–243). Chicago: University of Chicago Press.

Goffman, E. (1959). *The presentation of self in everyday life*. New York: Doubleday.

Goffman, E. (1961). *Asylums*. New York: Anchor.

Goffman, E. (1963). *Behavior in public places*. New York: Free Press.

Gofton, L. (1986). The rules of the table. In L. Gofton & J. McKenzie (Eds.), *The food consumer* (pp. 127–153). New York: John Wiley.

Goldman, R. (1992). *Reading ads socially*. New York: Routledge.

Goldschieder, F. K., & Waite, L. J. (1991). *New families, no families?: The transformation of the American home*. Berkeley: University of California Press.

Goldschmidt, W. (1974) [1946]. *As you sow: Three studies in the social consequences of agribusiness*. New York: Allenheld/Osmun.

Goldstein, M. S. J. (1992). *The health movement: Promoting fitness in America*. New York: Twayne.

Goldstone, J. (1991). *Revolution and rebellion in the early modern world*. Berkeley: University of California Press.

Goode, J. G., Curtis, K., & Theophano J. (1984). Meal formats, meal cycles, and menu negotiations in the maintenance of an Italian-American community. In M. Douglas (Ed.), *Food in the social order* (pp. 143–218). New York: Russell Sage Foundation.

Goodman, D., & Redclift, M. (1991). *Refashioning nature: Food, ecology, and culture.* New York: Routledge.

Goodwin, D. D., & Marlowe, J. (1990). Farm wives' labor force participation and earnings. *Rural Sociology*, 55, 25–43.

Goodwin, J. M., & Attias, R. (1994). Eating disorders in survivors of multimodal childhood abuse. In M. G. Winkler & L. B. Cole (Eds.), *Asceticism in contemporary culture* (pp. 23–35). New Haven: Yale University Press.

Goody, J. (1982). *Cooking, cuisine, and class: A study in comparative sociology.* New York: Cambridge University Press.

Gordon, Jr., A. M. (1983). The nutriture of Cubans: Historical perspective and nutritional analysis. *Cuban Studies*, 13, 1–40.

Gordon, R. A. (1990). *Anorexia and bulimia: Anatomy of a social epidemic.* Cambridge: Basil Blackwell.

Gould, M. (1987). *Revolution in the development of capitalism: The coming of the English revolution.* Berkeley: University of California Press.

Gramsci, A. (1971). *Selections from the prison notebooks.* New York: International Publishers.

Granovetter, M. (1973). The strength of weak ties. *American Journal of Sociology*, 78, 1360–1380.

Grant, J. P. (1991). *The state of the world's children 1991.* New York: Oxford University Press.

Grant, M. W. (1964). Rate of growth in relation to birth rank and family size. *British Journal of Preventative Social Medicine*, 18, 35–39.

Greely, A. (1974). *Ethnicity in the United States: A preliminary reconnaissance.* New York: John Wiley.

Gronow, J. (1991). Need, taste, and pleasure: Understanding food and consumption. In E. L. Furst, R. Prattala, M. Elestrom, L. Holm, & U. Kjaernes (Eds.), *Palatable worlds: Sociocultural food studies* (pp. 33–52). Oslow: Solum Vorlag.

Gross, D. R., & Underwood, B. A. (1971). Technological change and caloric costs: Sisal agriculture in N. E. Brazil. *American Anthropologist*, 73, 725–740.

Groth, III, E. (1991). Communicating with consumers about food safety and risk issues. *Food Technology*, 45, 248–253.

Guilkey, D. K., & Stewart, J. F. (1995). Infant feeding patterns and the marketing of infant foods in the Philippines. *Economic Development and Cultural Change*, 43, 369–399.

Guither, H. D. (1980). *The food lobbyists: Behind the scenes of food and agri-politics.* Lexington: Lexington Books.

Gusefield, J. (1991). Benevolent repression: Popular culture, social structure, and the control of drinking. In S. Barrows & R. Room (Eds.), *Drinking: Behavior and belief in modern history* (pp. 399–424). Berkeley: University of California Press.

Gusefield, J. (1992). Nature's body and the metaphors of food. In M. Lamont & M. Fournier (Eds.), *Cultivating differences: Symbolic boundaries and the making of inequality* (pp. 75–103). Chicago: University of Chicago Press.

Guseman, P. K., & Sapp, S. G. (1984). Demographic trends and consumer demand for agricultural products. *Southern Rural Sociology*, 1, 1–24.

Guseman, P. K., & Sapp., S. G. (1986). Regional trends in U.S. food consumption: Population scale, composition, and income effects. *Review of Regional Studies*, 1, 1–24.

Guseman, P. K., Bassenyemukasa, C., & Sapp, S. G. (1987). *Population size, composition, and income effects on per capita and aggregate beef consumption: An illustrative analysis (Department of Rural Sociology Tech.* Rep. No. 87–2). College Station: Texas A&M University, Texas Agricultural Experiment Station.

Gussow, J. D. (1990, August). *Dazed in the supermarket: Is this free choice?* Keynote address at the annual meeting for the Association for the Study of Food and Society, Philadelphia, PA.

Gvion-Rosenberg, L. (1988, August). *Cultural pluralism or culinary hegemony: The case of ethnic dishes: 1945–1987*. Paper presented at the annual meeting of the American Sociological Association, Atlanta, GA.

Gvion-Rosenberg, L. (1989, June). *Printing, hegemony, and cuisines: The story of vegetables: 1945–1987*. Paper presented at the annual meeting of the Association for the Study of Food and Society, Tucson, AZ.

Haas, J. E., & Drabek, T. E. (1973). *Complex organizations: A sociological perspective*. New York: Macmillan.

Habermas, J. (1976). *Legitimization crisis*. Boston: Beacon Press.

Hagerstrand, T. (1976). *Innovation diffusion as a spatial process*. Chicago: University of Chicago Press.

Hakim, P., & Solimano, G. (1978). *Development, reform, and malnutrition in Chile*. Cambridge: MIT Press.

Hall, E. (1993). Waitering/waitressing: Engendering the work of table service. *Gender and Society, 7*, 329–346.

Halpern, S. A. (1990). Medicalization as a professional process: Postwar trends in pediatrics. *Journal of Health and Social Behavior, 31*, 28–42.

Hamilton, S., Popkin, B. M., & Spicer, D. (1984). *Women and nutrition in the Third World*. South Hadley: Bergin/Garvey.

Hane, M. (1982). *Peasants, rebels, and outcastes: The underside of modern Japan*. New York: Pantheon.

Hansell, S., Sherman, G., & Mechanic, D. (1991). Body awareness and medical care utilization among older adults in an HMO. *Journal of Gerontology, 46*, S151–S159.

Hansen, J. M. (1991). *Gaining access: Congress and the farm lobby, 1919–1981*. Chicago: University of Chicago Press.

Harper, A. E. (1987). Dietary standards: Recommended dietary allowances in perspective. In C. C. Cook-Fuller (Ed.), *Nutrition 87/88. Annual editions* (pp. 54–58). Guilford: Dushkin.

Harris, M. (1974). *Cows, pigs, wars, and witches: The riddle of culture*. New York: Vintage Books.

Harris, M. (1979). *Cultural materialism: The struggle for a science of culture*. New York: Vintage Books.

Harris, M. (1985). *Good to eat: Riddles of food and culture*. New York: Simon/Schuster.

Harris, M., & Ross, E. B. (Eds.). (1987). *Food and evolution*. Philadelphia: Temple University Press.

Harris, N. (1990). The drama of consumer desire. In N. Harris (Ed.), *Cultural excursions: Marketing, appetites, and cultural tastes in modern America* (pp. 174–197). Chicago: University of Chicago Press.

Harriss, B. (1990). Food distribution, death, and disease in South Asia. In G. A. Harrison & J. C. Waterlow (Eds.), *Diet and disease in traditional and developing societies* (pp. 290–306). New York: Cambridge University Press.

Harvey, D. (1989). *The condition of postmodernity*. Cambridge: Basil Blackwell.

Hattox, R. S. (1985). *Coffee and coffeehouses: The origins of a social beverage in the Medieval Near East*. Seattle: University of Washington Press.

Hawkins, R. (1984). Employee theft in the restaurant trade: Forms of ripping off by waiters at work. *Deviant Behavior, 5*, 47–69.

Heffernan, W. D. (1972). Sociological dimensions of agricultural structures in the United States. *Sociologica Ruralis, 22*, 481–499.

Heffernan, W. D. (1984). Constraints in the U.S. poultry industry. In H. Schwarzweller (Ed.), *Research in rural sociology and development* (pp. 237–260). Greenwich: JAI Press.

Heffernan, W. D., & Constance, D. H. (1994). Transnational corporations and the globalization of the food system. In A. Bonnano, W. Friedland, L. Gouveia, & E. Mingione (Eds.), *From Columbus to ConAgra: The globalization of agriculture and food* (pp. 29–51). Lawrence: University Press of Kansas.

Heffernan, W. D., Constance, D., & Gronski, R. (1993, August). *Concentration of agricultural markets.* Paper presented at the annual meeting of the Rural Sociological Society, State College, PA.

Heick, W. H. (1991). *A propensity to protect: Butter, margarine, and the rise of urban culture in Canada.* Canada: Wilfrid Lawner University Press.

Herzlich, C., & Pierret, J. (1987) [1984]. *Illness and self in society.* Baltimore: Johns Hopkins University Press.

Hilgartner, S., & Bosk, C. L. (1988). The rise and fall of social problems: A public arena model. *American Journal of Sociology*, 94, 53–78.

Hinkle, R. C. (1980). *Founding theory of American sociology 1881–1915.* Boston: Routledge/Kegan Paul.

Hinton, M. A., Eppright, E., Chadderdon, H., & Wolins, L. (1963). Eating behavior and dietary intake of girls 12 to 14 years old. *Journal of the American Dietetics Association*, 43, 223–227.

Hirschman, A. O. (1976). *The passions and the interests: Political arguments for capitalism before its triumph.* Princeton: Princeton University Press.

Hirschl, T. A., & Rank, R. M. (1991). The effect of population density on welfare participation. *Social Forces*, 70, 225–235.

Hoban, T. J., & Kendall, P. A. (1993). *Consumer attitudes about food biotechnology.* Raleigh: North Carolina Cooperative Extension Service.

Hoban, T. J., Woodrum, E., & Czaja, R. (1992). Public opposition to genetic engineering. *Rural Sociology*, 57, 476–493.

Hochschild, A. (1989). *The second shift: Working parents and the revolution at home.* New York: Viking Press.

Homans, G. (1974). *Social behavior: Its elementary forms* (2nd ed.). New York: Harcourt/Brace/Jovanovich.

Hook, N. C., & Paolucci, B. (1970). The family as an ecosystem. *Journal of Home Economics*, 62, 315–318.

Hugill, P. J. (1993). *World trade since 1431: Geography, technology, and capitalism.* Baltimore: John Hopkins Press.

Ibarra, P. R., & Kitsuse, J. I. (1993). Vernacular constituents of moral discourse: An interactionist proposal for the study of social problems. In G. Miller & J. A. Holstein (Eds.), *Constructivist controversies: Issues in social problems theory* (pp. 21–54). New York: Aldine De Gruyter.

Ilmonen, K. (1991). Change and stability in Finnish eating habits. In E. L. Furst, R. Prattala, M. Ekstrom, L. Holm, & U. Kjaernes (Eds.), *Palatable worlds: Sociocultural food studies* (pp. 169–184). Oslo: Solum Vorlag.

Immink, M. D. C., & Viteri, F. E. (1981). Energy intake and productivity of Guatemalan sugarcane cutters: An empirical test of the efficiency wage hypothesis. *Journal of Development Economics*, 9, 251–271.

Inkeles, A., & Smith, D. H. (1974). *Becoming modern: Individual and society.* Princeton: Princeton University Press.

Jackson, L. A. (1992). *Physical appearance and gender: Sociological and sociocultural perspectives.* Albany: State University of New York Press.

Jankowiak, J. (1989). Huge staff mans German co-op. *The National Provisioner*, 201, 5–13.

Jessop, B. (1989). Capitalism, nation-state, and surveillance. In D. Held & J. B. Thompson (Eds.), *Social theory of modern societies* (pp. 103–128). New York: Cambridge University Press.

Jhally, S. (1987). *The codes of advertising: Fetishism and the political economy of meaning in the consumer society.* New York: Routledge.

Johnson, A. (1991). *Factory farming.* Cambridge: Basil Blackwell.

Johnson, C. (1966). *Revolutionary change.* Boston: Little/Brown.

Johnson, M. (1989). Feminism and the theories of Talcott Parsons. In R. A. Wallace (Ed.), *Feminism and sociological theory* (pp. 101–118). Newbury Park: Sage.

Johnson, P. J. (1983). Divorced mother's management of responsibilities: Conflicts between employment and child care. *Journal of Family Issues, 4,* 83–103.

Johnson, R. K., Smiciklas-Wright, H., Croutier, A. C., & Willits, F. K. (1992). Maternal employment and the quality of young children's diets: Empirical evidence based on the 1987–1988 Nationwide Food Consumption Survey. *Pediatrics, 90,* 245–249.

Jones, E. L. (1981). *The European miracle: Environments, economies, and geopolitics in the history of Europe and Asia.* New York: Cambridge University Press.

Jones, J. (1989). The Tuskegee syphilis experiment. In P. Brown (Ed.), *Perspectives in medical sociology* (pp. 538–549). Belmont: Wadsworth.

Jurska, A., & Busch, L. (1994). The production of knowledge and the production of commodities: The case of rapeseed techno-science. *Rural Sociology, 59,* 581–597.

Jussame, R. A., & Judson, D. H. (1992). Public perceptions about food safety in the United States and Japan. *Rural Sociology, 57,* 235–249.

Kalcik, S. (1984). Ethnic foodways in America: Symbol and the performance of identity. In L. Keller-Brown & K. Mussell (Eds.), *Ethnic and regional foodways in the United States* (pp. 37–65). Knoxville: University of Tennessee Press.

Kallen, D. J. (1971). Nutrition and society. *Journal of the American Medical Society, 215,* 94–100.

Kallen, D. J. (1973). Nutrition and the community. In D. Kallen (Ed.), *Nutrition, development and social behavior* (pp. 33–50). Washington, DC: National Institutes of Health, U.S. Department of Health, Education, and Welfare.

Kandel, D. B., Davies, M., & Raveis, V. H. (1985). The stressfulness of daily social roles for women: Marital, occupational, and household roles. *Journal of Health and Social Behavior, 26,* 64–78.

Kandel, R. F., & Pelto, G. H. (1980). The health food movement: Social revitalization or alternative health maintenance system. In N. W. Jerome, R. F. Kandel, & G. H. Pelto (Eds.), *Nutritional anthropology: Contemporary approaches to diet and culture* (pp. 327–363). Pleasantville: Redgrave.

Kaneko, L. (1993). Of rice and bread. In K. Aguero (Ed.), *Daily fare: Essays from the multicultural experience* (pp. 174–185). Athens: University of Georgia Press.

Kanter, R. M. (1977). *Men and women of the corporation.* New York: Basic Books.

Kaplan, H. B. (1986). *The social psychology of self referential behavior.* New York: Plenum.

Kaplan, H. B. (1991). Social psychology of the immune system: A conceptual framework and review of literature. *Social Science and Medicine, 33,* 909–923.

Kaplan, S. L. (1976). *Bread, politics, and political economy in the reign of Louis XV* (2 vol.). The Hague: M. Nijhoff.

Kaplan, S. L. (1982). The famine plot persuasion in eighteenth-century France. *Transactions of the American Philosophical Society, 72,* 1–79.

Kaplan, S. L. (1990). The state and the problem of dearth in the eighteenth-century France: The crisis of 1738–41 in Paris. *Food and Foodways, 4,* 16–59.

Katz, F. (1968). Integrative and adaptive use of autonomy: Worker autonomy in factories. In F. Katz (Ed.), *Autonomy and organization: The limits of social control.* New York: Random House.

Keith, P. M., & Schafer, R. B. (1991). *Relationships and well-being over the life stages.* New York: Praeger.

Kellman, M. (1987). *World hunger: A neo-Malthusian perspective.* New York: Praeger.

Kellner, D. (1989). *Jean Baudrillard: From Marxism to postmodernism and beyond.* Stanford: Stanford University Press.

Kellner, D. (1991). Popular culture and the construction of postmodern identities. In S. Lash & J. Friedman (Eds.), *Modernity and identity* (pp. 141–177). Cambridge: Basil Blackwell.

Kennedy, E. (1994). Health and nutrition effects of commercialization of agriculture. In J. von Braun & E. Kennedy (Eds.), *Agricultural commercialization, economic development, and nutrition* (pp. 79–99). Baltimore: John Hopkins University Press.

Kenny, M. (1986). *Biotechnology: The university-industrial complex.* New Haven: Yale University Press.

Keplinger, K. O. (1981). *The nutritional impact of domestic food programs in the United States.* Unpublished master's thesis. Texas A&M University, Department of Agricultural Economics, College Station.

Keys, A. J., Brozek, A., Henschel, O., Micklesen, G., & Taylor, H. L. (1950). *The biology of human starvation. Vol. II.* Minneapolis: University of Minnesota Press.

Kick, E. L. (1987). World system structure, national development, and the prospects for a socialist world order. In T. Boswell & A. Bergesen (Eds.), *America's changing role in the world-system* (pp. 127–156). New York: Praeger.

Kinsey, J. (1983). Working wives and the marginal propensity to consume food away from home. *American Journal of Agricultural Economics*, 65, 10–19.

Kintner, M., Boss, P., & Johnson, N. (1978). The relationship between dysfunctional family environments and family member food intake. *Journal of Marriage and the Family*, 43, 633–641.

Klopfer, L. (1993). Padang restaurants: Creating 'ethnic' cuisine in Indonesia. *Food and Foodways*, 5, 293–304.

Kloppenburg, Jr., J. R. (1988). *First the seed: The political economy of plant biotechnology, 1492–2000.* New York: Cambridge University Press.

Komlos, J. (1994). On the significance of anthropometric history. In J. Komlos (Ed.), *Stature, living standards, and economic development* (pp. 210–220). Chicago: University of Chicago Press.

Kucera, B. (1986). *The effects of family structure variables on the nutritional status of children: An empirical assessment.* Unpublished master's thesis, Texas A&M University, Department of Sociology, College Station.

Kucera, B., & McIntosh, W. A. (1991). Family size as a determinant of children's dietary intake: A dilution model approach. *Ecology of Food and Nutrition*, 25, 1–12.

Lamont, M. (1992). *Money, morals, and manners: The culture of the French and American upper-middle class.* Chicago: University of Chicago Press.

Langman, L. (1991). From pathos to panic: American character meets the future. In P. Wexler (Ed.), *Critical theory now* (pp. 165–241). New York: Falmer Press.

Lasch, C. (1977). *Haven in a heartless world: The family besieged.* New York: Basic Books.

Lasswell, T. G. (1965). *Class and stratum.* New York: Houghton Mifflin.

Latham, M. D. (1973). A historical perspective. In A. Berg, N. S. Scrimshaw, & D. L. Call (Eds.), *Nutrition, national development, and planning* (pp. 313–328). Cambridge: MIT Press.

Leder, D. (1990). *The absent body.* Chicago: University of Chicago Press.

Lee, J. (1989). Food neophobia: Major causes and treatments. *Food Technology*, 43, 62–73.

Leidner, R. (1993). *Fast food, fast talk: Service work and the routinization of everyday life.* Berkeley: University of California Press.

Leigh, J. P. (1983). Direct and indirect effects of education on health. *Social Science and Medicine*, 17, 227–234.

Leistritz, F. L., & Murdock, S. H. (1988). Financial characteristics of farms and of farm financial markets and policies in the United States. In S. H. Murdock & F. L. Leistritz (Eds.), *The farm financial crisis: Socioeconomic dimensions and implications for producers and rural areas* (pp. 13–28). Boulder: Westview Press.

Lenski, G., & Lenski, J. (1987). *Human societies: An introduction to macro-sociology (5th ed.).* New York: McGraw-Hill.

Leopold Center for Sustainable Agriculture. (1993). *Progress Report Vol.* 2. Ames: Iowa State University.

Leslie, J. (1995). Improving the nutrition of women in the Third World. In P. Pinstrup-Anderson, D. Pelletier, & H. Alderman (Eds.), *Child growth and nutrition in developing countries: Priorities for action* (pp. 117–138). Ithaca: Cornell University Press.

Levenstein, H. (1988). *Revolution at the table: The transformation of the American diet.* New York: Oxford University Press.

Levenstein, H. (1993). *Paradox of plenty: A social history of eating in modern America.* New York: Oxford University Press.

Levin, H. M., Pollitt, E., Galloway, R., & McGuire, J. (1993). Micronutrient deficiency disorders. In D. T. Jamison, W. H. Mosley, A. R. Measham, & J. L. Bobadilla (Eds.), *Disease control priorities in developing countries* (pp. 421–451). New York: Oxford University Press.

Lewin, K. (1943). Forces behind food habits and methods of change. In National Research Council (Eds.), *The problem of changing food habits* (Bulletin No. 108, pp. 35–65). Washington, DC: National Academy of Science.

Lewis, G. H. (1989). The Maine lobster as regional icon: Competing images over time and social class. *Food and Foodways, 3,* 303–316.

Lewis, M., & Feiring, C. (1982). Some American families at dinner. In L. M. Laosa & I. E. Sigel (Eds.), *Families as learning environments for children* (pp. 115–145). New York: Plenum.

Light, D. (1989). Corporate medicine for profit. In P. Brown (Ed.), *Perspectives in medical sociology* (pp. 294–308). Belmont: Wadsworth.

Lindberg, C. (1993). *Beyond charity: Reformation initiatives for the poor.* Minneapolis: Fortress Press.

Lipton, M. (1989). *New seeds and poor people.* Baltimore: Johns Hopkins University Press.

Livi-Bacci, M. (1991). *Population and nutrition: An essay on European demographic history.* New York: Oxford University Press.

Lloyd, C. (1988). *Explanations in social history.* New York: Basil Blackwell.

Lochhead, C. (1991). How hungry? How many? In C. C. Cook-Fuller (Ed.), *Nutrition 91/92* (pp. 210–212). Guilford: Duskin.

Logue, A. W. (1991). *The psychology of eating and drinking: An introduction (2nd ed.).* New York: W. H. Freeman.

Lorenz, F. O., Conger, R. D., & Montague, R. (1994). Doing worse and feeling worse: Psychological consequences of economic hardship. In R. D. Conger & G. H. Elder, Jr. (Eds.), *Families in troubled times: Adapting to change in rural America* (pp. 167–186). New York: Aldine De Gruyter.

Lunn, P. G. (1991). Nutrition, immunity, and infection. In R. Schofield, D. R., & A. Bideau (Eds.), *The decline of mortality in Europe* (pp. 131–145). New York: Oxford University Press.

MacClancy, J. (1992). *Consuming culture: Why you eat what you eat.* New York: Henry Holt.

MacDonald, M. (1977). *Food stamps and income maintenance.* New York: Academic Press.

Macy, M. W. (1991). Chains of cooperation: Threshold effects in collective action. *American Sociological Review, 56,* 475–493.

Malinowski, B. (1944). *A scientific theory of culture and other essays.* Chapel Hill: University of North Carolina Press.

Malthus, T. R. (1959) [1798]. *Population: The first essay.* Ann Arbor: University of Michigan Press.

Manderson, L. (1989). Political economy and the politics of gender: Maternal and child health in colonial Malaya. In P. Cohen & J. Purcal (Eds.), *The political economy of primary health care in Southeast Asia* (pp. 79–100). Canberra: Australian Developmental Studies Network, ASEAN Training Centre for Primary Health Care.

Maney, A. L. (1989). *Still hungry after all these years: Food assistance from Kennedy to Reagan*. New York: Greenwood Press.

Mann, M. (1986). *The sources of social power: Vol. 1. A history of power from the beginning to A.D. 1760*. New York: Cambridge University Press.

Mann, M. (1993). *The sources of social power: The rise of classes and nation-states, 1760–1914*. Vol. 2. New York: Cambridge University Press.

Mann, S. A. (1990). *Agrarian capitalism in theory and practice*. Chapel Hill: University of North Carolina Press.

Mann, S. A., & Dickinson, J. M. (1978). Obstacles to the development of a capitalist agriculture. *Journal of Peasant Studies*, 5, 466–481.

Mann, S. A., & Dickinson, J. M. (1980). State and agriculture in two eras of American capitalism. In F. Buttel & H. Newby (Eds.), *The rural sociology of advanced capitalist societies. Critical perspectives* (pp. 283–325). Montclair: Allanheld/ Osmun.

Marcus, J. (1993, May 5). Famine-relief organization to turn its attention to hungry in America. *The Eagle*, p. A1.

Marcuse, H. (1964). *One-dimensional man: Studies in the ideology of advanced industrial society*. Boston: Beacon Press.

Marmot, M., & Theorell, T. (1994). Social class and cardiovascular disease: The contribution of work. In P. Conrad & R. Kern (Eds.), *The sociology of health & illness: Critical perspectives* (4th ed., pp. 93–106). New York: St. Martin's Press.

Martindale, D. (1960). *The nature and types of sociological theory*. Boston: Houghton-Mifflin.

Marx, R. D. (1993). Depression and eating disorders. In A. Giannini & A. E. Selby (Eds.), *The eating disorders* (pp. 110–127). New York: Springer-Verlag.

Mascie-Taylor, C. G. N. (1990). The biology of social class. In C. G. N. Mascie-Taylor (Ed.), *Biosocial aspects of social class* (pp. 117–142). Oxford: Oxford University Press.

Matthews, R., Anderson, D., Chen, R. S., & Webb, T. (1990). Global climate and the origins of agriculture. In L. F. Newman, W. Crossgrove, R. W. Kates, R. Matthews, & S. Millman (Eds.), *Hunger in history: Food shortage, poverty, and deprivation* (pp. 3–24). Cambridge: Basil Blackwell.

Matossian, M. K. (1989). *Poisons of the past: Molds, epidemics, and history*. New Haven: Yale University Press.

Matras, J. (1979). Mechanisms and processes of societal growth. In A. H. Hawley (Ed.), *Societal growth: Processes and implications* (pp. 30–60). New York: Free Press.

Maurer, D. (1995). Meat as a social problem: Rhetorical strategies in the contemporary vegetarian literature. In D. Maurer & J. Sobal (Eds.), *Eating agendas: Food and nutrition as social problems* (pp. 143–163). New York: Aldine de Gruyter.

Maurer, D., & Sobal, J. (Eds.). (1995). *Eating agendas: Food and nutrition as social problems*. New York: Aldine de Gruyter.

McCracken, G. (1988). *Culture and consumption*. Bloomington: Indian University Press.

McIntosh, W. A. (1975). *Social indicators for monitoring the nutritional aspects of societal well-being*. Unpublished doctoral dissertation, Iowa State University, Department of Sociology, Ames.

McIntosh, W. A. (1995). World hunger as a social problem. In D. Maurer & J. Sobal (Eds.), *Eating agendas: Food and nutrition as social problems*. New York: Aldine de Gruyter.

McIntosh, W. A., & Evers, S. (1982). The role of women in the production of food and nutrition in less developed countries. In P. S. Horne (Ed.), *Women in international development* (pp. 27–51). Texas A&M University President's World University Series No. 2, College Station.

McIntosh, W. A., & Picou, J. S. (1985). Manpower training and the political economy of agriculture: CETA and Texas agriculture. *Social Science Quarterly*, 66, 46–57.

McIntosh, W. A., & Shifflett, P. A. (1981). *The impact of social structure and social attachments, future time perspective, and changing food habits on the nutrient intake of the elderly* (Final Report USDA Competitive Grant No. S901–0410–0126–0). College Station: Texas A&M University, Department of Sociology.

McIntosh, W. A., & Shifflett, P. A. (1984a). Dietary behavior, dietary adequacy, and religious social support: An exploratory study. *Review of Religious Research, 26,* 158–175.

McIntosh, W. A., & Shifflett, P. A. (1984b). Influence of social support systems on dietary intake of the elderly. *Journal of Nutrition for the Elderly,* 4, 5–18.

McIntosh, W. A., & Shifflett, P. (1993). *Characteristics of recipe innovators versus traditionalists.* Unpublished manuscript, Texas A&M University, Department of Sociology, College Station.

McIntosh, W. A., & Zey-Ferrell, M. (1986). Lending officers' decision to recommend innovative agricultural technology. *Rural Sociology, 51,* 471–489.

McIntosh, W. A., & Zey, M. (1989). Women as gatekeepers of food consumption: A sociological critique. *Food and Foodways, 3,* 317–332.

McIntosh, W. A., Klongan, G. E., & Wilcox, L. D. (1977). Theoretical issues and social indicators: A societal process approach. *Policy Sciences, 8,* 245–267.

McIntosh, W. A., Kubena, K. S., & Landmann, W. A. (1989a). *Social support, stress, and the aged's diet and nutrition.* Final report for the National Institute on Aging (Project No. RO1 AGO 04043). College Station: Texas A&M University, Department of Rural Sociology.

McIntosh, W. A., Shifflett, P. A., & Picou, J. S. (1989b). Social support, stress, strain, and the diet of the elderly. *Medical Care, 27,* 190–153.

McIntosh, W. A., Thomas, J. K., & Albrecht, D. (1990). A Weberian perspective on the adoption of value rational technology. *Social Science Quarterly, 55,* 848–860.

McIntosh, W. A., Kaplan, H. B., & Kubena, K. S. (1993a). Life events, social support, and immune response in elderly respondents. *International Journal of Aging and Human Development, 37,* 23–36.

McIntosh, W. A., Kubena, K. S., & Peterson, C. (1993b, June). *Predicting reductions in dietary fat from mass media exposures and health belief.* Paper presented at the annual meeting of the Association for the Study of Food and Society, Tucson, AZ.

McIntosh, W. A., Kubena, K. S., & Landmann, W. A. (1994a). *The effects of social support and stress on hematocrit and hemoglobin.* Unpublished paper. College Station: Texas A&M University, Department of Sociology.

McIntosh, W. A., Christenson, L. B., & Acuff, G. R. (1994b). Perceptions of risks of eating undercooked meat and the willingness to change cooking practices. *Appetite, 22,* 83–96.

McIntosh, W. A., Acuff, G. R., & Christenson, L. B. (1994c). Public perceptions of food safety. *Social Science Journal,* 31, 285–292.

McIntosh, W. A., Fletcher, R. D., Kubena, K. S., & Landmann, W. A. (1995). Factors affecting reasons for reducing red meat intake by elderly subjects. *Appetite,* 24, 219–230.

McIntosh, W. A., Kaplan, H., Kubena, K. S., Bateman, R., & Landmann, W. A. (1996). Platelet status, stress, and social support in the elderly. *Applied Social Science Journal,* 4.

McKenzie, J. (1986). An integrated approach with special reference to study of changing food habits in the United Kingdom. In C. Ritson, L. Gofton, & J. McKenzie (Eds.), *The food consumer* (pp. 155–170). New York: John Wiley.

McKeown, T. (1976). *The modern rise of population.* London: Edward Arnold.

McLaren, D. S. (1974). The great protein fiasco. *Lancet,* 2, 93–96.

McLaren, D. S. (1976a). Concepts and content of nutrition. In D. S. McLaren (Ed.), *Nutrition in the community: A textbook for public health workers* (pp. 3–12). New York: John Wiley.

McLaren, D. S. (1976b). Historical perspective of nutrition in the community. In D. S. McLaren (Ed.), *Nutrition in the community: A textbook for public health workers* (pp. 25–42). New York: John Wiley.

McMichael, P. (1994). Introduction: Agro-food system restructuring—unity in diversity. In P. Mc-Michael (Ed.), *The global restructuring of agro-food systems* (pp. 1–17). Ithaca: Cornell University Press.

McNaughton, J. P., Boyle, C. R., & Bryant, E. S. (1990). *Beef and pork consumers: Socioeconomic, personal and lifestyle characteristics* (Mississippi Agricultural Experiment Station Technical Bulletin No. 172). Starkville: Mississippi State University.

McNeil, W. H. (1976). *Plagues and peoples.* New York: Doubleday.

Meadows, D., Meadows, D. L., Randers, J., & Behrens, W. W., III. (1974). *The limits to growth.* New York: Universe Books.

Mebrahtu, S., Pelletier, D., & Pinstrup-Anderson, P. (1995). Agriculture and nutrition. In P. Pinstrup-Anderson, D. Pelletier, & H. Alderman (Eds.), *Child growth and nutrition in developing countries: Priorities for action* (pp. 220–242). Ithaca: Cornell University Press.

Mechanic, D. (1962). The concept of illness behavior. *Journal of Chronic Diseases, 15,* 189–194.

Mehrabian, A. (1987). *Eating characteristics and temperament: General measures and interrelationships.* New York: Springer-Verlag.

Meigs, A. S. (1984). *Food, sex, and pollution: A New Guinea religion.* New Brunswick: Rutgers University Press.

Mellor, J. W. (1966). *The economics of agricultural development.* Ithaca: Cornell University Press.

Meneig, D. W. (1986). *The shaping of America: A geographical perspective on 500 years of history: Volume I: Atlantic America, 1492–1800.* New Haven: Yale University Press.

Mennell, S. (1985). *All manner of food: Eating and taste in England and France from the Middle Ages to the present.* Oxford: Basil Blackwell.

Mennell, S., Murcott, A., & van Otterloo, A. H. (1992). The sociology of food: Eating, diet, and food. *Current Sociology, 40,* 1–148.

Merleau-Ponty, M. (1962). *Phenomenology of perception.* London: Routledge/Kegan Paul.

Mestrovic, S. G. (1990). *The Coming Fin de Siecle: An application of Durkheim's sociology to modernity and postmodernity.* New York: Routledge.

Mestrovic, S. G. (1992). *Durkheim and postmodern culture.* New York: Aldine De Gruyter.

Mestrovic, S. G., & Glassner, B. (1983). A Durkheimian hypothesis on stress. *Social Science and Medicine, 17,* 1315–1327.

Mexican food served in experiment aimed at spicing up school menus. (1994, September 17). *The Eagle,* p. A1.

Milikan, M. (1971). The relationship between population, food supply, and economic behavior. In N. S. Scrimshaw & A. Altshul (Eds.), *Amino acid fortification of protein foods* (pp. 26–40). Cambridge: MIT Press.

Miller, D. (1987). *Material culture and mass consumption.* Cambridge: Basil Blackwell.

Miller, J. G. (1978). *Living systems.* New York: McGraw Hill.

Miller, R. W. (1981). Production forces and the forces of change: A review of Cohen, G. A., *Karl Marx's theory of history: A defense. Philosophical Review, 90,* 91–117

Millman, S., & Kates, R. W. (1990). Toward understanding hunger. In L. F. Newman, W. Crossgrove, R. W. Kates, R. Matthews, & S. Millman (Eds.), *Hunger in history: Food shortage, poverty, and deprivation* (pp. 3–24). Cambridge: Basil Blackwell.

Minnis, P. E. (1985). *Social adaptation to food stress: A prehistoric southwestern example.* Chicago: University of Chicago Press.

Mintz, S. W. (1985). *Sweetness and power: The place of sugar in modern history.* New York: Viking Press.

Molm, L. D. (1990). Structure, action, and outcomes: The dynamics of power in social exchange. *American Sociological Review, 55,* 427–447.

Monk-Turner, E. (1990). Comparing advertisements in British and American women's magazines. *Social Science Research, 75,* 53–56.

Moon, B. E. (1991). *The political economy of basic human needs*. Ithaca: Cornell University Press.

Mooney, P. H. (1986). Class relations and class structure in the Midwest. In E. Havens, G. Hooks, P. H. Mooney, & M. J. Pfeffer (Eds.), *Studies in the transformation of agriculture* (pp. 206–251). Boulder: Westview Press.

Moore, W. E. (1974). *Social change* (2nd ed.). Englewood Cliffs: Prentice Hall.

Moos, R. H. (1974). *Family environment scale. Preliminary manual*. Palo Alto: Consulting Psychologist Press.

Morgan, D. (1979). *The merchants of grain*. New York: Viking Press.

Mosley, W. H., & Cowley, P. (1991). *The challenge of world health* (Population Reference Bureau. Vol. 46, No. 4.). Washington, DC: Population Reference Bureau.

Moss, D. (1978). Brain, body, and world: Body image and the psychology of the body. In R. S. Valle & M. King (Eds.), *Phenomenological alternatives for psychology* (pp. 63–82). New York: Oxford University Press.

Mothersbaugh, D. L., Hermann, R. O., & Warland, R. H. (1993). Perceived time pressure and recommended dietary practices: The moderating effects of knowledge of nutrition. *Journal of Consumer Affairs*, 27, 106–126.

Mukerji, C. (1983). *From graven images: Patterns of modern materialism*. New York: Columbia University Press.

Mullins, N. C. (1973). *Theories and theory groups in contemporary American sociology*. New York: Harper/Row.

Murcott, A. (Ed.). (1983a). *The sociology of food and eating*. Aldershot: Gower.

Murcott, A. (1983b). Cooking and the cooked. In A. Murcott (Ed.), *The sociology of food and eating* (pp. 178–193). Aldershot: Gower.

Murcott, A. (1986). You are what you eat—Anthropological factors influencing food choices. In C. Ritson, L. Gofton, J. McKenzie (Eds.), *The food consumer* (pp. 107–126). New York: John Wiley.

Murcott, A. (1988). Sociological and anthropological approaches to food and eating. *World Review of Nutrition and Dietetics*, 55, 1–40.

Murcott, A. (1993a). Talking of good food: An empirical study of women's conceptualizations. *Food and Foodways*, 5, 305–318.

Murcott, A. (1993b). Purity and pollution: Body management and the social place of infancy. In S. Scott & D. Morgan (Eds.), *Body matters: Essays on the sociology of the body* (pp. 122–134). Bristol: Falmer Press.

Murdoch, W. W. (1980). *The poverty of nations: The political economy of hunger and population*. Baltimore: Johns Hopkins University Press.

National Center for Health Statistics. (1985). *Health interview survey*. Hyattsville: Public Health Service.

National Center for Health Care Statistics. (1992). *Health, United States, 1991*. Hyattsville: Public Health Service.

Nayga., R. M., Jr., & Capps, O., Jr. (1994a). *Effect of socioeconomic and demographic factors on away-from-home and at-home consumption of selected nutrients* (TAEX Bulletin No. 1717). College Station: Texas Agricultural Experiment Station.

Nayga, R. M., Jr., & Capps, O., Jr. (1994b). *Meat product selection: An analysis for the away-from-home and at-home markets* (TAEX Bulletin No. 1718). College Station: Texas Agricultural Experiment Station.

Neimi, R. G., Mueller, J., & Smith, T. W. (1989). *Trends in public opinion: A compendium of survey data*. New York: Greenwood Press.

Nelson, M. C., & Svanberg, I. (1993). Coffee in Sweden: A question of morality, health, and economy. *Food and Foodways*, 5, 239–254.

Nisbet, R. (1969). *Social change and history*. New York: Oxford University Press.

Nisbet, R. (1972). Introduction: The problem of social change. In R. Nisbet (Ed.), *Social change* (pp. 1–45). New York: Harper Books.

Nicholson, N. K., & Esseks, J. D. (1978). The politics of food scarcities in developing countries. *International Organization*, 32, 679–719.

Offe, C. (1985). New social movements: Challenging the boundaries of institutional politics. *Social Research*, 52, 817–868.

Officials take women's child after learning she was breast feeding. (1992, February 4). *The Eagle*, p. A3.

Ogburn, W. F. (1950). *Social change*. New York: Viking Press.

Ogburn, W. F. (1964). *On culture and social change*. Chicago: University of Chicago Press.

Ogburn, W. F., & Thomas, D. S. (1922). The influence of the business cycle on certain social conditions. *Quarterly Journal of the American Statistical Association*, 18, 324–340.

O'Grada, C. (1989). *The great Irish famine*. Houndmills, England: Macmillan.

Ohnuki-Tierney, E. (1993). *Rice as self: Japanese identities through time*. Princeton: Princeton University Press.

Ollenburger, J. C., Grana, S. J., & Moore, H. A. (1989). Labor force participation of rural farm, rural nonfarm, and urban women: A panel update. *Rural Sociology*, 54, 533–550.

Omran, A. R. (1971). The epidemiologic transition: A theory of population change. *Milbank Memorial Quarterly*, 49, 509–538.

O'Neill, J. (1985). *Five bodies: The human shape of modern society*. Ithaca: Cornell University Press.

Orbach, S. (1979). *Fat is a feminist issue*. New York: Berkeley Press.

Oshima, H. T. (1967). Food consumption, nutrition, and economic development in Asian countries. *Economic Development and Cultural Change*, 15, 385–396.

Ostrow, J. M. (1990). *Social sensitivity: A study of habit and experience*. Albany: State University of New York Press.

Paarlberg, R. C. (1985). *Food trade and foreign policy: India, the Soviet Union, and the United States*. Ithaca: Cornell University Press.

Paige, J. M. (1975). *Agrarian revolution: Social movements and export agriculture in the underdeveloped world*. New York: Free Press.

Pan American Health Organization. (1992). *Health statistics from the Americas, 1992 edition*. Washington, DC: PAHO.

Panic, M. (1993). The impact of multinationals on national economic policies. In B. Burgenmeir & J. L. Mucchilli (Eds.), *Multinationals and Europe* (pp. 204–222). New York: Routledge.

Parsons, T. (1951). *The social system*. New York: Free Press.

Parsons, T. (1966). *Societies: Evolutionary and comparative perspectives*. Englewood Cliffs: Prentice Hall.

Parsons, T., & Bales, R. F. (1955). *Family, socialization, and interaction process*. Glencoe: Free Press.

Parsons, T., & Shils, E. A. (1951). *Toward a general theory of action*. New York: Harper/Row.

Parsons, T., & Smelser, N. J. (1956). *Economy and society*. Glencoe: Free Press.

Paules, G. F. (1991). *Dishing it out: Power and resistance among waitresses in a New Jersey restaurant*. Philadelphia: Temple University Press.

Paulin, G. D., & Weber, W. D. (1995). The effects of health insurance on consumer spending. *Monthly Labor Review*, 118, 34–54.

Perry, R. (1992). Colonizing the breast: Sexuality and maternity in eighteen-century England. In J. C. Fout (Ed.), *Forbidden history: The state, society, and the regulation of sexuality in modern Europe* (pp. 107–137). Chicago: University of Chicago Press.

Peters, G. R., & Rappaport, L. (Eds.). (1988). Food, nutrition, and aging: Behavioral perspectives [Special issue]. *American Behavioral Scientist*, 32, 1–88.

Phillips, D. R. (1990). *Health and health care in the Third World*. New York: Longman.

Physicians Committee for Responsible Medicine. (1990, November-December). *Guide to healthy eating*. Washington, D.C.

Piazza, A. (1986). *Food consumption and nutritional status in the PRC*. Boulder: Westview Press.

Picou, J. S., Wells, R. H., & Nyberg, K. L. (1978). Paradigms, theories, and methods in contemporary rural sociology. *Rural Sociology*, 43, 559–583.

Picou, J. S., Curry, E. W., & Wells, R. H. (1990). Paradigm shifts in the social sciences: Twenty years of research in rural sociology. *Rural Sociology*, 55, 91–100.

Pierson, C. (1991). *Beyond the welfare state? The political economy of welfare*. University Park: Pennsylvania State University Press.

Pillsbury, R. (1990). *From boarding house to bistro: The American restaurant then and now*. Boston: Urvin Hyman.

Piven, F. F., & Cloward, R. A. (1993). *Regulating the poor: The functions of public welfare* (rev. ed.). New York: Vintage Books.

Pollitt, E., & Leibel, R. (1980). Biological and social correlates of failure to thrive. In L. S. Greene & F. E. Johnston (Eds.), *Social and biological predictors of nutritional status, physical growth, and neurological development* (pp. 173–200). New York: Academic Press.

Polsky, A. J. (1991). *The rise of the therapeutic state*. Princeton: Princeton University Press.

Popkin, B. M. (1993). Nutritional patterns and transitions. *Population and Development Review*, 19, 138–157.

Popkin, B. M., & Lim-Ybanez, M. (1982). Nutrition and school achievement. *Social Science and Medicine*, 16, 53–61.

Popkin, B. M., & Solon, F. S. (1976). Income, time, the working mother, and child nutrition. *Environmental Health*, 22, 156–166.

Popkin, B. M., Haines, P. S., & Reidy, K. C. (1989). Food consumption of U. S. women: Patterns and determinants between 1977 and 1985. *American Journal of Clinical Nutrition*, 49, 1307–1319.

Popkin, B. M., Haines, P. S., & Paterson, R. (1992). Dietary changes among older Americans, 1977–87. *American Journal of Clinical Nutrition*, 55, 823–830.

Poppendieck, J. (1986). *Breadlines knee-deep in wheat: Food assistance in the Great Depression*. New Brunswick: Rutgers University Press.

Post, J. D. (1985). *Food shortage, climatic variability, and epidemic disease in preindustrial Europe: The mortality peak in the early 1740's*. Ithaca: Cornell University Press.

Povlsen, K. K. (1991). Food, fashion, and gender: Pictures of food in women's magazines. In E. L. Furst, R. Prattala, M. Ekstrom, L. Holm, & U. Kjaernes (Eds.), *Palatable worlds: Sociocultural food studies* (pp. 131–144). Oslo: Solum Vorlag.

Powers, M. (1991). Decay from within: The inevitable doom of the American saloon. In S. Barrows & R. Room (Eds.), *Drinking: Behavior and belief in modern history* (pp. 112–131). Berkeley: University of California Press.

Rabiee, F., & Geissler, C. (1992). The impact of maternal work load on child nutrition in rural Iran. *Food and Nutrition Bulletin*, 14, 43–48.

Rama, R. (1992). *Investing in food*. Paris: Organization for Economic Co-Operation and Development.

Rau, B. (1991). *From feast to famine: Official cures and grassroots remedies to Africa's food crisis*. Atlantic Highlands: Zed Books.

Reed, M. R., & Marchant, M. A. (1994). The behavior of U. S. food firms in international markets. In A. Bonnano, L. Busch, W. Friedland, L. Gouveia, & E. Mingione (Eds.), *From Columbus to ConAgra: The globalization of agriculture and food* (pp. 149–159). Lawrence: University Presses of Kansas.

Reid, A. (1988). *Southeast Asia in the age of commerce 1450–1680. Vol. I. The lands below the winds*. New Haven: Yale University Press.

Reilly, M. D. (1982). Working wives and convenience consumption. *Journal of Consumer Research*, 8, 407–417.

Reiter, E. (1991). *Making fast food: From the frying pan into the fryer.* Montreal: McGill-Queen's University Press.

Reskin, B. F., & Hartmann, H. I. (1986). *Women's work, men's work.* Washington, DC: National Academy Press.

Riecters, R., Alvin, S., & Dellenbayer, L. (1988). A cross-sectional analysis of consumer trends in red meat consumption. *Journal of Food Distribution,* 19, 1–10.

Riessman, C. K. (1994). Improving the health experiences of low income patients. In P. Conrad & R. Kern (Eds.), *The sociology of health and illness: Critical perspectives* (4th ed., pp. 424–437). New York: St. Martin's Press.

Ritzer, G. (1990). The current status of sociological theory: The new synthesis. In G. Ritzer (Ed.), *Frontiers of social theory: The new synthesis* (pp. 1–30). New York: Columbia University Press.

Ritzer, G. (1991). *Metatheorizing in sociology.* Lexington: Lexington Books.

Ritzer, G. (1993). *The McDonaldization of society.* Newbury Park: Pine Forge Press.

Rizvi, N. (1991). Socioeconomic and cultural factors affecting interhousehold food distribution in rural and urban Bangladesh. In A. Sharman, J. Theophano, K. Curtis, & E. Messer (Eds.), *Diet and domestic life in society* (pp. 91–118). Boulder: Westview Press.

Robbins, Jr., R. G. (1975). *Famine in Russia, 1891–1892: The Imperial government responds to a crisis.* New York: Columbia University Press.

Robinson, J. (1980). Housework technology and household work. In S. F. Berk (Ed.), *Women and household labor* (pp. 53–68). Beverly Hills: Sage.

Rodefeld, R. D. (1978). The causes of change in farm technology, size, and organizational structure. In R. D. Rodefeld, J. Flora, D. Voth, I. Fujimoto, & J. Converse (Eds.), *Change in rural America: Causes, consequences, and alteration* (pp. 217–237). St. Louis: C. V. Mosby.

Rodefeld, R. D., Flora, J., Voth, D., Fujimoto, I., & Converse, J. (Eds.). (1978). *Change in rural America: Causes, consequences, and alteration.* St. Louis: C. V. Mosby.

Rogers, E. M. (1983). *Diffusion of innovations* (3rd ed.). New York: Free Press.

Rogers, R. G., & Hackenberg, R. (1987). Extending epidemiologic transition theory: A new stage. *Social Biology,* 34, 234–243.

Rosenau, P. M. (1992). *Post-modernism and the social sciences: Insights, inroads, and intrusions.* Princeton: Princeton University Press.

Rosenberg, M. (1981). The self-concept: Social product and social force. In M. Rosenberg & R. H. Turner (Eds.), *Social psychology, sociological perspectives* (pp. 593–624). New York: Basic Books.

Rosenfeld, R. A. (1985). *Farm women, work, farm, and family in the United States.* Chapel Hill: University of North Carolina Press.

Rozin, P. (1987). Psychological perspectives on food: Preferences and avoidances. In M. Harris & E. B. Ross (Eds.), *Food and evolution: Toward a theory of human food habits* (pp. 181–205). Philadelphia: Temple University Press.

Rozin, P. (1988). Social learning about food by humans. In T. R. Zentall & B. G. Golef, Jr. (Eds.), *Social learning: Psychological and biological perspectives* (pp. 165–187). Hillsdale: Lawrence Erlbaum.

Rozin, P., & Fallon, A. E. (1987). A perspective on disgust. *Psychological Review,* 94, 23–41.

Ruzicka, L. T., & Lopez, A. D. (1990). The use of cause of death statistics for health status assessment: National and international experiences. *World Health Statistical Quarterly,* 43, 249–258.

Sachs, C. (1983). *The invisible farmers: Women in agricultural production.* Totowa: Rowman and Littlefield.

Sagen, L. (1987). *The health of nations: True causes of sickness and well-being.* New York: Basic Books.

Sahlins, M. (1976). *Cultural and practical reasons.* Chicago: University of Chicago Press.

Said, E. W. (1988). Michel Foucault, 1926–1984. In J. Arac (Ed.), *After Foucault: Humanistic knowledge, postmodern challenges* (pp. 1–10). New Brunswick: Rutgers University Press.

Samets, I. (1991). *Running out of food: The results of the community childhood hunger identification project in Suffolk County.* Albany: Nutrition Consortium of New York State.

Sanderson, S. K. (1990). *Social evolutionism: A critical history.* Cambridge: Basil Blackwell.

Sanjur, D. (1982). *Social and cultural perspectives in nutrition.* Englewood Cliffs: Prentice-Hall.

Sapp, S. G., & Harrod, W. J. (1989). Social acceptability and intention to eat beef: An expansion of the Fishbein-Ajzen model using reference group theory. *Rural Sociology, 54*, 420–438.

Schafer, R. B. (1978). Factors affecting food behavior and quality of husband's and wive's diets. *Journal of the American Dietetics Association, 72*, 138–145.

Schafer, R. B., & Bohlen, J. M. (1977). Exchange of conjugal power and control of family food consumption. *Home Economics Research Journal, 6*, 131–140.

Schafer, R. B., & Keith, P. M. (1981). Influences on food decisions across the family life cycle. *Journal of the American Dietetic Association, 78*, 144–148.

Schafer, R. B., & Schafer, E. A. (1989). Relationship between gender roles and food roles in the family. *Journal of Nutritional Education, 21*, 119–126.

Scheper-Hughes, N., & Lock, M. (1987). The mindful body: A prolegomenon to work in medical sociology. *Medical Anthropology, 1*, 6–41.

Schivelbusch, W. (1992). *Tastes of paradise: A social history of spices, stimulants, and intoxicants.* New York: Pantheon.

Schmitt, R. L. (1986). Embodies identities: Breasts as emotional reminders. In N. K. Denzin (Ed.), *Studies in symbolic interaction, 7 part A* (pp. 229–289). New York: JAI Press.

Scholliers, P. (1992). From the crisis of Flanders to Belgium's social question: Nutritional landmarks of transition in industrializing Europe. *Food and Foodways, 4*, 151–175.

Schudson, M. (1986). *Advertising, the uneasy persuasion: Its dubious impact on American society.* New York: Basic Books.

Schultz, T. W. (1967). Investing in human capital. In C. Sripati & C. W. Hultman (Eds.), *Problems of economic development* (pp. 1–15). Boston: D. C. Heath.

Schupter, J. A. (1950). *Capitalism, socialism, and democracy.* (3rd ed.). New York: Harper/Row.

Schwartz, H. (1986). *Never satisfied: A cultural history of diets, fantasies, and fat.* New York: Free Press.

Scott, J. C. (1976). *The moral economy of the peasant: Rebellion and subsistence in Southeast Asia.* New Haven: Yale University Press.

Scott, J. C. (1990). *Domination and the art of resistance: Hidden transcripts.* New Haven: Yale University Press.

Scott, T. R. (1990). The effect of physiological need on taste. In E. Capaldi & T. L. Powley (Eds.), *Taste, experience, and feeding* (pp. 46–61). Washington: American Psychological Association.

Scull, A. (1993). *The most solitary of afflictions: Madness and society in Britain, 1700–1900.* New Haven: Yale University Press.

Seavoy, R. E. (1986). *Famine in peasant societies.* Westport: Greenwood.

Sellerberg, A. M. (1991). In food we trust? Vitally necessary confidence and unfamiliar ways. In E. L. Furst, R. Prattala, M. Ekstrom, L. Holm, & U. Kjaernes (Eds.), *Palatable worlds: Sociocultural food studies* (pp. 193–202). Oslo: Solum Vorlag.

Sen, A. (1981). *Poverty and famine: An essay on entitlement and deprivation.* New York: Oxford University Press.

Senauer, B., Asp, E., & Kinsey, J. (1991). *Food trends and the changing consumer.* St. Paul: Egan Press.

Service, E. R. (1975). *Origins of the state and civilization: The process of cultural evolution.* New York: W. W. Norton.

Sewell, Jr., W. H. (1980). *Work and revolution in France: The language of labor from the old regime to 1948.* New York: Cambridge University Press.

Shepard, J. (1975). *The politics of starvation.* New York: Carnegie Endowment for International Peace.

Shifflett, P. A. (1980). *Future time perspective and food habits of the aged.* Unpublished doctoral dissertation, Texas A&M University, Department of Sociology, College Station.

Shifflett, P. A., & McIntosh, W. A. (1986–87). Food habits and future time: An exploratory study of age-appropriate food habits among the elderly. *International Journal of Aging and Human Development,* 24, 1–14.

Shilling, C. (1993). *The body and social theory.* Newburg Park: Sage.

Shiva, V. (1991). *The violence of the Green Revolution: Third World agriculture, ecology, and politics.* Atlantic Highlands: Zed Books.

Simmonds, D. (1990). What's next?: Fashion, foodies, and the illusion of freedom. In A. Tomlinson (Ed.), *Consumption, identity, and style: Marketing meanings and the packaging of pleasure* (pp. 121–138). New York: Routledge.

Simon, J. L. (1977). *The economics of population growth.* Princeton: Princeton University Press.

Simon, J. L., & Kahn, H. (1984). Introduction. In J. L. Simon & H. Kahn (Eds.), *The resourceful earth: A response to global 2000* (pp. 1–49). Cambridge: Basil Blackwell.

Simpson, I. H., Wilson, J., & Young, K. (1988). The sexual division of labor of farm household labor: A replication and extension. *Rural Sociology,* 53, 145–165.

Simpson, I. H., Wilson, J., & Jackson, R. A. (1992). The contrasting effects of social, organizational, and economic variables on farm production. *Work and Occupations,* 19, 237–254.

Sims, L. B., Paolucci, F., & Morris, P. (1972). A theoretical model for the study of nutritional status: An ecosystems approach. *Journal of Food and Nutrition,* 1,192–205.

Skinner, J. D., Ezell, J. M., Salvetti, N. N., & Penfield, M. P. (1985). Relationship between mother's employment and nutritional quality of adolescents' diets. *Home Economics Research Journal,* 13, 218–225.

Sklar, L. (1991). *Sociology of the global system.* Baltimore: Johns Hopkins University Press.

Skocpol, T. (1979). *States and social revolutions.* London: Cambridge University Press.

Skocpol, T. (1985). Bringing the state back: Strategies of analysis in current research. In P. B. Evans, D. Rueschemeyer, & T. Skocpol (Eds.), *Bringing the state back in* (pp. 3–41). New York: Cambridge University Press.

Skocpol, T., & Amenta, E. (1986). States and social policies. *Annual Review of Sociology,* 123, 131–157.

Skocpol, T., & Finegold, K. (1982). State capacity and economic intervention in the early New Deal. *Political Science Quarterly,* 97, 255–278.

Skocpol, T., & Orloff, A. S. (1986). Explaining the origins of welfare states: A comparison of Britain and the United States, 1880s-1920s. In G. Siegwart & N. Nowak (Eds.), *Approaches to social theory* (pp. 229–257). New York: Russell Sage Foundation.

Sloane, M. (1993, August 18). NBC peacock to make debut on cereal boxes. *The Eagle,* p. C2.

Slocum, W. L., & Nye, F. I. (1976). Provider and housekeeper roles. In F. I. Nye (Ed.), *Role structure and the analysis of the family* (pp. 81–100). Beverly Hills: Sage.

Smith, D. A., & White, D. R. (1992). Structure dynamics of the global economy: Network analysis of international trade 1965–1980. *Social Forces,* 70, 857–893.

Smith, D. E. (1987). *The everyday world as problematic: A feminist sociology.* Boston: Northeastern University Press.

Sobal, J. (1984a). Marriage, obesity, and dieting. *Marriage and Family Review,* 7, 115–139.

Sobal, J. (1984b). Group dieting, the stigma of obesity, and overweight adolescents: The contributions of Natalie Allon to the sociology of obesity. *Marriage and Family Review,* 7, 9–20.

Sobal, J. (1991a). Obesity and nutritional sociology: A model for coping with the stigma of obesity. *Clinical Sociology Review*, 9, 21–32.

Sobal, J. (1991b). Obesity and socioeconomic status: A framework for examining relationships between physical and social variables. *Medical Anthropology*, 13, 231–247.

Sobal, J. (1992). The practice of nutritional sociology. *Sociological Practice Review*, 3, 23–31.

Sobal, J. (1995). Medicalization and demedicalization of obesity. In D. Maurer & J. Sobal (Eds.), *Eating agendas: Food and nutrition as social problems* (pp. 67–90). New York: Aldine de Gruyter.

Sobal, J., & Maurer, D. (1995). Food, eating, and nutrition as social problems: An introduction and overview. In D. Maurer & J. Sobal (Eds.), *Eating agendas: Food and nutrition as social problems* (pp. 3–7). New York: Aldine de Gruyter.

Sobal, J., & Stunkard, A. J. (1989). Socioeconomic status and obesity: A review of the literature. *Psychological Bulletin*, 105, 260–275.

Sobal, J., Rauschenbach, B. S., & Frongillo, Jr., E. A. (1992). Marital status, fatness, and obesity. *Social Science and Medicine*, 35, 915–923.

Sobal, J., McIntosh, W. A., & Whit, W. (1993). Teaching the sociology of food, eating, and nutrition. *Teaching Sociology*, 21, 50–59.

Sobel, M. S. (1981). *Lifestyle and social structure: Concepts, definitions, and analysis*. New York: Academic Press.

Sokolov, R. (1991). *Why we eat what we eat: How the encounter between the New World and the Old changed the way everyone on the planet eats*. New York: Summit Books.

Sorokin, P. A. (1975) [1922]. *Hunger as a factor in human affairs*. Gainesville: University Presses of Florida.

Spencer, H. (1892). *Sociology, vol. 1*. New York: Appleton.

Spitzack, C. (1990). *Confessing excess: Women and the politics of body reduction*. Albany: State University of New York.

Spurling, L. (1977). *Phenomenology and the social world: The philosophy of Merleau-Ponty and its relation to the social sciences*. Boston: Routledge/Kegan Paul.

Stack, C. B. (1974). *All our kin: Strategies for survival in the black community*. New York: Harper/Row.

Staff. (1994, January 1). The big picture: R&I's 1994 foodservice industry forecast. *Restaurant & Institutions*, pp. 7–19.

Stanton, B. F. (1993). Recent changes in size and structure in American agriculture. In A. Hallam (Ed.), *Size, structure, and the changing face of American agriculture* (pp. 42–70). Boulder: Westview Press.

Staples, W. E. (1990). *Castles of our conscience: Social control and the American state, 1800–1985*. New Brunswick: Rutgers University Press.

State investigates East Texas chicken producer. (1994, September 25). *The Eagle*, p. A7.

Stavis, B. (1981). Ending famine in China. In R. V. Garcia & J. C. Esudero (Eds.), *Drought and man: Volume 2. The constant catastrophe: Malnutrition, famines, and drought* (pp. 112–139). New York: Pergamon Press.

Stimson, G., & Webb, B. (1989). Face-to-face interaction. In P. Browne (Ed.), *Perspectives in medical sociology* (pp. 519–529). Belmont: Wadsworth.

Stinchcombe, A. L. (1983). *Economic sociology*. New York: Academic Press.

Stokes, R. G., & Anderson, A. B. (1990). Disarticulation and human welfare in less developed countries. *American Sociological Review*, 55, 63–74.

Stone, G. P. (1962). Appearance and the self. In A. M. Rose (Ed.), *Human behavior and social processes* (pp. 86–118). Boston: Houghton-Mifflin.

Stonich, S. C. (1991). The political economy of environmental destruction: Food security in southern Honduras. In S. Whiteford and A. E. Ferguson (Eds.), *Harvest of want: Hunger and food security in Central America and Mexico* (pp. 45–74). Boulder: Westview Press.

Strasser, S. (1982). *Never done: A history of American housework.* New York: Pantheon.

Strasser, S. (1989). *Satisfaction guaranteed: The making of the American mass market.* New York: Pantheon.

Straus, J. (1986). Does better nutrition raise farm productivity? *Journal of Political Economy*, 94, 297–320.

Straus, R. (1957). The nature and status of medical sociology. *American Sociological Review*, 22, 200–204.

Streckel, R. (1994). Heights and health in the United States, 1710–1950. In J. Komlos (Ed.), *Stature, living standards, and economic development* (pp. 153–170). Chicago: University of Chicago Press.

Suchman, E. A. (1965). Social patterns of illness and medical care. *Journal of Health and Social Behavior*, 6, 2–16.

Susser, M., Watson, W., & Hopper, K. (1985). *Sociology in medicine* (3rd ed.). New York: Oxford University Press.

Sussman, G. D. (1982). *Selling mothers' milk: The wet-nursing industry in France, 1715–1914.* Urbana: University of Illinois Press.

Syme, S. L., & Berkman, L. F. (1976). Social class, susceptibility, and sickness. *American Journal of Epidemiology*, 104, 1–8.

Symons, M. (1991). *Eating into thinking: Explorations in the sociology of cuisine.* Unpublished doctoral dissertation, Flinders University, Department of Sociology, Adelaide, South Australia.

Symons, M. (1994). Simmel's gastronomic sociology: An overlooked essay. *Food and Foodways*, 5, 333–351. (Appendix: The sociology of the meal by George Simmel [1915]. M. Symons, trans.)

Synnott, A. (1993). *The body social: Symbolism, self, and society.* New York: Routledge.

Szasz, T. S. (1974). *The myth of mental illness* (Rev. ed.). New York: Harper/Row.

Tanner, J. M. (1994). Introduction: Growth in height as a mirror of the standard of living. In J. Komlos (Ed.), *Stature, living standards, and economic development* (pp. 16–28). Chicago: University of Chicago Press.

Terhune, K. W. (1974). *A review of the actual and expected consequences of family size.* Report to the Center for Population Research, National Institute of Child Health and Human Development (DHEW Pub. No. [N.I.H.], pp. 75–799).

Thomas, S. G., & Middleton, M. K. (1994). *Desertification: Exploding the myth.* New York: John Wiley.

Thompson, B. W. (1994). *A hunger so wide and deep: American women speak out on eating problems.* Minneapolis: University of Minnesota Press.

Thompson, E. P. (1971). The moral economy of the English growth in the eighteenth century. *Past and Present*, 50, 76–136.

Tickamayer, A., & Bokemeier, J. (1988). Sex differences in labor-market experiences. *Rural Sociology*, 53, 166–189.

Tilly, C. (1975a). Introduction. In C. Tilly (Ed.), *The formation of national states in western Europe* (pp. 3–83). Princeton: Princeton University Press.

Tilly, C. (1975b). Food supply and public order in modern Europe. In C. Tilly (Ed.), *The formation of national states in western Europe* (pp. 380–455). Princeton: Princeton University Press.

Tilly, C. (1992). *Coercion, capital, and European states, AD 990–1992.* New York: Cambridge University Press.

Tilly, C., Tilly, L., & Tilly, R. (1975). *The rebellious century 1830–1930.* Cambridge: Harvard University Press.

Tilly, L. (1983). Food entitlement, famine, and conflict. In R. I. Rotberg & T. K. Rabb (Eds.), *Hunger and history: The impact of changing food production on consumption patterns of society* (pp. 135–151). Cambridge: Cambridge University Press.

Timmer, C. P., Falcon, W. P., & Pearson, S. R. (1983). *Food policy analysis*. Baltimore: John Hopkins University Press.

Tobin, J. (1992). A Japanese French restaurant in Hawaii. In J. J. Tobin (Ed.), *Remade in Japan: Everyday life and consumer taste in a changing society* (pp. 159–175). New Haven: Yale University Press.

Todhunter, E. N. (1973). Food habits, faddism, and nutrition. *World Review of Nutrition and Dietetics*, 16, 286–317.

Torres, C. C. (1987). *Examining the applicability of formal organizational theory on voluntary organizations*. Unpublished doctoral dissertation, Texas A&M University, Department of Sociology, College Station.

Torres, C. C., McIntosh, W. A., & Zey, M. (1990). The effects of bureaucratization and commitment on resource mobilization in voluntary organizations. *Sociological Spectrum*, 11, 19–44.

Torres, C. C., Zey, M., & McIntosh, W. A. (1991). Effectiveness in voluntary organizations. An empirical assessment. *Sociological Focus*, 24, 157–174.

Torres, C. C., McIntosh, W. A., & Kubena S. (1992). Social network and social background characteristics of elderly who live and eat alone. *Journal of Aging and Health*, 4, 564–578.

Touliatos, J., Linholm, B. W., Weinberg, M. F., & Melbagene, R. (1984). Family and child correlates of nutrition knowledge and dietary quality in 10–13 year olds. *Journal of School Health*, 54, 247–249.

Touraine, A. (1995) [1992]. *Critique of modernity* (David Macy, trans.). Cambridge: Basil Blackwell.

Tripp, R. (1982). Fathers and traders: Some economic determinants of nutritional status in northern Ghana. *Food and Nutrition Bulletin*, 8, 3–11.

Tucker, K., & Sanjur, D. (1988). Maternal employment and child nutrition in Panama. *Social Science and Medicine*, 26, 605–612.

Turner, B. S. (1984). *The body and society: Explorations in social theory*. Oxford: Basil Blackwell.

Turner, B. S. (1987). *Medical power and social knowledge*. Beverly Hills: Sage.

Turner, B. S. (1992). *Regulating bodies: Essays in medical sociology*. New York: Routledge.

Turner, J. H. (1988). *A theory of social interaction*. Stanford: Stanford University Press.

Turner, J. H. (1991). *The structure of sociological theory*. Belmont: Wadsworth.

Twigg, J. (1979). Food for thought: Purity and vegetarianism. *Religion*, 9, 13–35.

United Nations Statistical Office. (1980). *World health statistics annual*. Geneva: World Health Organization.

United Nations Statistical Office. (1990). *World health statistics annual*. Geneva: World Health Organization.

U. S. Bureau of the Census. (1988). *Statistical abstract of the United States: 1987*. Washington, DC: U.S. Government Printing Office.

U. S. Bureau of the Census. (1994). *Statistical abstract of the United States: 1994*. Washington, DC: U.S. Government Printing Office.

U. S. Department of Commerce. (1994, January). *U.S. industrial outlook 1994*. Washington, DC: U.S. Government Printing Office.

van den Berghe, P. L. (1984). Ethnic cuisine: Culture in nature. *Ethnic and Racial Studies*, 7, 387–397.

Van Esterik, P. (1989). *Beyond the breast-bottle controversy*. New Brunswick: Rutgers University Press.

Van Esterik, P. (1992). From Marco Polo to McDonald's: Thai cuisine in transition. *Food and Foodways*, 5, 177–194.

Varnis, S. L. (1990). *Reluctant aid or aiding the reluctant?: U.S. food aid policy and Ethiopian famine relief*. New Brunswick: Transaction Books.

Veblen, T. (1953) [1899]. *The theory of the leisure class.* New York: New American Library.

Verbrugge, L. M. (1989). The twain meet: Empirical explanations of sex differences in health and mortality. *Journal of Health and Social Behavior,* 30, 282–304.

Victor, D. M., & Cralle, H. T. (1992). Value-laden knowledge and holistic thinking in agricultural research. *Agriculture and Human Values,* 9, 44–57.

Viteri, F. E. (1982). Nutrition and work performance. In N. S. Scrimshaw & M. B. Wallerstein (Eds.), *Nutrition policy implementation: Issues and experience* (pp. 3–13). New York: Plenum Press.

Vogt, T. M. (1988). Aging, stress, and illness: Psychobiological linkages. In M. G. Ory, R. P. Abeles, & P. D. Lipman (Eds.), *Aging, health, and behavior* (pp. 207–236). Newbury Park: Sage.

von Braun, J. (1994). Production, employment, and income effects of commercialization of agriculture. In J. von Braun & E. Kennedy (Eds.), *Agricultural commercialization, economic development, and nutrition* (pp. 37–64). Baltimore: Johns Hopkins University Press.

Wacquant, L. J. D. (1992). The structure and logic of Bourdieu's sociology. In P. Bourdieu & L. J. D. Wacquant (Eds.), *An invitation to reflexive sociology* (pp. 1–59). Chicago: University of Chicago Press.

Waitzkin, H. (1989). A critical theory of medical discourse: Ideology, social control, and the processing of social context in medical encounters. *Journal of Health and Social Behavior,* 30, 220–239.

Wallace, W. L. (1969). Overview of contemporary sociological theory. In W. L. Wallace (Ed.), *Sociological theory: An introduction* (pp. 1–59). Chicago: Aldine.

Wallace, W. L. (1983). *Principles of scientific sociology.* New York: Aldine.

Wallerstein, I. (1974). *The modern world-system: Capitalist agriculture and the origins of the European world-economy in the sixteenth century.* New York: Academic Press.

Wallerstein, I. (1980). *The modern world system II: Mercantilism and the consolidation of the European world-economy 1600–1750.* New York: Academic Press.

Wallerstein, M. (1980). *Food for war-food for peace. United States food aid in a global context.* Cambridge: MIT Press.

Walsh, J. P. (1991). The social context of technological change: The case of the retail food industry. *Sociological Quarterly,* 32, 447–468.

Walsh, J. P. (1993). *Supermarkets transformed.* New Brunswick: Rutgers University.

Walter, J. (1989). The serial economy of dearth in early modern England. In J. Walter & R. Schofield (Eds.), *Famine, disease, and the social order in early modern society* (pp. 75–128). New York: Cambridge University Press.

Walter, J., & Schofield, R. (1989). Famine, disease, and crisis mortality in early modern society. In J. Walter & R. Schofield (Eds.), *Famine, disease, and the social order in early modern society.* (pp. 1–73). New York: Cambridge University Press.

Walton, J. (1984). *Reluctant rebels: Comparative studies of revolution and underdevelopment.* New York: Columbia University Press.

Walton, J., & Seddon, D. (1994). *Free markets and food riots: The politics of global adjustment.* New York: Cambridge University Press.

Wandel, M., & Holmboe-Otterson, G. (1992). Maternal work, child feeding, and nutrition in rural Tanzania. *Food and Nutrition Bulletin,* 14, 49–54.

Wann, J. J., & Sexton, R. J. (1992). Imperfect competition in multiproduct food industries with application to pear processing. *American Agricultural Economics,* 74, 980–990.

Warner, W. L. (1963). *Yankee city.* New Haven: Yale University Press.

Warner, W. L., & Lunt, P. S. (1941). *The social life of modern community.* New Haven: Yale University Press.

Warner, W. L., & Lunt, P. S. (1947). *The status system of a modern community.* New Haven: Yale University Press.

Warnock, J. W. (1987). *The politics of hunger: The global food system.* Toronto: Methuen.

Watkins, S. C., & van de Walle, E. (1983). Nutrition, mortality, and population size: Malthus' court of last resort. In R. I. Rotberg & T. K. Rabb (Eds.), *Hunger and history: The impact of changing food production and consumption patterns on society* (pp. 72–129). New York: Cambridge University Press.

Way, K. (1993). *Anorexia nervosa and recovery. A hunger for meaning.* New York: Haworth Press.

Webb, P., von Braun, J., & Yohannes, Y. (1992). *Famine in Ethiopia: Policy implications of coping failure at national and household levels* (International Food Policy Research Report No. 92). Washington D.C.

Weber, M. (1968). *Economy and society* (2 vols.). New York: Bedminster Press.

Weismantel, M. J. (1988). *Food, gender, and poverty in the Ecuadorian Andes.* Philadelphia: University of Pennsylvania Press.

Weiss, B. (1980). Nutritional adaptation and cultural maladaptation: An evolutionary view. In N. W. Jerome, R. F. Kandel, & G. H. Pelto (Eds.), *Nutritional anthropology: Contemporary approaches to diet and culture* (pp. 147–179). Pleasantville: Redgrave.

Wells, R. H. (1980). *An empirical investigation of the paradigmatic structure of American sociology.* Unpublished doctoral dissertation, Texas A&M University, Department of Sociology, College Station.

Wells, R. H., & Picou, J. S. (1981). *American sociology: Theoretical and methodological structure.* Washington, DC: University Presses of America.

Wells, R. H., Miller, Jr., R. K., & Deville, K. S. (1983). Hunger as a global social phenomenon: A case of sociological neglect. *Humanity and Society, 7,* 338–372.

West, C., & Fenstermaker, S. (1993). Power, inequality, and the accomplishment of gender: An ethnomethodological view. In P. A. England (Ed.), *Theory on gender/feminism of theory* (pp. 151–174). New York: Aldine de Gruyter.

Whit, B., & Lockwood, Y. (1990). *Teaching food and society: A collection of syllabi and instructional material.* Grand Rapids: Aquinas College, Department of Sociology.

Whit, W. (1995). *Food and society: A sociological approach.* Dix Hills: General Hall.

Whiteford, M. B. (1991). From Gullo Pinto to "sacks snacks": Observations on dietary change in a rural Costa Rican village. In S. Whiteford & A. E. Ferguson (Eds.), *Harvest of want: Hunger and food security in Central America and Mexico* (pp. 127–140). Boulder: Westview Press.

Whiteford, S., & Ferguson, A. E. (1991). Social dimensions of food security and hunger: An overview. In S. Whiteford, & A. E. Ferguson (Eds.), *Harvest of want: Hunger and food security in Central America and Mexico* (pp. 1–21). Boulder: Westview Press.

Whyte, W. F. (1948). *Human relations in the restaurant industry.* New York: McGraw-Hill.

Wieglemann, G. (1974). Innovations in food and meals. *Folk Life: A Journal of Ethnological Studies, 12,* 20–30.

Wilkinson, R. G. (1973). *Poverty and progress: An ecological perspective on economic development.* New York: Praeger.

Williams, C. D. (1933). A nutritional disease associated with maize diet. *Archives of Disease in Children, 8,* 423–433.

Williams, R. G. (1991). Land, labor, and the crisis in Central America. In S. Whiteford & A. E. Ferguson (Eds.), *Harvest of want: Hunger and food security in Central America and Mexico* (pp. 23–44). Boulder: Westview Press.

Williams, R. G. (1994). *States and social evolution: Coffee and the rise of national governments in Central America.* Chapel Hill: University of North Carolina Press.

Williams, R. H. (1982). *Dream worlds: Mass consumption in late nineteenth-century France.* Berkeley: University of California Press.

Willis, S. (1991). *A primer for daily life.* New York: Routledge.

Wimberly, D. W. (1991a). Transnational corporate investment and food consumption in the Third World: A cross-national analysis. *Rural Sociology, 56,* 406–431.

Wimberly, D. W. (1991b). Investment dependency and alternative explanation of Third World mortality: A cross-national study. *American Sociological Review*, 55, 75–91.

Winner, L. (1977). *Autonomous technology: Technics out of control as a theme in political thought.* Cambridge: MIT Press.

Winson, A. (1993). *The intimate commodity: Food and the development of the agro-industrial complex in Canada.* Toronto: Garamond Press.

Wolf, E. R. (1969). *Peasant wars of the twentieth century.* New York: Harper/Row.

Wolf, E. R. (1982). *Europe and the people without history.* Berkeley: University of California Press.

Wolf, N. (1991). *The beauty myth: How images of beauty are used against women.* New York: William Morrow.

Wolinsky, F. D. (1980). *The sociology of health: Principles, professions, and issues.* Boston: Little/ Brown.

Woolhandler, S., Himmelstein, D. U., Silber, R., Bader, M., Harnly, M., & Jones, A. A. (1989). Medical care and mortality: Racial differences in preventable deaths. In P. Brown (Ed.), *Perspectives in medical sociology* (pp. 71–81). Belmont: Wadsworth.

World Bank. (1983). *World development report 1983.* New York: Oxford University Press.

World Bank. (1993). *World development report 1993. Investing in health.* New York: Oxford University Press.

World Health Organization (WHO). (1989). *World health statistics annual.* Geneva: World Health Organization.

World Health Organization (WHO). (1990). *Global estimates for health situation assessment and projections, 1990.* Geneva: Division of Epidemiological Surveillance and Health Situation and Trend Assessment, WHO.

Wray, J. D. (1971). Population pressure on families: Family size and child spacing. In Study Committee of the Office of the Foreign Secretary (Ed.), *Rapid population growth: Consequences and policy implications* (pp. 403–461). Washington, DC: National Academy of Sciences.

Wright, E. O. (1983). Giddens' critique of Marxism. *New Left Review*, 138, 111–135.

Wright, J. D., & Rossi, P. H. (1981). *Social science and natural hazards.* Cambridge: Abt Books.

Wrigley, E. A., & Schofield, R. S. (1981). *The population history of England, 1541–1871: A reconstruction.* Cambridge: Harvard University Press.

Wynne-Edwards, V. C. (1962). *Animal dispersion in relation to social behavior.* Edinburgh: Oliver/ Boyd.

Yamaji, S., & Ito, S. (1993). The political economy of rice in Japan. In L. Tweeten, C. L. Dishon, W. S. Chern, N. Imamura, & M. Morishima (Eds.), *Japanese and American agriculture: Tradition and progress in conflict* (pp. 349–365). Boulder: Westview Press.

Yates, R. D. S. (1990). War, food shortages, and relief measures in early China. In L. F. Newman, W. Crossgrove, R. W. Kates, R. Matthews, & S. Millman (Eds.), *Hunger in history: Food shortage, poverty, and deprivation* (pp. 147–177). Cambridge: Basil Blackwell.

Zablocki, B. D., & Kanter, R. M. (1976). The differentiation of life-styles. In A. Inkeles (Ed.), *Annual review of sociology* (pp. 269–298). Palo Alto: Annual Review.

Zeitlin, M., Ghassemi, H., & Mansour, M. (1990). *Positive deviance in child nutrition.* Tokyo: The United Nations University.

Zey-Ferrell, M., & McIntosh, W. A. (1987). Agricultural lending policies of commercial banks: Consequences of bank dominance and dependency. *Rural Sociology*, 52, 187–207.

Zey, M., & McIntosh, W. A. (1992). Predicting women's intent to eat beef: Normative versus attitudinal explanations. *Rural Sociology*, 57, 250–265.

Zey, M., Finlay, B., & McIntosh, W. A. (1986). *Working paper on family structure, labor force participation, and adolescent nutrition.* Texas A&M University, Department of Sociology, College Station.

Zuckerman, H. (1988). The sociology of science. In N. J. Smelser (Ed.), *Handbook of sociology* (pp. 519–574). Newbury Park: Sage.

Zwerdling, D. (1976). The food monopolies. In J. H. Skolnick & E. Currie (Eds.), *Crisis in American institutions* (3rd ed., pp. 43–50). Boston: Little/Brown.

INDEX